New Advances in Melanoma

New Advances in Melanoma

Editor

Lionel Larribère

MDPI • Basel • Beijing • Wuhan • Barcelona • Belgrade • Manchester • Tokyo • Cluj • Tianjin

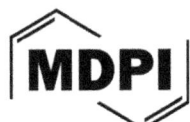

Editor
Lionel Larribère
Skin Cancer Unit
German Cancer Research Center (DKFZ)
Germany
University Medical Center Mannheim
Ruprecht-Karl University of Heidelberg
Germany

Editorial Office
MDPI
St. Alban-Anlage 66
4052 Basel, Switzerland

This is a reprint of articles from the Special Issue published online in the open access journal *Journal of Clinical Medicine* (ISSN 2077-0383) (available at: https://www.mdpi.com/journal/jcm/special_issues/melanoma_research).

For citation purposes, cite each article independently as indicated on the article page online and as indicated below:

LastName, A.A.; LastName, B.B.; LastName, C.C. Article Title. *Journal Name* **Year**, *Volume Number*, Page Range.

ISBN 978-3-0365-3453-4 (Hbk)
ISBN 978-3-0365-3454-1 (PDF)

© 2022 by the authors. Articles in this book are Open Access and distributed under the Creative Commons Attribution (CC BY) license, which allows users to download, copy and build upon published articles, as long as the author and publisher are properly credited, which ensures maximum dissemination and a wider impact of our publications.

The book as a whole is distributed by MDPI under the terms and conditions of the Creative Commons license CC BY-NC-ND.

Contents

About the Editor vii

Preface to "New Advances in Melanoma" ix

Lisa Linck-Paulus, Lisa Lämmerhirt, Daniel Völler, Katharina Meyer, Julia C. Engelmann, Rainer Spang, Norbert Eichner, Gunter Meister, Silke Kuphal and Anja Katrin Bosserhoff
Learning from Embryogenesis—A Comparative Expression Analysis in Melanoblast Differentiation and Tumorigenesis Reveals miRNAs Driving Melanoma Development
Reprinted from: *J. Clin. Med.* **2021**, *10*, 2259, doi:10.3390/jcm10112259 1

Lenka Kyjacova, Rafael Saup, Melanie Rothley, Anja Schmaus, Tabea Wagner, Anja Bößerhoff, Boyan K. Garvalov, Wilko Thiele and Jonathan P. Sleeman
Quantitative Detection of Disseminated Melanoma Cells by Trp-1 Transcript Analysis Reveals Stochastic Distribution of Pulmonary Metastases
Reprinted from: *J. Clin. Med.* **2021**, *10*, 5459, doi:10.3390/jcm10225459 21

Maria-Filothei Lazaridou, Chiara Massa, Diana Handke, Anja Mueller, Michael Friedrich, Karthikeyan Subbarayan, Sandy Tretbar, Reinhard Dummer, Peter Koelblinger and Barbara Seliger
Identification of microRNAs Targeting the Transporter Associated with Antigen Processing TAP1 in Melanoma
Reprinted from: *J. Clin. Med.* **2020**, *9*, 2690, doi:10.3390/jcm9092690 33

Maria Colombino, Carla Rozzo, Panagiotis Paliogiannis, Milena Casula, Antonella Manca, Valentina Doneddu, Maria Antonietta Fedeli, Maria Cristina Sini, Grazia Palomba, Marina Pisano, Paolo A. Ascierto, Corrado Caracò, Amelia Lissia, Antonio Cossu and Giuseppe Palmieri
Comparison of *BRAF* Mutation Screening Strategies in a Large Real-Life Series of Advanced Melanoma Patients
Reprinted from: *J. Clin. Med.* **2020**, *9*, 2430, doi:10.3390/jcm9082430 59

Sebastian Podlipnik, Cristina Carrera, Aram Boada, Nina Richarz, Joaquim Marcoval, Josep Ramon Ferreres, Domingo Bodet, Rosa María Martí, Sonia Segura, Mireia Sabat, Joan Dalmau, Mónica Quintana, Antoni Azon, Neus Curcó, Manel Formigon, María Rosa Olivella-Garcés, Pedro Zaballos, Joaquim Sola, Loida Galvany, Carola Baliu-Piqué, Marta Alegre, Paola Pasquali, Josep Malvehy and Susana Puig
Incidence of Melanoma in Catalonia, Spain, Is Rapidly Increasing in the Elderly Population. A Multicentric Cohort Study
Reprinted from: *J. Clin. Med.* **2020**, *9*, 3396, doi:10.3390/jcm9113396 73

Frédéric Soysouvanh, Serena Giuliano, Nadia Habel, Najla El-Hachem, Céline Pisibon, Corine Bertolotto and Robert Ballotti
An Update on the Role of Ubiquitination in Melanoma Development and Therapies
Reprinted from: *J. Clin. Med.* **2021**, *10*, 1133, doi:10.3390/jcm10051133 85

Hans Binder, Maria Schmidt, Henry Loeffler-Wirth, Lena Suenke Mortensen and Manfred Kunz
Melanoma Single-Cell Biology in Experimental and Clinical Settings
Reprinted from: *J. Clin. Med.* **2021**, *10*, 506, doi:10.3390/jcm10030506 105

Lionel Larribère and Jochen Utikal
NF1-Dependent Transcriptome Regulation in the Melanocyte Lineage and in Melanoma
Reprinted from: *J. Clin. Med.* **2021**, *10*, 3350, doi:10.3390/jcm10153350 127

About the Editor

Lionel Larribère defended his PhD in Life Science at the University of Nice, France. The research of his PhD and subsequent postdoc is focused on molecular mechanisms involved in the initiation and progression of melanoma cells. He spent several years as a senior investigator in the Dermato-Oncology department of the German Cancer Research Center (DKFZ) in Heidelberg. Currently, he is leading the Translational Oncology unit in the Department of Internal Medicine III at the SLK Clinic in Heilbronn, Germany.

Preface to "New Advances in Melanoma"

In this Special Issue, we focus on the latest advances in the fields of melanoma research and clinical diagnostics. The development of distant melanoma metastases, in the lungs for example, is a major cause of death, and the mechanisms underlying its development are still not completely understood. Kyjacova et al. proposed a method for Trp-1 transcript analysis by real-time PCR in a melanoma mouse model of lung metastasis. In another study, the role of miRNA in tumorigenesis was investigated by examining the precursors of melanocytes, the melanoblasts. Linck-Paulus et al. describe an miRNA signature, discovered by comparing the expression status of signature genes in melanoblasts and melanoma cells that play a major role in driving melanoma development. In the same line, comparison of RNAseq datasets from melanoblasts and metastatic melanoma cells led us to observe that major signaling pathways, such as of VEGF, senescence/secretome, endothelin, and cAMP/PKA, are likely to be upregulated upon NF1 loss of function in both situations (Larribere et al.). These data reinforce the utility of investigating gene regulation during embryogenesis to better understand tumorigenesis. Interestingly, it was also shown that an miRNA pair (miR-26-5p and miR-21-3p) are involved in the HLA class I-mediated immune escape by regulating the expression of components of the HLA class I antigen processing and presentation machinery (APM). These data might impact the discovery of new biomarkers for HLA class I low melanoma cells (Lazaridou et al.).

In the domain of clinical diagnostics, a study on the Catalonian melanoma population showed an increased incidence in the advanced age population, including a rapidly increasing trend of in situ melanoma and lentigo maligna subtype. In addition, BRAF mutations, which are present in 40% to 60% of melanomas, have been extensively used as a biomarker of the sensitivity to BRAF inhibitors for more than a decade. However, the accuracy in detecting BRAF mutations may lead to false-negatives depending on the detection method. To address this, Colombino et al. compared different screening strategies in a study of the Sardinian melanoma population and showed that real-time PCR and NGS were able to successfully detect additional BRAF mutant cases in comparison with conventional sequencing methods.

Finally, one review discussed the role of ubiquitination in melanoma development and therapies. Because each step of the ubiquitination process is pharmacologically targetable, increasing attention has been paid to its role in melanoma development as well as in the mechanisms of acquired therapy resistance (Soysouvanh et al.). In the other review, Binder et al. focuses on melanoma cellular heterogeneity and the utility of single-cell biology. This new technology has led, for example, to an improved understanding of mechanisms of resistance to checkpoint inhibitor therapy. It is also allowing a deeper comprehension of the transcriptional plasticity of metastatic melanoma cells.

Lionel Larribère
Editor

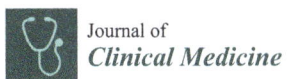

Article

Learning from Embryogenesis—A Comparative Expression Analysis in Melanoblast Differentiation and Tumorigenesis Reveals miRNAs Driving Melanoma Development

Lisa Linck-Paulus [1,†], Lisa Lämmerhirt [1,†], Daniel Völler [1], Katharina Meyer [2], Julia C. Engelmann [3], Rainer Spang [2], Norbert Eichner [4], Gunter Meister [4], Silke Kuphal [1] and Anja Katrin Bosserhoff [1,*]

[1] Institute of Biochemistry, Friedrich-Alexander-University Erlangen-Nürnberg, 91054 Erlangen, Germany; lisa.linck@fau.de (L.L.-P.); lisa.laemmerhirt@fau.de (L.L.); daniel.voeller@biontech.de (D.V.); silke.kuphal@fau.de (S.K.)
[2] Institute of Functional Genomics, University of Regensburg, 93053 Regensburg, Germany; katharina-meyer@gmx.de (K.M.); rainer.spang@klinik.uni-regensburg.de (R.S.)
[3] Department of Marine Microbiology and Biogeochemistry, NIOZ Royal Netherlands Institute for Sea Research, 1790 AB Den Burg, The Netherlands; julia.engelmann@nioz.nl
[4] Department of Biochemistry I, University of Regensburg, 93053 Regensburg, Germany; norbert.eichner@vkl.uni-regensburg.de (N.E.); gunter.meister@vkl.uni-regensburg.de (G.M.)
* Correspondence: anja.bosserhoff@fau.de
† These authors contributed equally to this work.

Citation: Linck-Paulus, L.; Lämmerhirt, L.; Völler, D.; Meyer, K.; Engelmann, J.C.; Spang, R.; Eichner, N.; Meister, G.; Kuphal, S.; Bosserhoff, A.K. Learning from Embryogenesis—A Comparative Expression Analysis in Melanoblast Differentiation and Tumorigenesis Reveals miRNAs Driving Melanoma Development. *J. Clin. Med.* **2021**, *10*, 2259. https://doi.org/10.3390/jcm10112259

Academic Editor: Lionel Larribère

Received: 13 April 2021
Accepted: 21 May 2021
Published: 24 May 2021

Publisher's Note: MDPI stays neutral with regard to jurisdictional claims in published maps and institutional affiliations.

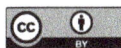

Copyright: © 2021 by the authors. Licensee MDPI, Basel, Switzerland. This article is an open access article distributed under the terms and conditions of the Creative Commons Attribution (CC BY) license (https://creativecommons.org/licenses/by/4.0/).

Abstract: Malignant melanoma is one of the most dangerous tumor types due to its high metastasis rates and a steadily increasing incidence. During tumorigenesis, the molecular processes of embryonic development, exemplified by epithelial–mesenchymal transition (EMT), are often reactivated. For melanoma development, the exact molecular differences between melanoblasts, melanocytes, and melanoma cells are not completely understood. In this study, we aimed to identify microRNAs (miRNAs) that promote melanoma tumorigenesis and progression, based on an in vitro model of normal human epidermal melanocyte (NHEM) de-differentiation into melanoblast-like cells (MBrCs). Using miRNA-sequencing and differential expression analysis, we demonstrated in this study that a majority of miRNAs have an almost equal expression level in NHEMs and MBrCs but are significantly differentially regulated in primary tumor- and metastasis-derived melanoma cell lines. Further, a target gene analysis of strongly regulated but functionally unknown miRNAs yielded the implication of those miRNAs in many important cellular pathways driving malignancy. We hypothesize that many of the miRNAs discovered in our study are key drivers of melanoma development as they account for the tumorigenic potential that differentiates melanoma cells from proliferating or migrating embryonic cells.

Keywords: miRNAs; melanoma; embryogenesis; melanoblasts

1. Introduction

Malignant melanoma is an aggressively metastatic tumor with a high incidence that has been increasing for years [1]. Especially patients with an advanced metastatic tumor stage still have a poor outcome [2]. Interestingly, melanoma has molecular features that are not found in other tumors [3]. Two aspects are of particular importance during melanoma development:

1. Melanoblasts, the precursors of melanocytes derived from the neural crest, exhibit several mechanisms during embryogenesis usually known from tumor cells, e.g., they actively migrate, adapt to different cellular environments, and "invade" the epidermis [4,5].

2. Melanoma cells can build stem-cell-like subpopulations that have the ability to differentiate into several cell lineages such as neural, mesenchymal, and endothelial cells [6–8].

These characteristic features show that melanoma cells can re-activate the pathways of neural crest differentiation and melanoblast migration, and thus reflect the high plasticity of malignant melanoma cells.

The neural crest, a transient component of the ectoderm, is located between the neural tube and epidermis during embryonal neural tube formation. Neural crest cells migrate during or shortly after neurulation, an embryological event characterized by the closure of the neural tube. Because of their great importance, they have been called the fourth germinal layer. Neural crest cells can differentiate into various cell types such as neurons and glial cells of the autonomic nervous system, some skeletal elements, and melanocytes [9]. There are two main migration pathways of neural crest cells: the ventral pathway and the dorsolateral pathway. Melanoblasts mainly migrate through the dorsolateral pathways between the somites and the ectoderm to their target region, the epidermis, where they then differentiate to melanocytes [4,5,10].

In addition to the high differentiation plasticity, malignant melanoma is characterized by being the tumor type with the highest mutation rate [11]. To date, however, only a few "drivers" of tumor development have been described in comparison to other cancers and all of those frequently mutated driver genes seem only to play a secondary role in the initiation of tumor metastasis [12].

microRNAs (miRNAs) are small non-coding RNAs that can regulate gene expression on a post-transcriptional level [13]. They are transcribed in the nucleus as long, double-stranded precursor molecules containing a characteristic stem-loop structure. Two mature, single-stranded miRNAs, which are complementary to each other and about 21 nucleotides long, are processed from the precursor by an intracellular enzymatic cascade. The location in the precursor molecule discriminates the annotation of the mature miRNA: the miRNA in the precursor arm with the 5′ end is called 5p, and the miRNA in the 3′ arm is called 3p [14]. One mature miRNA molecule binds to one of the four human Argonaute proteins to form the RNA-induced silencing complex (RISC). The RISC identifies target messenger RNAs (mRNAs) via complementary base pairing, interferes with their translation, and simultaneously mediates decay of the target mRNA by hydrolytic cleavage or via cellular degradation mechanisms [15]. miRNAs are deeply involved in the regulation of all important cellular processes and are the main contributor to the formation and progression of cancer [16]. In melanoma, many studies show that the expression of miRNAs is deregulated compared to normal human epidermal melanocytes and that deregulated miRNA expression is linked to important processes affecting tumor formation and progression [17–20]. The role of miRNAs during melanoblast differentiation and their involvement in de-differentiation processes that may drive tumor development, such as migration and invasion, is not well understood.

The aim of this study was to identify miRNAs that drive melanoma development and progression via a comparative analysis of miRNA expression in melanoblasts, differentiated melanocytes, and melanoma cells from primary tumors and metastases.

2. Materials and Methods

2.1. Cultivation of Melanocytes and De-Differentiation into Melanoblast-Related Cells

Normal human epidermal melanocytes (NHEM) were obtained from PromoCell (Heidelberg, Germany) or Lonza (Basel, Switzerland) and were derived from human neonatal foreskin tissue of Caucasian donors. The melanocytes were grown either in melanocyte serum-free M2 medium without PMA (phorbol myristate acetate) from PromoCell (Heidelberg, Germany) or in melanocyte serum-free medium with PMA from Lonza (Basel, Switzerland) at 37 °C and 5% CO_2. For de-differentiation, NHEM were grown for three passages and subsequently cultivated in a special melanoblast growth medium for 7 or 14 days to de-differentiate into melanoblast-related cells (MBrCs): MCBD 153 medium

(Sigma-Aldrich, Steinheim, Germany) containing 8% chelated fetal bovine serum (FBS), 2% normal FBS (PAA Laboratories, Pasching, Austria), 2 mM glutamine, 1.66 ng/mL cholera toxin B, 10 ng/mL SCF (Sigma-Aldrich, Steinheim, Germany), 100 nM endothelin-3 and 2.5 ng/mL bFGF. Chelated FBS was prepared by mixing 1.2 g of Chelex-100 (Sigma-Aldrich, Steinheim, Germany) per 40 mL of FBS for 1.5 h at 4 °C with gentle stirring. One sub-group of cells continued growing in PromoCell M2 medium (labeled as melanocytes in this study). The de-differentiation procedure of melanocytes to MBrCs is published by Cook et al. [21].

2.2. Melanoma Cell Culture

The melanoma cell lines Mel Juso (RRID:CVCL_1403), Mel Ei (RRID:CVCL_3978), Mel Wei (RRID:CVCL_3981), and Mel Ho (RRID:CVCL_1402) [22] were derived from primary cutaneous melanomas, whereas Mel Ju (RRID:CVCL_3979), Mel Im (RRID:CVCL_3980) [22], Hmb2 (RRID:CVCL_6646) [23], A375 (RRID:CVCL_0132) [24], 1205Lu (RRID:CVCL_5239) [25], and 501 Mel (RRID:CVCL_4633) [26] were derived from metastases of malignant melanomas. The cells were maintained in DMEM or RPMI-1640 medium (Sigma-Aldrich, Steinheim, Germany) supplemented with penicillin (400 units/mL), streptomycin (50 mg/mL), and 10% FBS (Sigma-Aldrich, Steinheim, Germany). Only RPMI was additionally supplemented with 0.2% sodium bicarbonate (Sigma-Aldrich, Steinheim, Germany). The melanoma cells were incubated in a humidified atmosphere containing 8% CO_2 at 37 °C in T75 cell culture flasks (Corning Incorporated, New York, NY, USA). They were split at a ratio of 1:5 every 3 days.

2.3. microRNA-Sequencing and Bioinformatic Sequence Data Analysis

microRNA-sequencing was performed on four different samples of NHEM from different passages, two independent replicates of MBrCs and the melanoma cell lines Mel Wei, Mel Ei, Mel Juso, Mel Ju, Mel Im, and Hmb2. Performance of sample preparation, miRNA profiling, and sequencing are described elsewhere [17]. miRNA-sequencing data of melanoma cells and NHEMs are already published [17]. For this study, all miRNA sequencing data were re-analyzed using current software and databases: preprocessing and counting against human miRNA listed in the miRbase database (http://www.mirbase.org; version 22 March 2018) was performed using the "miRDeep2" package [27] running with standard parameters as part of the Galaxy environment [28]. After transferring the resulting raw miRNA counts to R, normalization and differential expression analysis were performed using the "Deseq2" package [29].

The heatmaps of differentially expressed miRNAs were designed with Microsoft Excel® using a 3-color scale with red, white, and blue representing the minimum, median (50th percentile), and maximum, respectively. The colors encode log2FoldChange from Deseq2, and the highest and the lowest log2fold change are indicated respectively.

Principal component analysis (PCA) was performed using https://maayanlab.cloud/biojupies (accessed on 13 January 2021) [30]. Venn diagrams were calculated using the "VennDiagram" package in R and were illustrated with the venn.diagram function. The overlap was calculated using the calculate.overlap function. Figures were created using CorelDRAW® 2017 (64-Bit, Corel Corporation, Ottawa, ON, Canada).

Analysis of predicted target genes of miRNAs was performed using http://www.targetscan.org/vert_72, release 7.2 March 2018 [31]. Gene ontology enrichment analysis of predicted targets was performed with http://geneontology.org, release 1 January 2021 [32]. The STRING network analysis of miRNA target genes was performed using https://string-db.org, version 11.0b October 2020 [33] and presented using the stringApp in Cytoscape version 3.8.2 [34]. The STRING network shows known protein–protein associations from curated databases or experimentally determined, predicted interactions from gene neighborhood, gene fusions or co-occurrence and text mining, and co-expression or homology-based interactions. The minimum required interaction score was 0.4.

2.4. Gene Expression Microarray and Gene Set Enrichment Analysis (GSEA) of miRNA Target Genes

Gene expression microarray analysis was performed with three different replicates of MBrCs and the respective NHEM in the melanoma cell lines Mel Ho, A375, 501 Mel, and 1205 Lu. RNA was isolated with Rneasy® Mini Kit of Qiagen (Hilden, Germany) and was reverse-transcribed followed by hybridization to the Human Gene 1.0 ST Expression Array from Affymetrix (Santa Clara, CA, USA). Sample processing and Affymetrix microarray hybridization were carried out at the Genomics Core Unit: Center of Excellence for Fluorescent Bioanalytics (KFB, University of Regensburg, Regensburg, Germany). Signal intensities were summarized to Affymetrix probe_set level using 'rma' within the Bioconductor package oligo [35], and packages pd.hugene.1.0.st.v1 and hugene10sttranscriptcluster [36]. Probe_sets with an Entrez identifier were retained (21,995 genes) for further analyses. We used the non-parametric empirical Bayes approach of Combat [37] to remove the donor effects of MBrCs and the corresponding NHEM and ranked differentially expressed genes between melanoblasts and melanocytes versus melanoma cell lines by fold change using limma [38]. This ranked gene list was used for Gene Set Enrichment Analysis with the GSEA software version 4.0.3 (https://www.gsea-msigdb.org/gsea/index.jsp) [39,40]. For GSEA analysis, the C3 collection of the molecular signature database was used (MSigDB version 7.2, https://www.gsea-msigdb.org/gsea/msigdb/collection_details.jsp#MIRDB) with special attention to the miRDB gene set collection consisting of MirTarget high-confidence predicted human miRNA target genes [41] and the MIR Legacy geneset containing genes with 7-nucleotide miRNA-binding motifs of miRNAs cataloged in v7.1 of miRBase (http://www.mirbase.org, version 7.1, October 2005). For calculation of the false discovery rate (FDR), a pre-ranked GSEA analysis using one single gene set with targets of the respective miRNA was performed.

2.5. Isolation and Reverse Transcription of miRNAs from Mammalian Cells

The isolation and purification of miRNAs were performed using the miRNeasy Mini Kit from Qiagen (Hilden, Germany) according to the manufacturer. For the reverse transcription, the miScript II RT Kit from Qiagen (Hilden Germany) was used. In this study, 500 ng of miRNA were reversed transcribed into micDNA according to the manufacturer's specification.

2.6. Quantitative RT-PCR with miRNA

The qRT-PCR was performed on a *LightCycler®* 480 System from Roche (Mannheim, Germany). For the determination of the relative expression of miRNAs in melanocytes (at least $n = 3$), MBrCs (at least $n = 3$) and different melanoma cell lines (at least $n = 9$), from primary melanoma and melanoma metastasis, the *miScript SYBR® Green* PCR Kit of Qiagen (Hilden, Germany) was used. The snRNA U6 was taken as a reference for the relative determination of miRNAs. For qRT-PCR, a 25 µL reaction was used containing 2 µL of transcribed miRNA, 12.5 µL of miScript SYBR Green, 2.5 µL of the respective miScript Primer Assay (Qiagen, Hilden, Germany), 2.5 µL of miScript Universal primer (Qiagen), and 5.5 µL RNase-free water. The following PCR program containing 60 cycles was used: 4.4 °C/s to 95 °C 15 min (initial denaturation); 2.2 °C/s to 94 °C 15 s (denaturation); 2.2 °C/s to 55 °C 30 s (annealing); 4.4 °C/s to 70 °C 30 s (amplification); 4.4 °C/s to 72 °C 1 s (measurement); 4.4 °C/s to 95 °C 5 s, 2.2 °C/s to 65 °C 1 min, and 0.11 °C/s to 97 °C (melting point analysis); and 2.2 °C/s to 40 °C 30 s (end). The PCR reaction was evaluated by melting curve analysis. Statistical analysis was performed via the software GraphPad Prism 5.04 (Version 5.0.4.533, GraphPad Software Inc., San Diego, CA, USA).

3. Results

3.1. miRNAs Differentially Expressed Only in Melanoma Cells but Not in NHEMs and Melanoblasts Drive Tumor Development

To identify the unknown miRNAs and their respective target molecules, which are important for the development or progression of melanoma, we followed the idea of "learning from embryology". To deduce tumor-relevant molecular mechanisms from comparison with embryonic development, two hypotheses are plausible:

1. Genes and miRNAs, which are equally expressed in melanoma and melanoblasts but differently in melanocytes, are the relevant decisive factors for melanoma development; or
2. genes and miRNAs differentially expressed in melanoma compared to melanocytes and melanoblasts are key drivers of melanoma development and progression because these are stabilizing the tumor phenotype. This second hypothesis implicates that hypothesis 1 "only" focuses on genes, which are involved in differentiation/dedifferentiation processes but not in forcing tumor progression.

Using an experimental system first described by Rick Sturm's group [21], we dedifferentiated melanocytes into melanoblast-related cells (MBrC) using a cytokine cocktail (SCF, End-3, and bFGF) [5]. miRNA expression of MBrCs was compared to the respective normal human epidermal melanocytes (NHEMs) and melanoma cell lines derived from primary tumors (Mel Wei, Mel Ei, and Mel Juso) as well as from melanoma metastases (Mel Ju, Mel Im, and Hmb2) by miRNA sequencing.

We first analyzed the data using a principal component analysis (PCA). The PCA shows similar miRNA expression for NHEMs and MBrCs but considerable differences in melanoma (Figure 1A). Interestingly, the PCA supports the second hypothesis. It indicates that miRNAs are mainly equally expressed during melanoblast to melanocyte development but differentially regulated during tumor progression and thus may drive malignancy.

To further analyze this hypothesis, differential expression analysis of miRNAs was performed between all groups (MBrCs vs. NHEMs, MBrCs vs. primary tumor cell lines (PT), NHEMs vs. primary tumor-derived cell lines, and MBrCs vs. metastasis-derived cell lines (MET)) and illustrated in a heatmap (Figure 1B). The figure shows a noteworthy group of miRNAs, which are equally expressed in MBrCs and NHEMs, but strongly upregulated in melanoma cell lines (Figure 1B, indicated by arrow). These specific miRNAs follow the second hypothesis for learning from embryology and their in-depth analyses could provide molecular information about melanoma development.

To analyze this group of miRNAs in more detail, we filtered miRNA expression data for only miRNAs that were significantly differentially expressed (p-value < 0.05) in MBrCs vs. melanoma (primary tumor or metastasis-derived melanoma cell lines) but simultaneously not significantly regulated in MBrCs vs. NHEMs (p-value > 0.05). The miRNAs that fulfill these conditions are visualized in a Venn diagram (Figure 1C). The analysis provided 89 miRNAs that were significantly regulated in both, primary tumor and metastasis-derived melanoma cell lines, compared to MBrCs and NHEMs.

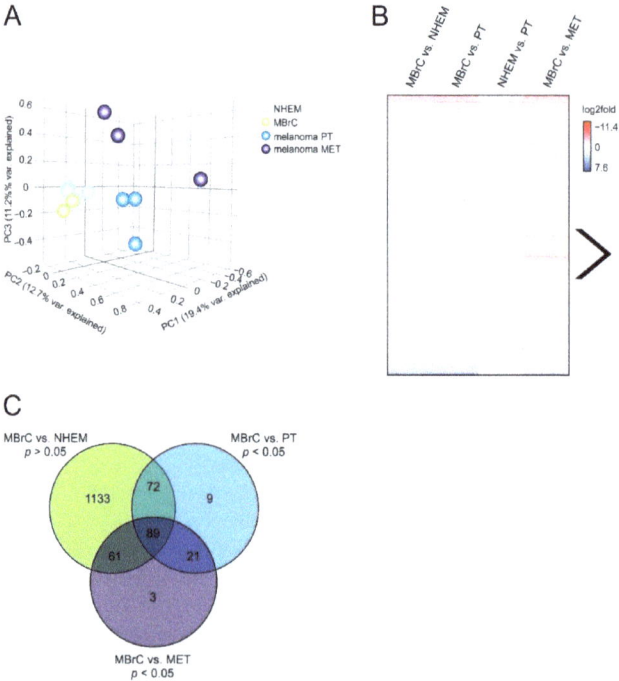

Figure 1. miRNA sequencing in NHEMs, MBrCs, and melanoma cell lines reveals a group of miRNAs, which are strongly regulated only in melanoma. (**A**) Principal component analysis of miRNA-seq data plot of the first three principal components (PCs). Samples with related gene expression profiles are closer in the three-dimensional embedding. Each sphere represents an RNA-seq sample, and replicates are shown in the same color: NHEM ($n = 4$), MBrC ($n = 2$), melanoma primary tumor (PT) cell lines Mel Juso, Mel Wei and Mel Ei, melanoma metastasis (MET) cell lines Mel Im, Mel Ju and Hmb2. (**B**) Differential gene expression analysis of miRNA-seq data in the indicated sample pairs is shown as a heatmap of log2fold values. The arrow indicates miRNAs, which are equally expressed in MBrCs and NHEMs but strongly upregulated in melanoma cell lines. (**C**) Venn diagram of miRNAs that are not significantly differentially expressed in MBrCs vs. NHEMs (p-value > 0.05) but significantly differentially expressed (p-value < 0.05) in MBrCs vs. melanoma primary tumor (PT) or metastasis-derived (MET) melanoma cell lines.

In the following, we analyzed whether these 89 miRNAs have a function in melanoma development. First, we visualized the differential expression analysis of those 89 miRNAs in a heatmap (Figure 2). A major part (63%) of those 89 miRNAs was upregulated in melanoma compared to MBrCs and 33% of the miRNAs were downregulated. In the following chapters, we separately focus on the upregulated and downregulated miRNAs, to elaborate whether they represent a group of regulators that play an important role during tumor progression.

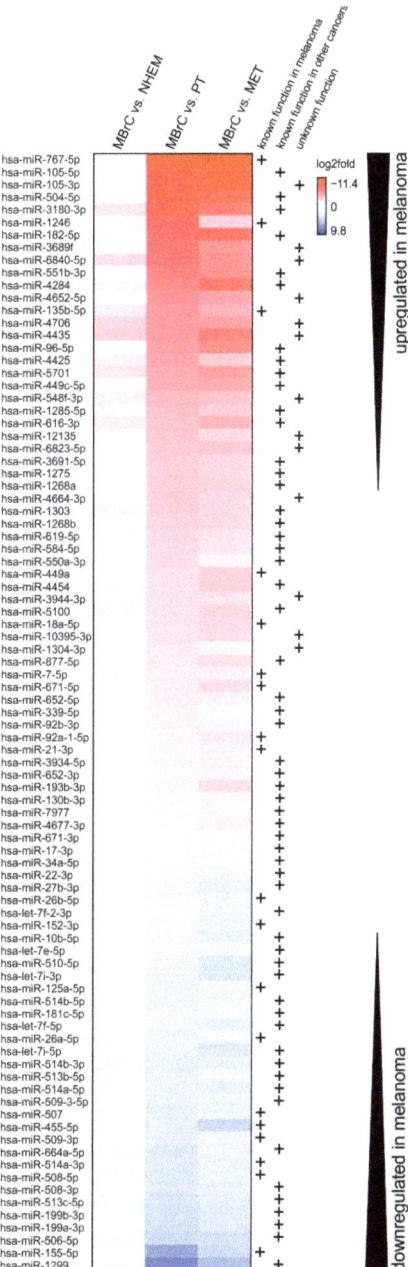

Figure 2. Significantly differentially expressed miRNAs in melanoma cells. Heatmap of log2fold values of all miRNAs that were not regulated in MBrCs vs. NHEMs ($p > 0.05$), but differentially expressed ($p < 0.05$) in MBrCs vs. melanoma primary tumor (PT), and MBrCs vs. melanoma metastasis-derived (MET) cell lines. miRNAs, which were upregulated in melanoma compared to MBrCs are shown in red, and miRNAs downregulated in melanoma are shown in blue. Both are indicated by black arrows. Mentions in the literature of functional relevance of the respective miRNA in melanoma or other cancers are depicted by +.

3.2. miRNAs Significantly Upregulated in Melanoma Cells Compared to MBrCs and NHEMs Regulate Important Target Genes Driving Tumorigenesis

For some of the miRNAs, which we found most strongly upregulated in melanoma cells compared to MBrCs and NHEMs, a functional role in melanoma development has already been described (see Figure 2, e.g., [42,43]). In addition, most of these miRNAs have known target genes with described functions in other cancers but no melanoma-associated role is known today, for example, miR-105 and miR-4284 [44,45]. Interestingly, miRNAs without known function to date are strongly upregulated in melanoma cell lines.

To elucidate the role of the upregulated miRNAs for the development of melanoma more deeply, we examined predicted target genes of the two most strongly upregulated miRNAs in melanoma cells, miR-767-5p and miR-105-5p using targetscan (http://www.targetscan.org/vert_72, release 7.2 March 2018 [31]). miR-767-5p and miR-105-5p share 1662 predicted target genes (Figure 3A). A gene ontology (GO) enrichment analysis of those targets showed, amongst others, a significant enrichment of genes involved in the Wnt signaling pathway (Supplementary Table S1) (http://geneontology.org, release 1 January 2021 [32]).

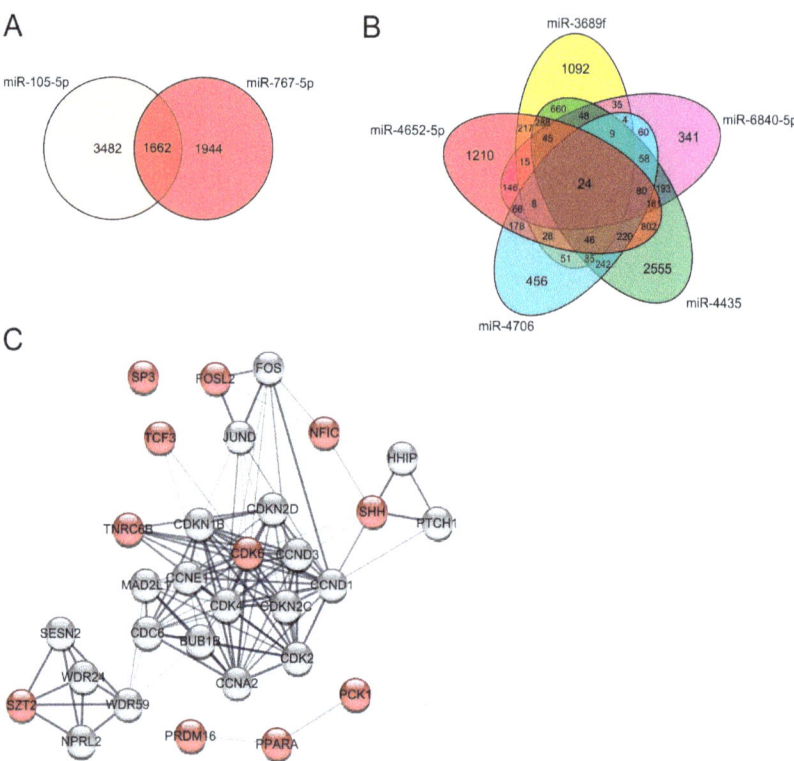

Figure 3. Target gene analysis of strongly upregulated miRNAs in melanoma compared to MBrCs and NHEMs. (**A**) Venn diagram of predicted targets of miR-105-5p and miR-767-5p. (**B**) Venn diagram of predicted target genes of miR-3689f, miR-6840-5p, miR-4652-5p, miR-4706, and miR-4435. (**C**) STRING network analysis of selected target genes of the 24 shared target genes of miR-3689f, miR-6840-5p, miR-4652-5p, miR-4706, and miR-4435 (red), and additional genes involved in the network (grey).

Other miRNAs that were strongly upregulated in melanoma cells compared to MBrCs and NHEMs, which are not described to have a functional role in melanoma or other cancers yet, were miR-3689f, miR-6840-5p, miR-4652-5p, miR-4706, and miR-4435 (see Figure 2).

A target gene analysis of those five miRNAs provided an enrichment of genes, e.g., involved in neuron development, response to cAMP, homophilic cell adhesion via plasma membrane adhesion molecules, protein localization to the plasma membrane and the cell periphery, actin cytoskeleton organization, regulation of BMP signaling pathway, endothelial cell differentiation, and negative regulation of developmental growth (Supplementary Table S1).

Further, we examined the shared predicted target genes of those five unknown miRNAs (Figure 3B). miR-3689f, miR-6840-5p, miR-4652-5p, miR-4706, and miR-4435 share 24 target genes. We analyzed those targets in a STRING network analysis (https://string-db.org, version 11.0b October 2020 [33]) (Figure 3C). Interestingly, all five miRNAs regulate targets that belong to a network with cyclin-D1 (CCND1), cyclin-E1 (CCNE1), cyclin-dependent kinase 4 inhibitor C (CDKN2C), and cyclin-A2 (CCNA2), and are strongly implicated in G1/S cell cycle transition and cell cycle regulation. Further, many shared target genes of these five miRNAs are important transcription factors such as FOSL2, NFIC, TCF3, and SP3. Additionally, PPARA, SHH, SZT2 were also determined to be shared target genes. PPARA, the peroxisome proliferator-activated receptor alpha, is a central regulator of lipid metabolism and can also function as a transcription factor. SHH, the sonic hedgehog protein, strongly interacts with its receptor PTCH1 and the hedgehog-interacting protein HHIP. The interaction between SHH and PTHC1 plays an important role during tumor growth and the regulation of apoptosis [46]. SZT2 is part of the KICSTOR complex, which regulates the amino acid-sensing part of the mTORC1 signaling pathway being required for many processes during cell proliferation and survival and often deregulated in cancer [47]. In conclusion, shared target genes of miR-3689f, miR-6840-5p, miR-4652-5p, miR-4706, and miR-4435 and their role for cell proliferation and survival implicates a so far unknown role of those five strongly upregulated miRNAs in melanoma development.

To further analyze our second hypothesis that especially genes, which are only deregulated in melanoma development but not differentially expressed during embryonal differentiation drive tumor development, we examined gene expression array data of genes differentially regulated comparing melanoma cells to MBrCs and NHEMs. To detect important miRNAs regulating these genes, gene set enrichment analysis (GSEA) was performed. We used gene sets containing predicted binding sites of miRNAs and compared them to a ranked list of genes from the gene expression array ranging from significantly upregulated genes in melanoma cells compared to MBrCs and NHEMs to significantly downregulated genes.

The GSEA analysis reveals that many target genes of the observed upregulated miRNAs are significantly downregulated in melanoma cells compared to MBrCs and NHEMs. The miRNAs miR-767-5p, miR-105-5p, mir-96-5p, miR-4425, miR-182-5p, and miR-3689f were analyzed in more detail (Figure 4).

miR-767-5p and miR-105-5p are the two most strongly upregulated miRNAs in melanoma cells compared to MBrCs (see Figure 2). The GSEA analysis showed a strong downregulation of their target genes in melanoma cells compared to MBrCs and NHEMs (Figure 4A,B) supporting our hypothesis that those miRNAs are important regulators of melanoma development. miR-96-5p, miR-4425, and miR-182-5p are known to regulate essential target genes in other tumor types [48–50]. Our data show significant downregulation of target genes of those miRNAs in melanoma cell lines compared to NHEM and MBrC (Figure 4A,C–E) implicating their important role also in melanoma. The role of miR-3689f is so far completely unknown in melanoma or other cancers. We found, on the one hand, a significant and strong upregulation of this miRNA in melanoma cells compared to MBrCs and NHEMs (Figure 2), and on the other hand, a significant downregulation of its target genes in melanoma (Figure 4F).

The similar expression of those miRNAs in NHEMs and MBrCs but strong upregulation in melanoma and the identified significant downregulation of their target genes in melanoma cells strongly supports our hypothesis. Therefore, those miRNAs have a significant share in driving the tumorigenic phenotype of melanoma.

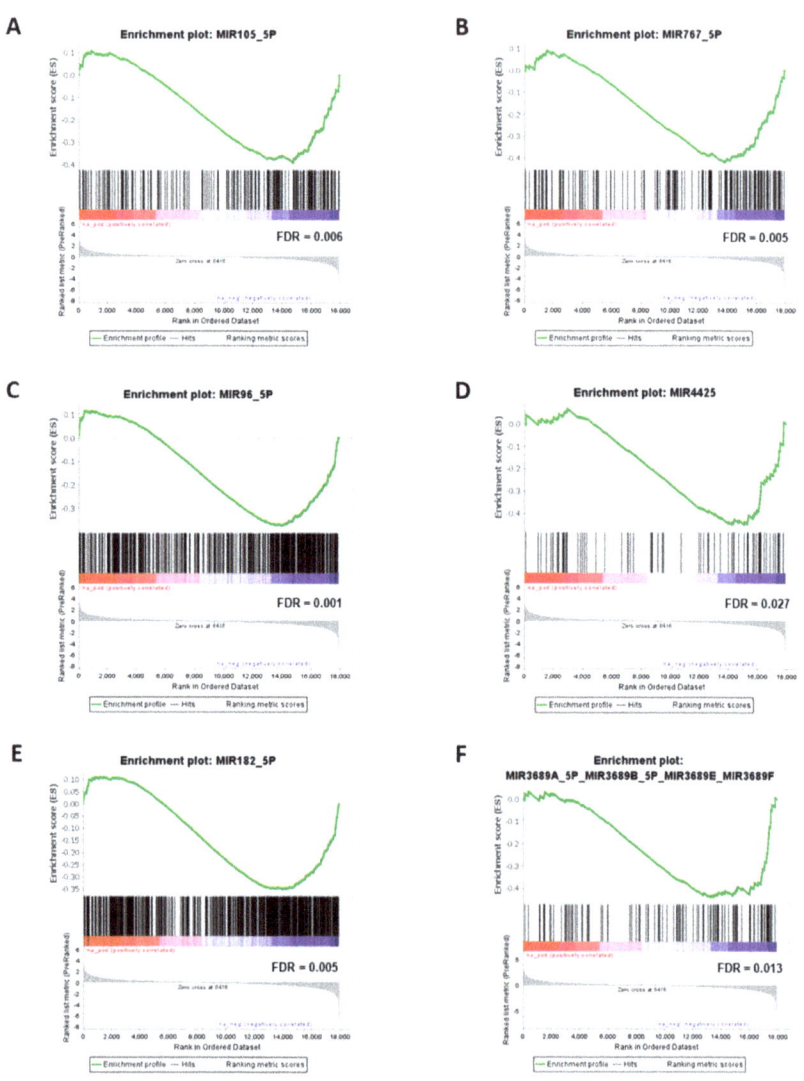

Figure 4. Significant downregulation of miRNA target genes in melanoma cells. Enrichment plot for (**A**) miR-105-5p, (**B**) miR-767-5p, (**C**) miR-96-5p, (**D**) miR-4425, (**E**) miR-182-5p, and (**F**) miR-3689F. Profile of the running enrichment score (green) and positions of gene set members of the respective miRNA target genes on the rank-ordered list of genes differentially regulated in melanoma cells compared to MBrCs and NHEMs identified by gene expression array analysis. Genes upregulated in melanoma are shown on the left side of the graph in red, genes downregulated in melanoma on the right side in blue.

3.3. miRNAs Significantly Downregulated in Melanoma Cells Compared to MBrCs and NHEMs Are Implicated in the Regulation of Tumorigenic Pathways

Focusing on those miRNAs that are significantly downregulated in melanoma vs. MBrCs and NHEMs yields in miRNAs that have already been described as implicated in melanoma development or have described functional roles in other cancers (see Figure 2, e.g., [51–54]). Interestingly, our analysis discovered many miRNAs of the so-called miR-506–514 cluster (miR-506, miR-508, miR-509, miR-513, and miR-514) as strongly and significantly downregulated in melanoma cells compared to MBrCs and NHEMs. The miR-506–514 cluster has been previously shown to be overexpressed in melanoma patient biopsies and cell lines and to promote melanoma growth [55]. To, therefore, confirm our miRNA expression data obtained by RNA-seq, we additionally performed qRT-PCR-based expression analysis of selected miRNAs of this miRNA cluster (Figure 5).

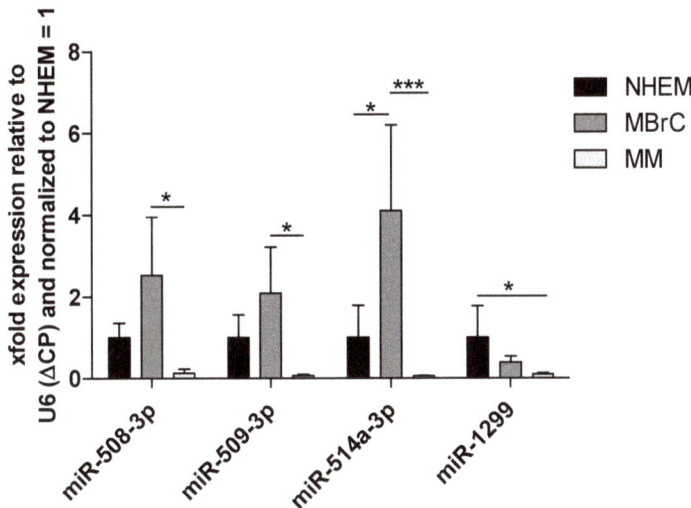

Figure 5. QRT-PCR shows a strong downregulation of miRNAs of the miR-506–514 cluster and miR-1299. Analysis of miR-508-3p, miR-509-3p, miR-514a-3p, and miR-1299 expression in normal human epidermal melanocytes (NHEM), melanoblast-related cells (MBrC), and at least 6 different melanoma cell lines (MM) via qRT-PCR. Bars represent mean + SEM, statistical significance was calculated using one-way ANOVA and subsequent Tukey's Multiple Comparison Test with ΔCP values before normalization to NHEM and is indicated as * $p \leq 0.05$ and *** $p \leq 0.001$.

Significant downregulation of miR-508-3p, miR-509-3p, and miR-514a-3p in melanoma cell lines compared to MBrCs can be observed, confirming the RNA-seq expression results. In addition, we could also show a strong downregulation of miR-1299. These data support the reliability of our RNA-seq analysis.

Although the most strongly downregulated miRNAs in melanoma compared to MBrCs obtained in our analysis were already described in the literature, most of those miRNAs have only known functional roles in other tumors but no association with melanoma development until now [54,56]. miRNAs with unknown function in melanoma are miR-1299, miR-199b-3p, and miR-664a-5p. We analyzed predicted target genes of those three miRNAs and found 99 shared targets (Figure 6A). GO term analysis of those 99 shared target genes showed significant enrichment of genes involved in stem cell proliferation, embryonic skeletal system morphogenesis, embryonic skeletal system development, and negative regulation of translation (Supplementary Table S1).

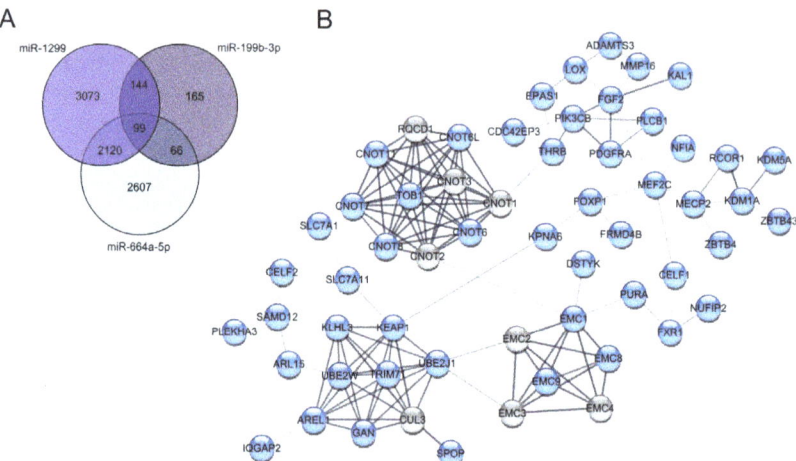

Figure 6. Target gene analysis of strongly downregulated miRNAs in melanoma compared to MBrCs and NHEMs. (**A**) Venn diagram of shared predicted targets of miR-1299, miR-199b-3p and miR-664a-5p. (**B**) STRING network analysis of selected target genes of the 99 shared targets of miR-1299, miR-199b-3p, and miR-664a-5p (blue), which belong to one network and additional genes involved in the network (grey).

Additional 144 shared targets of miR-1299 and miR-199b-3p include genes involved in developmental growth and embryo development.

Additionally, we analyzed the 99 shared targets of miR-1299, miR-199b-3p, and miR-664a-5p in a STRING network analysis to get an overview of how the target genes are related to each other (Figure 6B). The STRING analysis of the targets shows several clusters of connected genes.

The first gene cluster includes general CCR4-NOT transcription complex subunits (CNOT), which are involved in gene silencing by miRNA, transcriptional regulation, and negative regulation of the cell cycle [57]. The next target gene cluster includes the endoplasmic reticulum (ER) membrane protein complex subunits (EMC1-4, 8, and 9). These genes are known to be involved in protein folding. Another target gene cluster consists of the following genes: KLHL3, KEAP1, UBE2W, UBE2J1, TRIM71, AREL1, SPOP, CUL3, and GAN (Figure 6B). CUL3, KEAP1, and TRIM 71, for example, are involved in embryonic development. Additionally, some of these proteins are involved in proteasomal degradation via ubiquitination. The next cluster contains the genes KDM5A, KDM1A, ZBTB43, ZBTB4, MECP2, and RCOR1. These genes have the molecular function of transcription regulator activity in common. Moreover, KDM1A, KDM5A, and MECP2 are involved in embryonic development. The genes in the last cluster, PLCB1, PIK3B, PDGFRA, FGF2, and KAL1, are involved in developmental processes as well, with FGF2, PDGFRA, and PIK3CB being involved in embryonal development. Moreover, FGF2, PDGFRA, and PIK3CB play a role in the regulation of the actin cytoskeleton. Interestingly, FGF2 and PIK3CB are known to be involved in the activation of the mitogen-activated protein kinase (MAPK) activity. In summary, the STRING analysis provides a reliable overview of potentially important target genes that miR-1299, miR-199b-3p, and miR-664a have in common. The loss of these three miRNAs and the resulting upregulation of the described target genes might play a significant role in melanoma development and progression.

3.4. miRNAs Differentially Expressed in Only Metastasis-Derived Melanoma Cell Lines Compared to Melanoblasts Provide Information about Metastasis Processes

As previously shown, there are 89 miRNAs, which are significantly regulated during early tumor development (primary tumor cell lines) and stay highly expressed during tumor progression (metastasis-derived cell lines). The analysis also resulted in 61 miRNAs that are significantly differentially expressed (*p*-value < 0.05) only in MBrCs vs. metastasis-derived melanoma cell lines (see Figure 1B,C). Further focusing on these 61 miRNAs, based on strong miRNA regulation only in metastasis-derived cell lines (log2fold MET vs. PT > 1 or < −1) and absence of regulation during early tumorigenesis (log2fold MBrC vs. PT > −1 and simultaneously < 1), resulted in 17 miRNAs fulfilling the criteria (Figure 7A). Several of those miRNAs are already known to play a role during the development and metastasis of melanoma or other cancers (see Figure 7A, e.g., [58–60]). To determine if unknown miRNAs of this list (Figure 7A) have a specific impact on tumor metastasis, we analyzed those miRNAs in more detail.

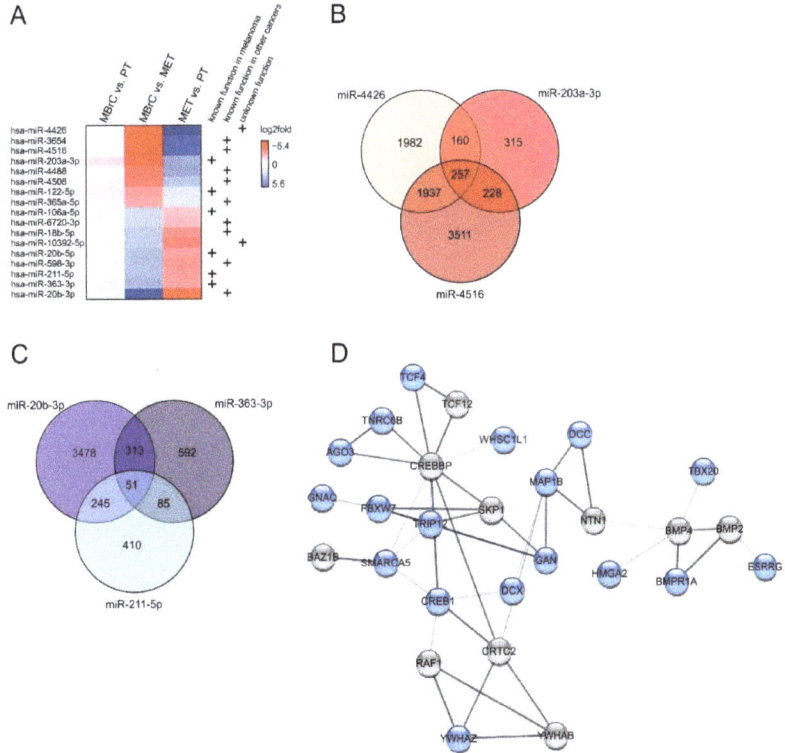

Figure 7. miRNAs are significantly regulated in only metastasis-derived melanoma cell lines. (**A**) miR-NAs that are not regulated in MBrCs vs. NHEMs (*p* > 0.05) and only significantly differentially expressed (*p* < 0.05) in MBrCs vs. melanoma metastasis-derived (MET) cell lines with log2fold in MET vs. PT > 1 or < −1 and in MBrC vs. PT > −1 and simultaneously < 1. Mentions in the literature of functional relevance of the respective miRNA in melanoma or other cancers are indicated (+). (**B**) Venn diagram of shared predicted targets of upregulated miR-4426, miR-203a-3p, and miR-4516. (**C**) Venn diagram of shared predicted targets of downregulated miR-20b-3p, miR-363-3p, and miR-211-5p. (**D**) STRING network analysis of connected target genes of the 51 shared targets of miR-20b-3p, miR-363-3p, and miR-211-5p (blue) and additionally involved genes (grey).

Predicted target genes of the most strongly upregulated miRNA, miR-4426, which is so far unknown in cancer (Figure 7A), are implicated in the canonical Wnt signaling pathway, positive regulation of locomotion, positive regulation of cell migration, and positive regulation of cell motility (Supplementary Table S1).

miR-4426 shares 417 targets with miR-203a-3p (Figure 7B), a miRNA known in melanoma as a biomarker for metastatic melanoma [61], but the functional role of this miRNA is unknown so far. These target genes are involved in the regulation of transmembrane receptor protein serine/threonine kinase signaling pathway, cell population proliferation, and positive regulation of cell differentiation (Supplementary Table S1). Targets of miR-203a-3p alone are related to the BMP signaling pathway, mesenchymal cell development, and neural crest cell differentiation.

Further, miR-4426 shares 2194 predicted target genes with miR-4516 that are supposed to be important for positive regulation of blood vessel endothelial cell migration.

miR-4426, miR-4516, and miR-203-3p share 257 targets, and some of them are significantly involved in the regulation of developmental processes, internal protein amino acid acetylation, and histone acetylation implicating a role of these miRNAs into epigenetic regulatory processes.

The most strongly downregulated miRNA in metastasis-derived cell lines compared to primary tumor cell lines and MBrCs is miR-20b-3p (Figure 7A). Predicted target genes of this miRNA are implicated in cell cycle and nervous system development (Supplementary Table S1). miR-363-3p, which is also strongly downregulated, has predicted target genes that are involved in actin polymerization-dependent cell motility and adherens junction assembly.

miR-20b-3p and miR-363-3p share 51 predicted target genes with miR-211-5p (Figure 7C) that are significantly involved in neuron migration. The strong downregulation of those three miRNAs in only metastasis-derived melanoma cell lines indicates a specific role of those miRNAs in migratory processes. A STRING network analysis of selected target genes of those 51 shared targets shows 28 interacting genes (Figure 7D). The genes CREB1, RAF1, YWHAB, YWHAZ, and CRTC2 are involved in the KEGG pathway of PI3K-Akt signaling. It is known that dysregulation of the PI3K-Akt signaling pathway is related to a poor treatment outcome in melanoma [62]. Additionally, CREBBP and SKP1 are involved in the TGF-beta signaling pathway. TGF-beta is known to play a role in melanoma progression and growth [63]. Moreover, target genes of miR-20b-3p, miR-363-3p, and miR-211-5p strongly interact with BMP4 and BMP2, which are involved in the positive regulation of the epithelial to mesenchymal transition. In summary, the string analysis implicates that target genes of miR-20b-3p, miR-363-3p, and miR-211-5p are involved in important processes of melanoma metastasis and progression.

4. Discussion

In this study, we examined the expression profile of miRNAs in various stages of development from melanoblasts to melanocytes to melanoma. RNA-sequencing and subsequent bioinformatical analyses revealed that miRNAs are mainly equally expressed in embryonic development from MBrCs to NHEMs, but strongly deregulated during the development of melanoma. We hypothesize that those miRNAs are the key drivers of malignancy as they account for the tumorigenic potential that differentiates melanoma cells from proliferating or migrating embryonic cells.

Several of those miRNAs identified in our study are already well described in the literature as important regulators of melanoma development. An example is some members of the well-characterized let-7 miRNA-family, which we found as strongly downregulated in melanoma cells compared to MBrCs and NHEMs. It is known that let-7 miRNAs function as important tumor suppressors in melanoma [64]. An overexpression in melanoma of, e.g., let-7b leads to a decreased level of cell cycle regulators like cyclin D1 and cyclin D3 [65]. Moreover, the loss of let-7a leads to an upregulation of ITGB3 indicating involvement in melanoma development and progression [66]. Further, miR-1246, which we found as strongly upregulated in melanoma cells in our study, is known to act as an oncogene in melanoma via influencing cell viability and migration and promoting BRAF inhibitor resistance [43,67]. The differential expression analysis in our study confirmed the regulation of those prominent tumor-promoting miRNAs in melanoma indicating the reliability of our gained results.

In addition, our study also showed a strong downregulation of the miRNAs miR-506, miR-508, miR-509, miR-513, and miR-514, which belong to a miRNA cluster called miR-506–514. This cluster has been previously shown to be overexpressed in melanoma patient biopsies and cell lines and to promote melanoma growth [55]. miR-514a-3p was further described to regulate the tumor suppressor NF1 and to be involved in BRAF inhibitor sensitivity in melanoma [68]. Interestingly, in our study, many miRNAs belonging to the miR-506–514 cluster are strongly downregulated in melanoma cells compared to MBrCs and NHEMs. The downregulation could be confirmed via qPCR in independent samples, implicating an interesting new and controversial role of this miRNA cluster in melanoma development.

Many of the miRNAs, which we detected as significantly regulated in melanoma, are already described in the literature as relevant for the development of other cancers [69,70] or are known to be dysregulated in melanoma, but without a distinctly described molecular function [17,71]. The analysis of their potential target genes and involved pathways in our study allows interesting conclusions to be drawn about their role in melanoma tumorigenesis. For example, miR-767 and miR-105, the two most strongly upregulated miRNAs in melanoma cells in our study, both belong to a group of genes, normally inactivated by DNA methylation in somatic tissues [72]. Hypomethylation during cancer development can lead to activation of such genes whose expression is normally restricted to embryonic development, so-called "cancer-germline" genes. miR-767 and miR-105 have been shown to be genomically located in a "cancer germline" gene that is aberrantly activated in melanoma cell lines and tissues [72]. Additionally, miR-767-5p is also upregulated in different other cancer types such as thyroid cancer or hepatocellular carcinoma [73,74]. Further, our study shows a strong downregulation of target genes of miR-767 and miR-105 in melanoma cells. It is known from the literature that miR-767 drives tumorigenesis in other cancers via repression of the tumor suppressors TET1 and TET3, which are responsible for the transformation of 5-methylcytosines to 5-hydroxymethylcytosines (5hmC) in DNA [72]. It is known from pancreatic cancer that a low TET1 expression and subsequent low 5hmC content lead to low survival of patients because of high tumor cell proliferation and metastasis [75]. This is due to loss of the TET1 mediated inhibition of both the canonical and non-canonical Wnt signaling, which leads to increased EMT in tumors with low TET1 expression [75]. A possible misregulation of the Wnt signaling pathway was also observed in this study for shared putative target genes of miR-767 and miR-105. For melanoma, it is also known that the Wnt signaling pathway is often dysregulated [76]. Additionally, Wnt signaling plays a role in the migration of neural crest cells (NCC) and multipotent precursor cells [77,78]. In our study, regulation of target genes associated with Wnt signaling was also observed for several other miRNAs, which are significantly regulated in only metastasis-derived melanoma cell lines, such as miR-4426, miR-203a-3p, and miR-211-5p. This indicates that those genes play an important role throughout the whole process of tumor development and are selectively regulated by numerous miRNAs in different tumor stages.

The results indicate that the newly detected deregulated miRNAs in our study play a significant role during both melanoma development and metastasis. The connection of those miRNAs with the Wnt signaling pathway is so far not described and can be a promising target for future analyses.

Next to the Wnt signaling pathway, our study discloses many other important signaling pathways where targets of the analyzed deregulated miRNAs are involved in. For example, in melanoma cells strongly upregulated miR-3689f, miR-6840-5p, miR-4652-5p, miR-4706, and miR-4435 share the target FOSL2, a transcription factor that dimerizes with JUN and binds to AP-1 sites. It is known from other cancers, that FOSL2 is activated by the ERK1/2 kinase leading to the transcription of SNAI2, which plays an important role in tumor metastasis via activation of epithelial-to-mesenchymal transition (EMT) [79]. Further target genes involved in EMT have been observed for many other miRNAs shown as dysregulated in melanoma cells in our study, underlining the important role of this process in tumor development and especially for tumor cell migration.

In addition, our study shows a regulation of miR-20b-3p, miR-363-3p, and miR-211-5p in only metastasis-derived melanoma cells (see Figure 7C,D) leading to an upregulation of, amongst others, BMP4 and BMP2. BMP4 is known to be regulated by LIF (leukemia inhibitory factor), which might be involved in melanoma-induced bone metastasis [80,81]. It is also known from the literature, that in melanoma the establishment of drug resistance has some signaling pathway activation in common with cell lineage development, e.g., genes associated with the ERK1/2 or the BMP signaling pathway [82]. In our study, many identified regulated miRNAs are related to these pathways, therefore, it can be concluded that the MBrC in vitro model is not only useful to detect alterations in miRNA expression according to melanoma development but may also improve comprehending the expression profiles of drug-resistant melanomas.

For some of the newly identified miRNAs in our study, which are deregulated only in melanoma cells compared to MBrCs and NHEMs, a distinct connection of their associated target genes with specific developmental processes was observed. For example, for the strongly downregulated miR-1299, miR-199b-3p, and miR-664a-5p, which have no described function in melanoma so far. The results indicate that a loss of those miRNAs during melanoma development could result in a dysregulation of fine-tuning of developmental genes that regulate normal embryonic development and may lead to uncontrolled proliferation.

Thus, our study revealed many significantly regulated miRNAs, which are related to important pathways involved in melanoma development and progression. The connection between the newly identified miRNAs and their target genes could be the main contributor to the tumorigenicity of melanoma, which has not been investigated so far.

Many properties of embryonic cells, such as proliferation, migration, and invasion also play an important role during tumorigenesis and especially in metastasis. In our study, we examined miRNAs, which are only regulated in metastasis-derived melanoma cell lines compared to MBrCs and NHEMs to detect target genes and mechanisms that may drive the metastatic phenotype. We identified in total 89 miRNAs being significantly regulated in primary tumor and metastasis-derived cell lines. In contrast, only a few miRNAs were significantly regulated in metastasis-derived cell lines but not in primary tumor cell lines. This indicates that the most important changes leading to melanoma tumorigenesis on the miRNA level seem to already take place at the beginning of tumor development. Interestingly, our study revealed that many processes being regulated by targets of miRNAs that are upregulated in metastasis-derived melanoma cells, such as the Wnt signaling pathway or the BMP signaling pathway. These are also regulated by other miRNAs, which are already upregulated in primary tumor-derived melanoma cells. This indicates that those pathways play an important role throughout the whole process of tumor development and are selectively regulated by numerous miRNAs in different tumor stages.

5. Conclusions

This study revealed a strong and significant regulation of many miRNAs in melanoma cell lines compared to healthy cells but a similar expression profile of miRNAs during melanoblast to melanocyte development. Our analyses support our hypothesis that those miRNAs drive tumorigenesis and represent the decisive difference to comparable processes of proliferation or migration during embryonic development. Following this hypothesis, we identified many miRNAs, which were not described during melanoma development so far, but whose target gene analysis and comparison to known target genes from other cancers implicate a promising role as tumor driving candidates. This study lays the foundation for further interesting analyses of those novel miRNAs that may play a crucial role in the development and progression of malignant melanoma.

Supplementary Materials: The following supplementary materials are available online at https://www.mdpi.com/article/10.3390/jcm10112259/s1, Table S1: Gene ontology enrichment analysis of miRNA target genes.

Author Contributions: Conceptualization of the manuscript was done by L.L.-P., L.L., S.K. and A.K.B.; L.L. and D.V. performed the experiments; L.L.-P. and L.L. did the GSEA, Venn diagram, heatmap and STRING analysis and designed the figures; N.E. and G.M. did the bioinformatical analysis of the miRNA-seq data; K.M., J.C.E. and R.S. performed the processing of the gene expression microarray data; L.L.-P., L.L., S.K. and A.K.B. wrote the manuscript; All authors have read and agreed to the published version of the manuscript.

Funding: The work was funded by the Wilhelm Sander Foundation (2018.113 to A.K.B.).

Institutional Review Board Statement: Not applicable.

Informed Consent Statement: Not applicable.

Data Availability Statement: miRNA-sequencing data are deposited in the Gene Expression Omnibus (GEO) database under the accession number GSE174334.

Acknowledgments: We would like to thank Stefan Fischer for his kind support in bioinformatical questions.

Conflicts of Interest: The authors declare no conflict of interest.

References

1. Leiter, U.; Eigentler, T.; Garbe, C. Epidemiology of skin cancer. In *Sunlight, Vitamin D and Skin Cancer*; Springer: Berlin/Heidelberg, Germany, 2014; pp. 120–140.
2. Garbe, C.; Peris, K.; Hauschild, A.; Saiag, P.; Middleton, M.; Bastholt, L.; Grob, J.-J.; Malvehy, J.; Newton-Bishop, J.; Stratigos, A.J. Diagnosis and treatment of melanoma. European consensus-based interdisciplinary guideline—Update 2016. *Eur. J. Cancer* **2016**, *63*, 201–217. [CrossRef] [PubMed]
3. Shain, A.H.; Bastian, B.C. From melanocytes to melanomas. *Nat. Rev. Cancer* **2016**, *16*, 345. [CrossRef] [PubMed]
4. Thomas, A.J.; Erickson, C.A. The making of a melanocyte: The specification of melanoblasts from the neural crest. *Pigment Cell Melanoma Res.* **2008**, *21*, 598–610. [CrossRef] [PubMed]
5. Bosserhoff, A.K.; Ellmann, L.; Kuphal, S. Melanoblasts in culture as an in vitro system to determine molecular changes in melanoma. *Exp. Dermatol.* **2011**, *20*, 435–440. [CrossRef] [PubMed]
6. Fang, D.; Nguyen, T.K.; Leishear, K.; Finko, R.; Kulp, A.N.; Hotz, S.; Van Belle, P.A.; Xu, X.; Elder, D.E.; Herlyn, M. A tumorigenic subpopulation with stem cell properties in melanomas. *Cancer Res.* **2005**, *65*, 9328–9337. [CrossRef] [PubMed]
7. Brocker, E.B.; Magiera, H.; Herlyn, M. Nerve growth and expression of receptors for nerve growth factor in tumors of melanocyte origin. *J. Investig. Dermatol.* **1991**, *96*, 662–665. [CrossRef] [PubMed]
8. Hendrix, M.J.; Seftor, E.A.; Hess, A.R.; Seftor, R.E. Vasculogenic mimicry and tumour-cell plasticity: Lessons from melanoma. *Nat. Rev. Cancer* **2003**, *3*, 411–421. [CrossRef]
9. Vandamme, N.; Berx, G. From neural crest cells to melanocytes: Cellular plasticity during development and beyond. *Cell. Mol. Life Sci.* **2019**, *76*, 1919–1934. [CrossRef]
10. Le Douarin, N.; LeDouarin, N.M.; Kalcheim, C. *The Neural Crest*; Cambridge University Press: Cambridge, UK, 1999.
11. Watson, I.R.; Wu, C.-J.; Zou, L.; Gershenwald, J.E.; Chin, L. Genomic classification of cutaneous melanoma. In Proceedings of the AACR 106th Annual Meeting 2015, Philadelphia, PA, USA, 18–22 April 2015.
12. Tímár, J.; Vizkeleti, L.; Doma, V.; Barbai, T.; Rásó, E. Genetic progression of malignant melanoma. *Cancer Metastasis Rev.* **2016**, *35*, 93–107. [CrossRef]
13. Kim, V.N.; Han, J.; Siomi, M.C. Biogenesis of small RNAs in animals. *Nat. Rev. Mol. Cell Biol.* **2009**, *10*, 126–139. [CrossRef]
14. Starega-Roslan, J.; Koscianska, E.; Kozlowski, P.; Krzyzosiak, W.J. The role of the precursor structure in the biogenesis of microRNA. *Cell. Mol. Life Sci.* **2011**, *68*, 2859–2871. [CrossRef] [PubMed]
15. Meister, G. Argonaute proteins: Functional insights and emerging roles. *Nat. Rev. Genet.* **2013**, *14*, 447–459. [CrossRef]
16. Iorio, M.; Croce, C. microRNA dysregulation in cancer: Diagnostics, monitoring and therapeutics. A comprehensive review. *EMBO Mol. Med.* **2012**, *4*, 143–159.
17. Linck, L.; Liebig, J.; Voeller, D.; Eichner, N.; Lehmann, G.; Meister, G.; Bosserhoff, A. microRNA-sequencing data analyzing melanoma development and progression. *Exp. Mol. Pathol.* **2018**, *105*, 371–379. [CrossRef] [PubMed]
18. Mueller, D.W.; Rehli, M.; Bosserhoff, A.K. miRNA expression profiling in melanocytes and melanoma cell lines reveals miRNAs associated with formation and progression of malignant melanoma. *J. Investig. Dermatol.* **2009**, *129*, 1740–1751. [CrossRef]
19. Ding, N.; Wang, S.; Yang, Q.; Li, Y.; Cheng, H.; Wang, J.; Wang, D.; Deng, Y.; Yang, Y.; Hu, S. Deep sequencing analysis of microRNA expression in human melanocyte and melanoma cell lines. *Gene* **2015**, *572*, 135–145. [CrossRef]

20. Stark, M.S.; Tyagi, S.; Nancarrow, D.J.; Boyle, G.M.; Cook, A.L.; Whiteman, D.C.; Parsons, P.G.; Schmidt, C.; Sturm, R.A.; Hayward, N.K. Characterization of the melanoma miRNAome by deep sequencing. *PLoS ONE* **2010**, *5*, e9685. [CrossRef] [PubMed]
21. Cook, A.L.; Donatien, P.D.; Smith, A.G.; Murphy, M.; Jones, M.K.; Herlyn, M.; Bennett, D.C.; Leonard, J.H.; Sturm, R.A. Human melanoblasts in culture: Expression of BRN2 and synergistic regulation by fibroblast growth factor-2, stem cell factor, and endothelin-3. *J. Investig. Dermatol.* **2003**, *121*, 1150–1159. [CrossRef]
22. Johnson, J.P.; Demmer-Dieckmann, M.; Meo, T.; Hadam, M.R.; Riethmüller, G. Surface antigens of human melanoma cells defined by monoclonal antibodies. I. Biochemical characterization of two antigens found on cell lines and fresh tumors of diverse tissue origin. *Eur. J. Immunol.* **1981**, *11*, 825–831. [CrossRef]
23. Siracký, J.; Blasko, M.; Borovanský, J.; Kovarik, J.; Svec, J.; Vrba, M. Human melanoma cell lines: Morphology, growth, and alpha-mannosidase characteristics. *Neoplasma* **1982**, *29*, 661–668.
24. Giard, D.J.; Aaronson, S.A.; Todaro, G.J.; Arnstein, P.; Kersey, J.H.; Dosik, H.; Parks, W.P. In vitro cultivation of human tumors: Establishment of cell lines derived from a series of solid tumors. *J. Natl. Cancer Inst.* **1973**, *51*, 1417–1423. [CrossRef] [PubMed]
25. Cornil, I.; Theodorescu, D.; Man, S.; Herlyn, M.; Jambrosic, J.; Kerbel, R. Fibroblast cell interactions with human melanoma cells affect tumor cell growth as a function of tumor progression. *Proc. Natl. Acad. Sci. USA* **1991**, *88*, 6028–6032. [CrossRef] [PubMed]
26. Marincola, F.M.; Shamamian, P.; Alexander, R.B.; Gnarra, J.R.; Turetskaya, R.L.; Nedospasov, S.A.; Simonis, T.B.; Taubenberger, J.K.; Yannelli, J.; Mixon, A. Loss of HLA haplotype and B locus down-regulation in melanoma cell lines. *J. Immunol.* **1994**, *153*, 1225–1237.
27. Friedländer, M.R.; Mackowiak, S.D.; Li, N.; Chen, W.; Rajewsky, N. miRDeep2 accurately identifies known and hundreds of novel microRNA genes in seven animal clades. *Nucleic Acids Res.* **2012**, *40*, 37–52. [CrossRef] [PubMed]
28. Afgan, E.; Baker, D.; Batut, B.; Van Den Beek, M.; Bouvier, D.; Čech, M.; Chilton, J.; Clements, D.; Coraor, N.; Grüning, B.A. The Galaxy platform for accessible, reproducible and collaborative biomedical analyses: 2018 update. *Nucleic Acids Res.* **2018**, *46*, W537–W544. [CrossRef] [PubMed]
29. Love, M.; Anders, S.; Huber, W. Moderated estimation of fold change and dispersion for RNA-seq data with DESeq2. *Genome Biol.* **2014**, *15*, 550. [CrossRef]
30. Torre, D.; Lachmann, A.; Ma'ayan, A. BioJupies: Automated generation of interactive notebooks for RNA-Seq data analysis in the cloud. *Cell Syst.* **2018**, *7*, 556–561.e3. [CrossRef]
31. Agarwal, V.; Bell, G.W.; Nam, J.-W.; Bartel, D.P. Predicting effective microRNA target sites in mammalian mRNAs. *eLife* **2015**, *4*, e05005. [CrossRef]
32. Ashburner, M.; Ball, C.A.; Blake, J.A.; Botstein, D.; Butler, H.; Cherry, J.M.; Davis, A.P.; Dolinski, K.; Dwight, S.S.; Eppig, J.T. Gene ontology: Tool for the unification of biology. *Nat. Genet.* **2000**, *25*, 25–29. [CrossRef]
33. Szklarczyk, D.; Gable, A.L.; Lyon, D.; Junge, A.; Wyder, S.; Huerta-Cepas, J.; Simonovic, M.; Doncheva, N.T.; Morris, J.H.; Bork, P. STRING v11: Protein–protein association networks with increased coverage, supporting functional discovery in genome-wide experimental datasets. *Nucleic Acids Res.* **2019**, *47*, D607–D613. [CrossRef]
34. Shannon, P.; Markiel, A.; Ozier, O.; Baliga, N.S.; Wang, J.T.; Ramage, D.; Amin, N.; Schwikowski, B.; Ideker, T. Cytoscape: A software environment for integrated models of biomolecular interaction networks. *Genome Res.* **2003**, *13*, 2498–2504. [CrossRef] [PubMed]
35. Carvalho, B.S.; Irizarry, R.A. A framework for oligonucleotide microarray preprocessing. *Bioinformatics* **2010**, *26*, 2363–2367. [CrossRef] [PubMed]
36. Huber, W.; Carey, V.J.; Gentleman, R.; Anders, S.; Carlson, M.; Carvalho, B.S.; Bravo, H.C.; Davis, S.; Gatto, L.; Girke, T. Orchestrating high-throughput genomic analysis with Bioconductor. *Nat. Methods* **2015**, *12*, 115–121. [CrossRef] [PubMed]
37. Leek, J.; Johnson, W.; Parker, H.; Jaffe, A.; Storey, J. SVA detailed instruction. *Bioinformatics* **2012**, *28*, 882–883. [CrossRef] [PubMed]
38. De la Nava, J.G.; van Hijum, S.; Trelles, O. Saturation and quantization reduction in microarray experiments using two scans at different sensitivities. *Stat. Appl. Genet. Mol. Biol.* **2004**, *3*, 11. [CrossRef]
39. Mootha, V.K.; Lindgren, C.M.; Eriksson, K.-F.; Subramanian, A.; Sihag, S.; Lehar, J.; Puigserver, P.; Carlsson, E.; Ridderstråle, M.; Laurila, E. PGC-1α-responsive genes involved in oxidative phosphorylation are coordinately downregulated in human diabetes. *Nat. Genet.* **2003**, *34*, 267–273. [CrossRef]
40. Subramanian, A.; Tamayo, P.; Mootha, V.K.; Mukherjee, S.; Ebert, B.L.; Gillette, M.A.; Paulovich, A.; Pomeroy, S.L.; Golub, T.R.; Lander, E.S. Gene set enrichment analysis: A knowledge-based approach for interpreting genome-wide expression profiles. *Proc. Natl. Acad. Sci. USA* **2005**, *102*, 15545–15550. [CrossRef]
41. Chen, Y.; Wang, X. miRDB: An online database for prediction of functional microRNA targets. *Nucleic Acids Res.* **2020**, *48*, D127–D131. [CrossRef]
42. Hu, Y.; Wang, Q.; Zhu, X.-H. miR-135b is a novel oncogenic factor in cutaneous melanoma by targeting LATS2. *Melanoma Res.* **2019**, *29*, 119–125. [CrossRef]
43. Yu, Y.; Yu, F.; Sun, P. microRNA-1246 Promotes Melanoma Progression through Targeting FOXA2. *Oncotargets Ther.* **2020**, *13*, 1245. [CrossRef]
44. Shang, J.; Yu, G.; Ji, Z.; Wang, X.; Xia, L. miR-105 inhibits gastric cancer cells metastasis, epithelial-mesenchymal transition by targeting SOX9. *Eur. Rev. Med. Pharm. Sci.* **2019**, *23*, 6160–6169.

45. Li, Y.; Shen, Z.; Jiang, H.; Lai, Z.; Wang, Z.; Jiang, K.; Ye, Y.; Wang, S. microRNA-4284 promotes gastric cancer tumorigenicity by targeting ten-eleven translocation 1. *Mol. Med. Rep.* **2018**, *17*, 6569–6575. [CrossRef] [PubMed]
46. Bissey, P.-A.; Mathot, P.; Guix, C.; Jasmin, M.; Goddard, I.; Costechareyre, C.; Gadot, N.; Delcros, J.-G.; Mali, S.M.; Fasan, R. Blocking SHH/Patched interaction triggers tumor growth inhibition through Patched-induced apoptosis. *Cancer Res.* **2020**, *80*, 1970–1980. [CrossRef] [PubMed]
47. Laplante, M.; Sabatini, D. mTOR signaling in growth control and disease. *Cell* **2012**, *149*, 274–293. [CrossRef] [PubMed]
48. Qin, W.-Y.; Feng, S.-C.; Sun, Y.-Q.; Jiang, G.-Q. miR-96-5p promotes breast cancer migration by activating MEK/ERK signaling. *J. Gene Med.* **2020**, *22*, e3188. [CrossRef]
49. Lu, J.; Zhou, Y.; Zheng, X.; Chen, L.; Tuo, X.; Chen, H.; Xue, M.; Chen, Q.; Chen, W.; Li, X. 20(S)-Rg3 upregulates FDFT1 via reducing miR-4425 to inhibit ovarian cancer progression. *Arch. Biochem. Biophys.* **2020**, *693*, 108569. [CrossRef]
50. Cao, M.-Q.; You, A.-B.; Zhu, X.-D.; Zhang, W.; Zhang, Y.-Y.; Zhang, S.-Z.; Zhang, K.-w.; Cai, H.; Shi, W.-K.; Li, X.-L. miR-182-5p promotes hepatocellular carcinoma progression by repressing FOXO3a. *J. Hematol. Oncol.* **2018**, *11*, 1–12.
51. Gao, J.; Zeng, K.; Liu, Y.; Gao, L.; Liu, L. LncRNA SNHG5 promotes growth and invasion in melanoma by regulating the miR-26a-5p/TRPC3 pathway. *OncoTargets Ther.* **2019**, *12*, 169. [CrossRef]
52. Li, Y.; Wang, P.; Wu, L.-L.; Yan, J.; Pang, X.-Y.; Liu, S.-J. miR-26a-5p inhibit gastric cancer cell proliferation and invasion through mediated Wnt5a. *OncoTargets Ther.* **2020**, *13*, 2537. [CrossRef]
53. Zhou, X.; Yan, T.; Huang, C.; Xu, Z.; Wang, L.; Jiang, E.; Wang, H.; Chen, Y.; Liu, K.; Shao, Z. Melanoma cell-secreted exosomal miR-155-5p induce proangiogenic switch of cancer-associated fibroblasts via SOCS1/JAK2/STAT3 signaling pathway. *J. Exp. Clin. Cancer Res.* **2018**, *37*, 1–15. [CrossRef]
54. Dabbah, M.; Attar-Schneider, O.; Zismanov, V.; Tartakover Matalon, S.; Lishner, M.; Drucker, L. Letter to the Editor: miR-199b-3p and miR-199a-3p are isoforms with identical sequence and established function as tumor and metastasis suppressors. *J. Leukoc. Biol.* **2017**, *101*, 1069. [CrossRef] [PubMed]
55. Streicher, K.L.; Zhu, W.; Lehmann, K.P.; Georgantas, R.W.; Morehouse, C.A.; Brohawn, P.; Carrasco, R.A.; Xiao, Z.; Tice, D.A.; Higgs, B.W.; et al. A novel oncogenic role for the miRNA-506-514 cluster in initiating melanocyte transformation and promoting melanoma growth. *Oncogene* **2012**, *31*, 1558–1570. [CrossRef] [PubMed]
56. Cao, S.; Li, L.; Li, J.; Zhao, H. miR-1299 Impedes the Progression of Non-Small-Cell Lung Cancer Through EGFR/PI3K/AKT Signaling Pathway. *OncoTargets Ther.* **2020**, *13*, 7493. [CrossRef] [PubMed]
57. Behm-Ansmant, I.; Rehwinkel, J.; Doerks, T.; Stark, A.; Bork, P.; Izaurralde, E. mRNA degradation by miRNAs and GW182 requires both CCR4: NOT deadenylase and DCP1: DCP2 decapping complexes. *Genes Dev.* **2006**, *20*, 1885–1898. [CrossRef]
58. Cui, T.; Bell, E.H.; McElroy, J.; Becker, A.P.; Gulati, P.M.; Geurts, M.; Mladkova, N.; Gray, A.; Liu, K.; Yang, L. miR-4516 predicts poor prognosis and functions as a novel oncogene via targeting PTPN14 in human glioblastoma. *Oncogene* **2019**, *38*, 2923–2936. [CrossRef]
59. Hao, T.; Li, C.; Ding, X.; Xing, X. microRNA-363-3p/p21 (Cip1/Waf1) Axis Is Regulated by HIF-2α in Mediating Stemness of Melanoma Cells. *Neoplasma* **2019**, *66*, 427–436. [CrossRef]
60. Xue, M.; Tao, W.; Yu, S.; Yan, Z.; Peng, Q.; Jiang, F.; Gao, X. lncRNA ZFPM2-AS1 promotes proliferation via miR-18b-5p/VMA21 axis in lung adenocarcinoma. *J. Cell. Biochem.* **2020**, *121*, 313–321. [CrossRef]
61. Wang, J.; Tao, Y.; Bian, Q. miRNA and mRNA expression profiling reveals potential biomarkers for metastatic cutaneous melanoma. *Expert Rev. Anticancer Ther.* **2021**, *21*, 557–567. [CrossRef]
62. Chamcheu, J.C.; Roy, T.; Uddin, M.B.; Banang-Mbeumi, S.; Chamcheu, R.-C.N.; Walker, A.L.; Liu, Y.-Y.; Huang, S. Role and therapeutic targeting of the PI3K/Akt/mTOR signaling pathway in skin cancer: A review of current status and future trends on natural and synthetic agents therapy. *Cells* **2019**, *8*, 803. [CrossRef]
63. Busse, A.; Keilholz, U. Role of TGF-β in melanoma. *Curr. Pharm. Biotechnol.* **2011**, *12*, 2165–2175. [CrossRef]
64. Linck-Paulus, L.; Hellerbrand, C.; Bosserhoff, A.K.; Dietrich, P. Dissimilar Appearances Are Deceptive–Common microRNAs and Therapeutic Strategies in Liver Cancer and Melanoma. *Cells* **2020**, *9*, 114. [CrossRef] [PubMed]
65. Schultz, J.; Lorenz, P.; Gross, G.; Ibrahim, S.; Kunz, M. microRNA let-7b targets important cell cycle molecules in malignant melanoma cells and interferes with anchorage-independent growth. *Cell Res.* **2008**, *18*, 549–557. [CrossRef]
66. Müller, D.; Bosserhoff, A.-K. Integrin β 3 expression is regulated by let-7a miRNA in malignant melanoma. *Oncogene* **2008**, *27*, 6698–6706. [CrossRef] [PubMed]
67. Kim, J.-H.; Ahn, J.-H.; Lee, M. Upregulation of microRNA-1246 is associated with BRAF inhibitor resistance in melanoma cells with mutant BRAF. *Cancer Res. Treat. Off. J. Korean Cancer Assoc.* **2017**, *49*, 947. [CrossRef]
68. Stark, M.S.; Bonazzi, V.F.; Boyle, G.M.; Palmer, J.M.; Symmons, J.; Lanagan, C.M.; Schmidt, C.W.; Herington, A.C.; Ballotti, R.; Pollock, P.M.; et al. miR-514a regulates the tumour suppressor NF1 and modulates BRAFi sensitivity in melanoma. *Oncotarget* **2015**, *6*, 17753–17763. [CrossRef]
69. Dong, X.; Chang, M.; Song, X.; Ding, S.; Xie, L.; Song, X. Plasma miR-1247-5p, miR-301b-3p and miR-105-5p as potential biomarkers for early diagnosis of non-small cell lung cancer. *Thorac. Cancer* **2021**, *12*, 539–548. [CrossRef] [PubMed]
70. Jin, L.; Zhang, Z. Serum miR-3180-3p and miR-124-3p may Function as Noninvasive Biomarkers of Cisplatin Resistance in Gastric Cancer. *Clin. Lab.* **2020**, *66*. [CrossRef]

71. Valentini, V.; Zelli, V.; Gaggiano, E.; Silvestri, V.; Rizzolo, P.; Bucalo, A.; Calvieri, S.; Grassi, S.; Frascione, P.; Donati, P. miRNAs as potential prognostic biomarkers for metastasis in thin and thick primary cutaneous melanomas. *Anticancer Res.* **2019**, *39*, 4085–4093. [CrossRef]
72. Loriot, A.; Van Tongelen, A.; Blanco, J.; Klaessens, S.; Cannuyer, J.; van Baren, N.; Decottignies, A.; De Smet, C. A novel cancer-germline transcript carrying pro-metastatic miR-105 and TET-targeting miR-767 induced by DNA hypomethylation in tumors. *Epigenetics* **2014**, *9*, 1163–1171. [CrossRef]
73. Jia, M.; Li, Z.; Pan, M.; Tao, M.; Wang, J.; Lu, X. LINC-PINT Suppresses the Aggressiveness of Thyroid Cancer by Downregulating miR-767-5p to Induce TET2 Expression. *Mol. Ther. Nucleic Acids* **2020**, *22*, 319–328. [CrossRef]
74. Zhang, L.; Geng, Z.; Wan, Y.; Meng, F.; Meng, X.; Wang, L. Functional analysis of miR-767-5p during the progression of hepatocellular carcinoma and the clinical relevance of its dysregulation. *Histochem. Cell Biol.* **2020**, *154*, 231–243. [CrossRef] [PubMed]
75. Wu, J.; Li, H.; Shi, M.; Zhu, Y.; Ma, Y.; Zhong, Y.; Xiong, C.; Chen, H.; Peng, C. TET1-mediated DNA hydroxymethylation activates inhibitors of the Wnt/β-catenin signaling pathway to suppress EMT in pancreatic tumor cells. *J. Exp. Clin. Cancer Res.* **2019**, *38*, 1–17. [CrossRef]
76. Gajos-Michniewicz, A.; Czyz, M. WNT signaling in melanoma. *Int. J. Mol. Sci.* **2020**, *21*, 4852. [CrossRef] [PubMed]
77. Kaur, A.; Webster, M.R.; Marchbank, K.; Behera, R.; Ndoye, A.; Kugel, C.H.; Dang, V.M.; Appleton, J.; O'Connell, M.P.; Cheng, P. sFRP2 in the aged microenvironment drives melanoma metastasis and therapy resistance. *Nature* **2016**, *532*, 250–254. [CrossRef]
78. Regad, T. Molecular and cellular pathogenesis of melanoma initiation and progression. *Cell. Mol. Life Sci.* **2013**, *70*, 4055–4065. [CrossRef] [PubMed]
79. Yin, J.; Hu, W.; Fu, W.; Dai, L.; Jiang, Z.; Zhong, S.; Deng, B.; Zhao, J. HGF/MET regulated epithelial-mesenchymal transitions and metastasis By FOSL2 in non-small cell lung cancer. *OncoTargets Ther.* **2019**, *12*, 9227. [CrossRef] [PubMed]
80. Kuphal, S.; Wallner, S.; Bosserhoff, A.K. Impact of LIF (leukemia inhibitory factor) expression in malignant melanoma. *Exp. Mol. Pathol.* **2013**, *95*, 156–165. [CrossRef]
81. Maruta, S.; Takiguchi, S.; Ueyama, M.; Kataoka, Y.; Oda, Y.; Tsuneyoshi, M.; Iguchi, H. A role for leukemia inhibitory factor in melanoma-induced bone metastasis. *Clin. Exp. Metastasis* **2009**, *26*, 133. [CrossRef] [PubMed]
82. Larribère, L.; Kuphal, S.; Sachpekidis, C.; Hüser, L.; Bosserhoff, A.; Utikal, J. Targeted therapy-resistant melanoma cells acquire transcriptomic similarities with human melanoblasts. *Cancers* **2018**, *10*, 451. [CrossRef]

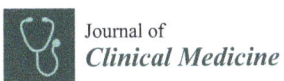

Article

Quantitative Detection of Disseminated Melanoma Cells by Trp-1 Transcript Analysis Reveals Stochastic Distribution of Pulmonary Metastases

Lenka Kyjacova [1], Rafael Saup [1], Melanie Rothley [1,2], Anja Schmaus [1,2], Tabea Wagner [1], Anja Bosserhoff [3], Boyan K. Garvalov [1], Wilko Thiele [1,2] and Jonathan P. Sleeman [1,2,*]

[1] Department of Microvascular Biology and Pathobiology, European Center for Angioscience (ECAS), Medical Faculty Mannheim, University of Heidelberg, D-68167 Mannheim, Germany; lenka.kyjacova@gmail.com (L.K.); Rafael.Saup@medma.uni-heidelberg.de (R.S.); melanie.rothley@kit.edu (M.R.); anja.schmaus@partner.kit.edu (A.S.); Tabea.Wagner@medma.uni-heidelberg.de (T.W.); Boyan.Garvalov@medma.uni-heidelberg.de (B.K.G.); Wilko.Thiele@medma.uni-heidelberg.de (W.T.)

[2] Institute for Biological and Chemical Systems-Biological Information Processing (IBCS-BIP), Karlsruhe Institute of Technology (KIT)-Campus North, D-76344 Karlsruhe, Germany

[3] Institute of Biochemistry, Faculty of Medicine, Friedrich-Alexander University Erlangen-Nürnberg (FAU), D-91054 Erlangen, Germany; anja.bosserhoff@fau.de

* Correspondence: jonathan.sleeman@medma.uni-heidelberg.de; Tel.: +49-621-383-71595

Abstract: A better understanding of the process of melanoma metastasis is required to underpin the development of novel therapies that will improve patient outcomes. The use of appropriate animal models is indispensable for investigating the mechanisms of melanoma metastasis. However, reliable and practicable quantification of metastases in experimental mice remains a challenge, particularly if the metastatic burden is low. Here, we describe a qRT-PCR-based protocol that employs the melanocytic marker Trp-1 for the sensitive quantification of melanoma metastases in the murine lung. Using this protocol, we were able to detect the presence of as few as 100 disseminated melanoma cells in lung tissue. This allowed us to quantify metastatic burden in a spontaneous syngeneic B16-F10 metastasis model, even in the absence of visible metastases, as well as in the autochthonous Tg($Grm1$)/$Cyld^{-/-}$ melanoma model. Importantly, we also observed an uneven distribution of disseminated melanoma cells amongst the five lobes of the murine lung, which varied considerably from animal to animal. Together, our findings demonstrate that the qRT-PCR-based detection of Trp-1 allows the quantification of low pulmonary metastatic burden in both transplantable and autochthonous murine melanoma models, and show that the analysis of lung metastasis in such models needs to take into account the stochastic distribution of metastatic lesions amongst the lung lobes.

Keywords: Trp-1; metastasis; melanoma; animal models; lung; mice

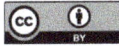

1. Introduction

Malignant cutaneous melanoma is characterized by early dissemination and subsequent metastatic colonization of multiple organs [1]. One of the most frequent sites of metastasis is the lung, with around 18% of melanoma patients developing metastatic pulmonary foci during follow-up [2,3], which is associated with a 1-year survival rate of 57% [4].

Experimentally, the process of melanoma metastasis is usually investigated using rodent models. However, accurate quantification of organ metastases in these models remains a significant challenge. Traditionally, visible superficial metastases are enumerated post mortem. However, metastases need to be relatively large to be quantified, and metastatic foci growing within the organ, that are not visible from the surface, will not contribute to the quantification. To circumvent these problems, organs are often also examined histologically. However, this is a laborious process, particularly if metastases are rare and entire organs must be sectioned to provide a systematic assessment of metastatic burden [5]. Immune cell infiltrates or perivascular areas may also be misidentified histologically as micrometastases [5]. Moreover, an unequal distribution of metastatic foci within a particular organ may lead to misleading quantification results with such histological methods. For example, the mouse lung has five lobes; if pulmonary metastasis is evaluated in only a single lobe, or if metastasis is quantified through multiple methods that each use a different lobe, then a skewed or misleading quantification may ensue if metastatic foci are not equally distributed throughout all of the lung lobes.

Several imaging technologies facilitate the evaluation of metastasis formation in specific organs, either longitudinally within living animals, or ex vivo post mortem. Photonic imaging methods based on fluorescence or bioluminescence have been widely employed, and while they offer a number of important advantages, they are also subject to a number of major limitations. Photon attenuation as a function of depth and of the heterogeneous optical properties of tissues can result in loss of signal and non-linear results, and signal scattering by tissues limits spatial resolution [6]. In addition, the luciferase proteins that catalyze the bioluminescence reaction, as well as fluorescent reporter proteins, such as GFP, can trigger immune responses in immunocompetent animals, leading to the elimination of luciferase- or GFP-expressing cells, and the suppression of metastasis formation [7–9]. Moreover, oxygen and ATP are required for the generation of a bioluminescence signal, and as tumor tissues are often hypoxic, this can significantly attenuate the signal generated [10]. Other imaging approaches, such as magnetic resonance imaging (MRI), X-ray computed tomography (CT), or positron emission tomography (PET) can be used for imaging and quantification of metastases, but are limited in their sensitivity and require specialized and costly equipment.

Therefore, there is a need for methods that allow reliable detection and quantification of overt metastases, micrometastases and disseminated tumor cells. PCR-based approaches have the potential to fulfil these requirements, if marker genes are expressed, specifically in metastatic cells and not in the tissues in which metastases develop [11–18]. Tyrosine-related proteins 1 and 2 (Trp-1 and Trp-2) are involved in the synthesis of melanin (reviewed in [19,20]), which is characteristic for cells of melanocytic origin. Accordingly, Trp-1 and Trp-2 transcripts are absent from most non-melanocytic tissues [21], but are expressed in melanocytes, in melanomas and their metastases, and by many different melanoma cell lines [17,22,23], including the well-established and widely used B16 cell line [22,24]. Therefore, Trp-1 and Trp-2 represent potentially useful markers for the detection of disseminated melanoma cells, over and above any endogenous expression from melanocytes in the tissue concerned [17].

Here, we describe the development of a protocol for the detection of melanoma cells in the lung of experimental mice, based on quantification of tyrosine-related protein 1 (Trp-1) expression by qRT-PCR, which can be used to quantify melanoma metastases in murine spontaneous metastasis and autochthonous models. In addition to allowing metastatic burden to be evaluated, even where overt metastases are not present, our results also show that pulmonary metastases are not equally distributed amongst the lobes of the murine lung in individual animals, indicating that the quantification of pulmonary metastasis in murine models must take this heterogeneous distribution into account.

2. Materials and Methods
2.1. Cell Lines

The RheoSwitch inducible expression system [25] was introduced into B16-F10 cells. The resulting B16-RheoSwitch (B16-RS) cells were cultivated in DMEM containing 4.5 g/L glucose (Gibco/Thermo Fisher Scientific, Dreieich, Germany), 10% fetal bovine serum (Sigma Aldrich, Taufkirchen, Germany), and 1% penicillin/streptomycin (Gibco/Thermo Fisher Scientific). The cells were confirmed to be mycoplasma negative.

2.2. Ex Vivo Admixture Experiments

Murine lung tissue was admixed with 1×10^2–1×10^6 B16-RS cells transfected with RheoSwitch constructs, which enable the induced expression of the immediate early gene Ier2, and was dissociated mechanically in TRIzol, using metal beads with a TissueLyser II (QIAGEN, Hilden, Germany) for 5 min at 30 Hz, with the holder pre-cooled to $-20\ ^\circ\text{C}$. In some experiments, individual lung lobes were admixed with 1×10^2–1×10^5 B16-RS cells. All samples were immediately processed for qRT-PCR analysis.

2.3. Quantitative Real Time PCR (qRT-PCR)

Total RNA was isolated using TRIzol reagent (Thermo Fisher Scientific), following the manufacturer's instructions. RNA (1–2 µg) was treated with RNase-free DNase I (Thermo Fisher), followed by EDTA deactivation for 10 min at 65 $^\circ$C. First strand cDNA was synthesized with random hexamer primers, using dNTP mix and RevertAid H Minus Reverse transcriptase (Thermo Fisher Scientific, Dreieich, Germany). qRT-PCR was performed in a Stratagene Mx3500P qPCR machine (Agilent, Waldbronn, Germany), using SYBR Select Master Mix, containing SYBR Green dye (Applied Biosystems/Thermo Fisher Scientific, Dreieich, Germany) or GoTaq qPCR Master Mix (Promega, Walldorf, Germany). The relative quantity of cDNA was estimated using the $\Delta\Delta$CT method, and data were normalized to ribosomal protein 60S acidic ribosomal protein P0 (RPLP0). For the experiments in which Trp-1 levels in spontaneous metastases were quantified (Figures 2C and 3C), the data were additionally normalized to the mean Trp-1 signal in lungs of non-tumor-bearing mice, which was set at 1. The PCR program parameters were: 1 cycle of initial denaturation (95 $^\circ$C, 2 min), followed by 40 cycles consisting of 95 $^\circ$C for 15 s and 60 $^\circ$C for 1 min, and a final cycle consisting of 95 $^\circ$C for 1 min, 55 $^\circ$C for 30 s, and 95 $^\circ$C for 30 s.

The following forward and reverse primers, purchased from metabion (Steinkirchen, Germany), were used for qRT-PCR: RPLP0: 5′-GGA CCC GAG AAG ACC TCC TT-3′, 5′-GCA CAT CAC TCA GAA TTT CAA TGG-3′; Trp-1: 5′-GCT GGA GAG AGA CAT GCA GGA-3′, 5′-AGT GCA GAC ATC GCA GAC GTT-3′. Trp-2: 5′- TTA CGC CGT TGA TCT GTC AGA G-3′, 5′-TTG CGA AGC CTT CTG TAT TGA A-3′; RheoActivator element (RA): 5′-ACG CGC TAG ACG ATT TCG AT-3′, 5′- TCA AAC CCC TCA CCT CTG GA-3′.

2.4. Animals

C57Bl/6J mice were obtained from Charles Rivers Laboratories (Sulzfeld, Germany) and C57Bl/6JOlaHsd (C57BL/6J) mice were purchased from Envigo (Horst, Netherlands). C57Bl/6J;Tg(Grm1)/Cyld$^{-/-}$ mice [26] were used with the permission of Prof. Suzie Chen, who originally established the Tg(Grm1) line [27].

Mice were kept in groups of 4 in type III Makrolon filtertop cages (Tecniplast, Hohenpeißenberg, Germany) containing SAFE fs14 bedding (J. Rettenmaier & Söhne, Rosenberg, Germany). Rat/mouse extruded food (ssniff, Soest, Germany) and sterilized water acidified with HCl (pH: 2.8–3.1) was provided ad libitum. The specific-pathogen-free area was kept at 20 $^\circ$C and 30–60% humidity on a 7:00–20:00 light cycle. The health status of the animals in the facility was routinely assessed by a commercial veterinarian laboratory (mfd Diagnostics, Wendelsheim, Germany) with serological examinations every three months (epizootic diarrhea of infant mice, mouse hepatitis virus, murine norovirus, minute virus of mice, Theiler´s encephalomyelitis virus, and *Pasteurella pneumotropica*) or annually (*Clostridium piliforme*, Mousepox, lymphocytic choriomeningitis virus, mouse adenovirus type 1 and type 2, *Mycoplasma pulmonis*, pneumonia virus of mice, Reovirus type 3, and Sendai virus).

2.5. Spontaneous Metastasis Assay

C57Bl/6 mice (9 weeks old) were injected with 1×10^5 OPN-deficient B16-RS cells transfected with RheoSwitch constructs that enable the induced expression of the immediate early gene Ier2. The cells were resuspended in 100 µL PBS and injected s.c. into the flank. The data presented in this study are part of an experiment where 50 mg/kg of pharmacologically inert diacylhydrazine RheoSwitch ligand (Exclusive Chemistry Ltd., Obninsk, Russia) was administered i.p. daily to induce the expression of Ier2, starting from day 5 following cell transplantation. Control mice received an equivalent volume of DMSO vehicle. Tumor size was measured regularly in three dimensions using a caliper. The animals were sacrificed when the tumor size reached 2 cm in one dimension or if they became moribund. Lungs were explanted post mortem, inspected for visible metastases, photographed, and then flash frozen in liquid nitrogen. The frozen lungs were kept at $-80\ °C$ until RNA isolation. For RNA isolation, the frozen lungs were transferred into TRIzol, and further processed as described above.

2.6. Autochthonous Metastasis Model

C57Bl/6J;Tg($Grm1$)/$Cyld^{-/-}$ transgenic animals were monitored once a week for the development of melanocytic lesions and melanoma growth. Mice aged 1 year were euthanized, lungs were explanted post mortem, inspected for visible metastases, photographed, and flash frozen in liquid nitrogen. The frozen lungs were kept at $-80\ °C$ until RNA isolation. For RNA isolation, the frozen lungs were transferred into TRIzol, and further processed as described above. For qRT-PCR analysis, half of each lung lobe was pooled into one sample. C57BL/6J mice aged 6 months and 1 year were used as controls.

2.7. Hematoxylin-Eosin Staining

Paraffin sections on glass slides were deparaffinized with three 5 min changes of RotiHistol and a descending series of 100%-96%-80%-70% ethanol. The slides were immersed for 30 s in Mayer's hemalum solution (Merck) and washed for 10 min in running tap water for bluing. Staining with a 0.5% alcoholic eosin-Y solution (Merck, Darmstadt, Germany) was followed by a short wash in tap water, dehydration in an ascending series of 70%-80%-96%-100%-100% ethanol, three 5 min changes of Roti-Histol, and embedding in Eukitt mounting medium (Merck).

2.8. Statistical Analysis

Results are represented as the mean +SEM. Graphs for qRT-PCR experiments represent data from a minimum of 3 biological replicates, with each biological replicate being executed in 2 technical replicates. For multiple group analysis, one-way ANOVA was used in Prism 7 (GraphPad Software, San Diego, CA, USA).

3. Results

3.1. Trp-1 and Trp-2 Transcript Levels Correlate with Melanoma Cell Numbers Admixed with Lung Tissue Ex Vivo

To allow easy and unambiguous quantification of melanoma metastatic burden, we determined the utility of Trp-1 and Trp-2 as melanoma cell markers, using the murine lung as a model organ. To this end, we first tested if the expression of Trp-1 and Trp-2 transcripts detected by qRT-PCR correlated with the number of B16-RS melanoma cells admixed with lung tissue. The presence of the RheoSwitch construct in the B16-RS cells enabled us to amplify and detect the RheoActivator element, which served as a tumor cell-specific marker, and was normalized to the expression of the 60S acidic ribosomal protein P0 (RPLP0), used as a house-keeping gene. We found that the level of RheoActivator signal detected by qPCR correlated with the number of admixed B16-RS cells in a linear manner, with a coefficient of determination of 0.92 (Figure 1). Similarly, Trp-1 and Trp-2 transcript levels also correlated with the number of admixed B16-RS cells, with comparable coefficients of determination for a linear correlation (Figure 1). The sensitivities of detection for both Trp-1 and Trp-2 were similarly high, since as few as 100 cells could be clearly detected by both markers (Figure 1). As the expression of Trp-1 was found to be higher than the expression of Trp-2, in further experiments, we focused on Trp-1 in order to optimize the detection of small numbers of tumor cells.

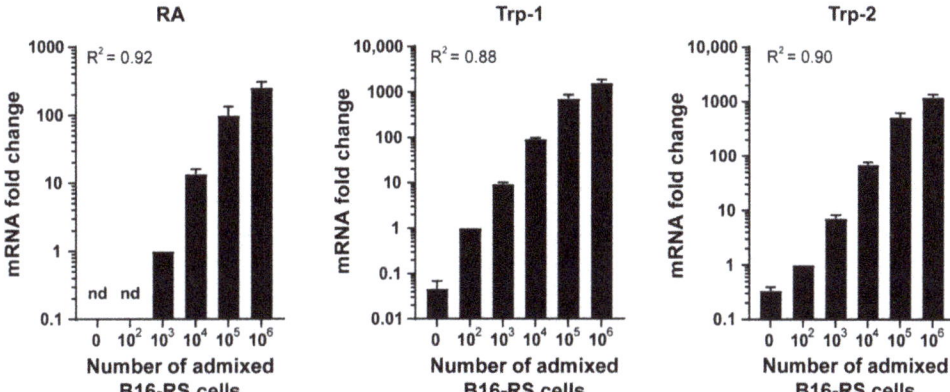

Figure 1. Trp-1 expression correlates with melanoma cell numbers admixed with lung tissue ex vivo. Metastatic load detection ex vivo. qRT-PCR analysis of RheoActivator (RA), Trp-1, and Trp-2 in murine lung tissue (1:1) admixed with 1×10^2–1×10^6 B16-RS cells. Data were normalized to RPLP0 and to the signal of 10^3 cells (RS) or 10^2 cells (Trp-1 and Trp-2) and represent mean + SEM, $n = 3$. R^2: coefficient of determination. n.d.: not detected.

Murine lungs consist of five individual lung lobes (right cranial lobe, right middle lobe, right caudal lobe, accessory lobe, and left lobe [28]) that differ in size (Figure 2A). To our knowledge, the incidence and distribution of metastases in each lobe has not been investigated so far. In order to determine whether Trp-1 expression might be useful to address this question for melanoma cells, we next assessed if the correlation between Trp-1 levels and melanoma cell number is maintained between the different lung lobes. To this end, different numbers of melanoma cells were admixed with individual lung lobes, and Trp-1 levels were then quantified and normalized to RPLP0. We observed a linear correlation with nearly identical coefficients of determination (0.84–0.86) for all lung lobes (Figure 2B). Together, these data show that Trp-1 transcription can be used as a quantifiable measure of the number of melanoma cells in all lung lobes.

3.2. B16-RS Lung Metastases Are Distributed Stochastically between the Lobes of the Mouse Lung

Next, we performed a spontaneous metastasis experiment with B16-RS cells in vivo, and investigated the utility of the qRT-PCR-based quantification of Trp-1 to determine metastatic burden in lung lobes where no visible overt metastases were present, as well as whether lung metastases were distributed equally amongst the lung lobes. To this end, B16-RS cells were subcutaneously injected into the flank of syngeneic mice. The animals were sacrificed once the primary tumors reached a diameter of 2 cm in one dimension. The lungs were then isolated, dissected, and the individual lobes were analyzed, first by eye for macroscopically visible metastases, and then via qRT-PCR for Trp-1 expression. We found that Trp-1 expression was highest in those lobes that showed overt macroscopically visible metastases (Figure 2C). Furthermore, a significant metastatic burden could be detected in specific lung lobes, even when no visible surface metastases were present (Figure 2C). Moreover, metastases were randomly distributed amongst the different lung lobes, and varied considerably from animal to animal, with some lobes being free of detectable tumor cells, while other lobes in the same animal had a high metastatic burden 3.3. Trp-1 Quantification Is a Sensitive Method for Detecting Pulmonary Metastases in Mice That Develop Autochthonous Melanoma.

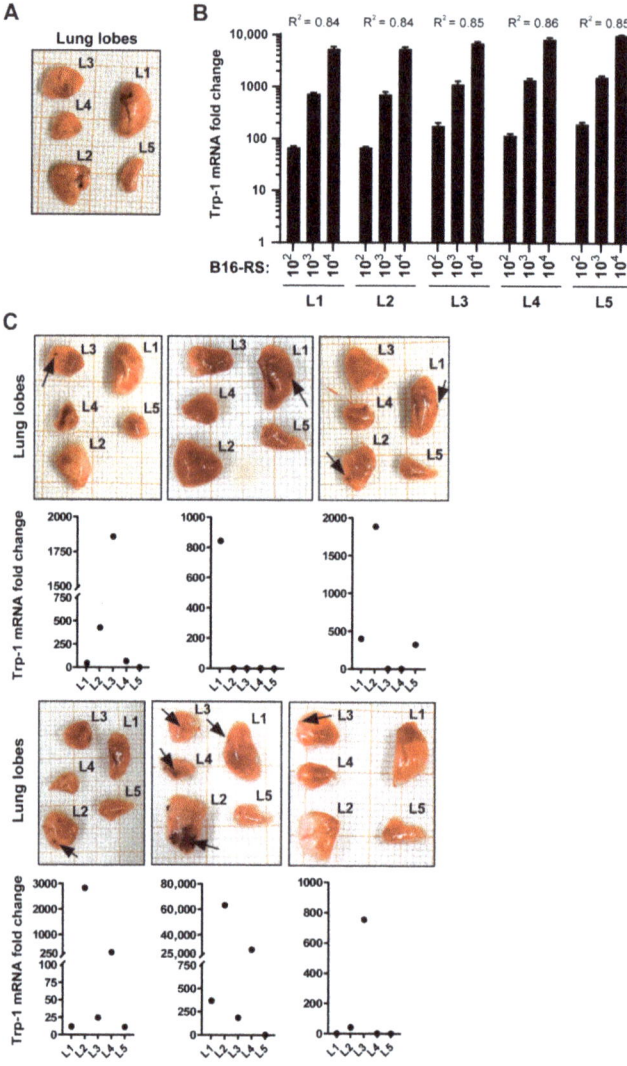

Figure 2. Trp-1 transcript levels correlated with metastatic burden in the lungs of experimental mice in a syngeneic mouse B16 model. (**A**) Representative image of a murine lung with isolated lung lobes: left lobe (L1), right caudal lobe (L2), right cranial lobe (L3), right middle lobe (L4), and accessory lobe (L5). Note that the arrangement of the lobes reflects the anatomical position, whereas the numbering corresponds to the size of the lobes, from largest to smallest. (**B**) qRT-PCR analysis of Trp-1 in samples containing 1×10^2–1×10^4 B16-RS cells admixed with individual lobes (L1–L5). Data were normalized to RPLP0 and to the mean Trp-1 signal in lobes without B16-RS cells. The graph shows mean Trp-1 expression + SEM, $n = 3$. R^2: coefficient of determination. (**C**) B16-RS cells (1×10^5) were injected subcutaneously into syngeneic mice ($n = 6$), and treated with either DMSO as a vehicle control (3 animals; top row) or RSL (3 animals; bottom row). The mice were sacrificed once the tumors reached a diameter of 2 cm in one dimension. Lungs were explanted and inspected for visible metastases. Trp-1 expression in the individual lobes was determined by qRT-PCR. Lung lobes with visible metastases (black arrows) are shown together with the corresponding Trp-1 expression in each of the five individual lung lobes (labelled L1 to L5, as in panel A), detected by qRT-PCR. Data were normalized to RPLP0 and to the mean Trp-1 signal in lobes of non-tumor-bearing mice.

Tg(*Grm1*)/*Cyld*$^{-/-}$ mice autochthonously developed melanoma mainly on the tail and ears (Figure 3A), due to an increased expression of the metabotropic glutamate receptor 1 (GRM1) under the control of the melanocyte specific Dct (Trp-2) promoter, and a lack of the tumor suppressor cylindromatosis (CYLD) [26]. The mice developed metastases in lymph nodes [26] and lung (Figure 3B,C). To assess the sensitivity of Trp-1 as a marker for quantifying pulmonary metastases in this context, we isolated lungs of Tg(*Grm1*)/*Cyld*$^{-/-}$ mice, documented macroscopically visible metastases, and tested their correlation with the expression levels of Trp-1 transcripts. Trp-1 expression in the lungs of C57Bl/6 wild type mice served as a baseline control. High Trp-1 expression in the lungs of Tg(*Grm1*)/*Cyld*$^{-/-}$ mice corresponded with the occurrence of visible metastases (Figure 3C). Lower levels of Trp-1 were also detected in lung lobes in which no visible metastases were present (Figure 3C), indicating that our protocol is sufficiently sensitive to detect disseminated tumor cells and micrometastases before they become macroscopically visible.

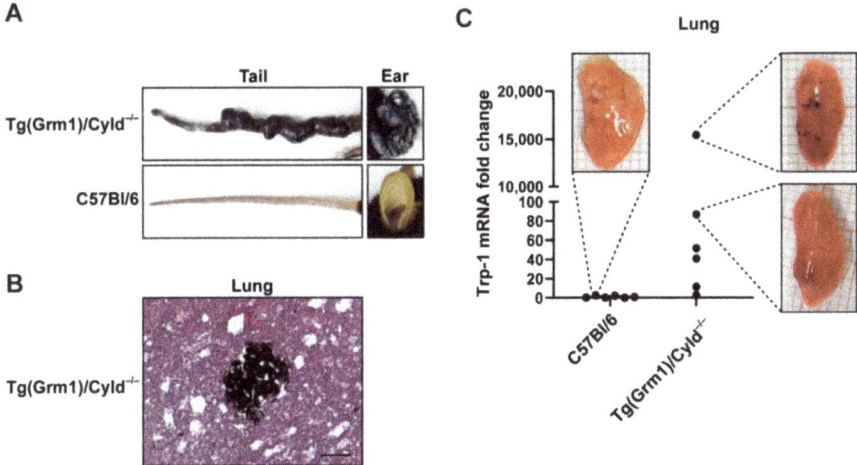

Figure 3. Quantitative detection of melanoma micrometastases in Tg(*Grm1*)/*Cyld*$^{-/-}$ transgenic mice. (**A**) Representative picture of melanomas detected on the tail and ear of 1-year-old C57Bl/6;Tg(*Grm1*)/*Cyld*$^{-/-}$ transgenic mice compared to C57Bl/6 control. (**B**) Hematoxylin/eosin (HE) staining of lung tissue from a C57Bl/6;Tg(*Grm1*)/*Cyld*$^{-/-}$ mouse containing a melanotic micrometastatic nodule. Scale bar, 500 µm. (**C**) qRT-PCR analysis of Trp-1 expression in lungs from C57Bl/6;Tg(*Grm1*)/*Cyld*$^{-/-}$ mice in comparison to C57Bl/6 controls. Data were normalized to RPLP0 and to the mean Trp1-1 signal in the C57Bl/6 controls; $n = 6$. The images show lung lobe L1 for the indicated data points.

4. Discussion

Here, we described a protocol for the detection and quantification of melanoma metastases in the murine lung, based on quantification of Trp-1, a glycoprotein involved in melanin synthesis that is expressed in melanoma cells. This method allowed for the detection and quantification of low metastatic burden in both transplantable and autochthonous models of melanoma pulmonary metastasis, even in the absence of overt superficial metastases. Furthermore, our data showed that pulmonary metastases were stochastically distributed amongst the different lobes of the murine lung, an observation that has important ramifications for the accurate quantification of metastatic burden in experimental animal models.

A number of qRT-PCR-based approaches for the detection and quantification of metastases in rodent models have been described. After xenografting of human tumor cells into immunocompromised mice, quantification based on the amplification of DNA sequences that are specific to humans has been employed [11,12,14]. In systems where tumor cells have been genetically modified, qRT-PCR-based quantification of the transgene can be used for the evaluation of metastatic burden, as exemplified by transfected genes that encode for neomycin resistance [13], mCherry [17], and luciferase [18]. Comparatively few endogenous tumor-cell markers offer sufficient specificity and sensitivity for qRT-PCR-based quantification. Examples include GP-100 [15], Trp-1 [17], Trp-2 [15,17], Grm1 [29], and Her-2 [16]. These qRT–based protocols have been validated after either intravenous injection of tumor cells [14,15,18], or after orthotopic or subcutaneous implantation of tumor cells [11–14,16–18]. Here, we show that qRT-PCR-based analysis of Trp-1 transcription can also be used to quantify low pulmonary metastatic burden in the Tg($Grm1$)/$Cyld^{-/-}$ autochthonous melanoma model, extending the range of metastasis models for which qRT-PCR-based strategies can be used.

Compared to other methods for the quantification of pulmonary melanoma metastases, the qRT-PCR-based approaches we described here offer a number of important advantages. The method facilitates a rapid, sensitive and accurate assessment of metastatic burden that is not possible with conventional visual inspection or histology-based methods. Furthermore, much lower levels of metastatic burden can be detected, compared to photonic imaging methods, as qRT-PCR is up to 10 times more sensitive than bioluminescence imaging [18,30]. Moreover, primary tumors often grow rapidly in spontaneous metastasis assays, which can require the termination of experiments before metastases have had time to develop fully, and can severely limit the utility of specific animal models for studying the process of metastasis. The sensitivity of the qRT-PCR-based quantification of Trp-1 means that metastatic burden can still be assessed at early stages of metastasis formation, extending the utility of these animal models. In addition, the sensitivity of the qRT-PCR method means that metastatic burden can be quantified when primary tumors are relatively small, reducing animal suffering. Similarly, the utility of Trp-1 quantification for the sensitive detection of metastasis in autochthonous melanoma models that we reported here means that metastasis formation can be assessed at an earlier stage, accelerating the time to endpoint analysis, thereby increasing experimental throughput. The method also facilitates assessment of metastasis formation in models in which rapid primary tumor growth necessitates termination of the experiment before overt visible metastases can be detected.

Although quantification of Trp-1 expression offers important advantages compared to other methods for quantifying metastatic burden, there are also a number of limitations. In contrast to live imaging techniques, qRT-PCR-based approaches allow only end-point analysis and no longitudinal assessment of metastasis in the same animal over time. Compared to quantification of superficial metastases or histology-based techniques, spatial information is lost, and it is not possible to determine whether a qRT-PCR signal is derived from a few large metastases or multiple small ones. Trp-1 expression may also be reduced in amelanotic melanoma metastases. Although amelanotic lesions can retain Trp-1 and Trp-2 expression [22,31], we have observed only very low Trp-1 expression in amelanotic lesions derived from YUMM melanoma cells ([32]). It has been shown that the expression of Trp-1 can be downregulated in invasive melanoma cells and in some melanoma metastases [20,33], and similar findings have been reported for Trp-2 [34]. Thus, reduced Trp-1 (or Trp-2) expression may limit the sensitivity of detection that can be achieved with our approach in some contexts. Nevertheless, Trp-1 protein expression has been demonstrated in the majority of melanoma metastases [35] and higher Trp-1 mRNA levels in skin and lymph node metastases have been correlated with worse clinical outcome for melanoma patients [36]. Furthermore, it was shown that in many cases Trp-1 protein cannot be detected in melanoma metastases even when its mRNA is expressed [36], which has been attributed to inhibition of Trp-1 translation by miR-155 [37]. Thus, the use of Trp-1 mRNA as a marker of disseminated melanoma cells could be possible even in metastases that are amelanotic or negative for Trp-1 by immunostaining.

Although we have focused on pulmonary metastasis in this study, the PCR-based quantification of Trp-1 can potentially also be used to quantify metastatic burden in other organs. Endogenous expression of Trp-1 in some organs may, however, limit the efficacy or sensitivity of such an approach. For example, Trp-1 and Trp-2 are expressed in the brain, but at much lower levels than those found in melanoma cells [38,39]. In addition, expression of Trp-1 in non-cutaneous melanocytes can generate some background signal in organs colonized by them, including the lung [40]. However, the endogenous Trp-1 levels in these organs are typically also much lower than those observed in melanoma cells, as demonstrated by our own results (Figure 2B,C and Figure 3C) and public datasets [40]). On the other hand, the approach we describe is likely to have limited utility for the detection of cutaneous dissemination of melanoma, due to the high numbers of Trp-1-expresing melanocytes in the skin.

Here, we report a dramatic animal-to-animal variation in the distribution of metastatic burden amongst the different lobes in the murine lung. This will have a pronounced impact on the reliability and accuracy of methods that assess pulmonary metastasis formation based on tissue sampling procedures, such as those that analyze metastasis formation in only a single lung lobe. The stochastic distribution of metastatic burden amongst the different lung lobes we observed strongly increases the risk that inappropriately high or low values for metastatic burden will be obtained for a given animal using these sampling methods, particularly in experimental settings in which few metastatic lesions develop. In turn, this will significantly increase variance in the experimental data, requiring the use of larger numbers of animals if statistically significant differences between experimental groups are to be obtained. Furthermore, non-concordant data may be obtained when, for example, one lobe is used for histology and another lobe is used for RNA-based analysis. Thus, analysis of pulmonary metastasis needs to take into account the distribution of metastatic lesions amongst the lung lobes, for which the qRT-PCR-based quantification we present here offers significant advantages.

Author Contributions: Conceptualization: J.P.S. and L.K.; Methodology: L.K. and R.S.; Investigation: L.K., R.S., M.R., A.S. and T.W.; Data curation: L.K. and B.K.G.; Resources: A.B.; Writing: L.K., B.K.G., W.T. and J.P.S.; Visualization: L.K., B.K.G. and W.T.; Project administration: W.T.; Supervision: J.P.S.; Funding Acquisition: J.P.S. All authors have read and agreed to the published version of the manuscript.

Funding: This work was supported by grants to J.P.S. from the Deutsche Forschungsgemeinschaft (DFG, German Research Foundation)–Project number 259332240/RTG 2099, and from the European Union (HEALTH-F2-2008-201662), under the auspices of the FP7 collaborative project TuMIC.

Institutional Review Board Statement: Animal experiments were performed according to German legal requirements and were approved by the local regulatory authorities (approval numbers AZ35-9185.81/G-134/17 and AZ 35-9185.81/G-155/18).

Data Availability Statement: The primary data presented in this study are available on request from the corresponding author(s).

Acknowledgments: We are very thankful to Selma Huber, Sabine Müller, and Amra Noa for their assistance with the animal experiments. We thank Annette Gruber and Sven Roßwag for their excellent technical support.

Conflicts of Interest: The authors declare no conflict of interest.

References

1. Braeuer, R.R.; Watson, I.R.; Wu, C.J.; Mobley, A.K.; Kamiya, T.; Shoshan, E.; Bar-Eli, M. Why is melanoma so metastatic? *Pigment Cell Melanoma Res.* **2014**, *27*, 19–36. [CrossRef] [PubMed]
2. Younes, R.; Abrao, F.C.; Gross, J. Pulmonary metastasectomy for malignant melanoma: Prognostic factors for long-term survival. *Melanoma Res.* **2013**, *23*, 307–311. [CrossRef]
3. Soliman, M.; Petrella, T.; Tyrrell, P.; Wright, F.; Look Hong, N.J.; Lu, H.; Zezos, P.; Jimenez-Juan, L.; Oikonomou, A. The clinical significance of indeterminate pulmonary nodules in melanoma patients at baseline and during follow-up chest CT. *Eur. J. Radiol. Open* **2019**, *6*, 85–90. [CrossRef]
4. Borghesi, A.; Tironi, A.; Michelini, S.; Scrimieri, A.; Benetti, D.; Maroldi, R. Two synchronous lung metastases from malignant melanoma: The same patient but different morphological patterns. *Eur. J. Radiol. Open* **2019**, *6*, 287–290. [CrossRef] [PubMed]

5. Chang, J.; Erler, J.T. Quantification of Lung Metastases from In Vivo Mouse Models. *Adv. Exp. Med. Biol.* **2016**, *899*, 245–251. [CrossRef]
6. Ntziachristos, V.; Ripoll, J.; Wang, L.V.; Weissleder, R. Looking and listening to light: The evolution of whole-body photonic imaging. *Nat. Biotechnol.* **2005**, *23*, 313–320. [CrossRef]
7. Steinbauer, M.; Guba, M.; Cernaianu, G.; Kohl, G.; Cetto, M.; Kunz-Schughart, L.A.; Geissler, E.K.; Falk, W.; Jauch, K.W. GFP-transfected tumor cells are useful in examining early metastasis in vivo, but immune reaction precludes long-term tumor development studies in immunocompetent mice. *Clin. Exp. Metastasis* **2003**, *20*, 135–141. [CrossRef]
8. Baklaushev, V.P.; Kilpelainen, A.; Petkov, S.; Abakumov, M.A.; Grinenko, N.F.; Yusubalieva, G.M.; Latanova, A.A.; Gubskiy, I.L.; Zabozlaev, F.G.; Starodubova, E.S.; et al. Luciferase Expression Allows Bioluminescence Imaging But Imposes Limitations on the Orthotopic Mouse (4T1) Model of Breast Cancer. *Sci. Rep.* **2017**, *7*, 7715. [CrossRef] [PubMed]
9. Banan, B.; Beckstead, J.A.; Dunavant, L.E.; Sohn, Y.; Adcock, J.M.; Nomura, S.; Abumrad, N.; Goldenring, J.R.; Fingleton, B. Development of a novel murine model of lymphatic metastasis. *Clin. Exp. Metastasis* **2020**, *37*, 247–255. [CrossRef]
10. Moriyama, E.H.; Niedre, M.J.; Jarvi, M.T.; Mocanu, J.D.; Moriyama, Y.; Subarsky, P.; Li, B.; Lilge, L.D.; Wilson, B.C. The influence of hypoxia on bioluminescence in luciferase-transfected gliosarcoma tumor cells in vitro. *Photochem. Photobiol. Sci.* **2008**, *7*, 675–680. [CrossRef]
11. Becker, M.; Nitsche, A.; Neumann, C.; Aumann, J.; Junghahn, I.; Fichtner, I. Sensitive PCR method for the detection and real-time quantification of human cells in xenotransplantation systems. *Br. J. Cancer* **2002**, *87*, 1328–1335. [CrossRef]
12. Schneider, T.; Osl, F.; Friess, T.; Stockinger, H.; Scheuer, W.V. Quantification of human Alu sequences by real-time PCR–an improved method to measure therapeutic efficacy of anti-metastatic drugs in human xenotransplants. *Clin. Exp. Metastasis* **2002**, *19*, 571–582. [CrossRef] [PubMed]
13. Eckhardt, B.L.; Parker, B.S.; van Laar, R.K.; Restall, C.M.; Natoli, A.L.; Tavaria, M.D.; Stanley, K.L.; Sloan, E.K.; Moseley, J.M.; Anderson, R.L. Genomic analysis of a spontaneous model of breast cancer metastasis to bone reveals a role for the extracellular matrix. *Mol. Cancer Res.* **2005**, *3*, 1–13. [PubMed]
14. Malek, A.; Catapano, C.V.; Czubayko, F.; Aigner, A. A sensitive polymerase chain reaction-based method for detection and quantification of metastasis in human xenograft mouse models. *Clin. Exp. Metastasis* **2010**, *27*, 261–271. [CrossRef]
15. Sorensen, M.R.; Pedersen, S.R.; Lindkvist, A.; Christensen, J.P.; Thomsen, A.R. Quantification of B16 melanoma cells in lungs using triplex Q-PCR–a new approach to evaluate melanoma cell metastasis and tumor control. *PLoS ONE* **2014**, *9*, e87831. [CrossRef]
16. Abt, M.A.; Grek, C.L.; Ghatnekar, G.S.; Yeh, E.S. Evaluation of Lung Metastasis in Mouse Mammary Tumor Models by Quantitative Real-time PCR. *J. Vis. Exp.* **2016**, e53329. [CrossRef]
17. Schwartz, H.; Blacher, E.; Amer, M.; Livneh, N.; Abramovitz, L.; Klein, A.; Ben-Shushan, D.; Soffer, S.; Blazquez, R.; Barrantes-Freer, A.; et al. Incipient Melanoma Brain Metastases Instigate Astrogliosis and Neuroinflammation. *Cancer Res.* **2016**, *76*, 4359–4371. [CrossRef] [PubMed]
18. Deng, W.; McLaughlin, S.L.; Klinke, D.J. Quantifying spontaneous metastasis in a syngeneic mouse melanoma model using real time PCR. *Analyst* **2017**, *142*, 2945–2953. [CrossRef]
19. del Marmol, V.; Beermann, F. Tyrosinase and related proteins in mammalian pigmentation. *FEBS Lett.* **1996**, *381*, 165–168. [CrossRef]
20. Ghanem, G.; Fabrice, J. Tyrosinase related protein 1 (TYRP1/gp75) in human cutaneous melanoma. *Mol. Oncol.* **2011**, *5*, 150–155. [CrossRef]
21. Wang, R.F.; Robbins, P.F.; Kawakami, Y.; Kang, X.Q.; Rosenberg, S.A. Identification of a gene encoding a melanoma tumor antigen recognized by HLA-A31-restricted tumor-infiltrating lymphocytes. *J. Exp. Med.* **1995**, *181*, 799–804. [CrossRef]
22. Orlow, S.J.; Hearing, V.J.; Sakai, C.; Urabe, K.; Zhou, B.K.; Silvers, W.K.; Mintz, B. Changes in expression of putative antigens encoded by pigment genes in mouse melanomas at different stages of malignant progression. *Proc. Natl. Acad. Sci. USA* **1995**, *92*, 10152–10156. [CrossRef]
23. Chu, W.; Pak, B.J.; Bani, M.R.; Kapoor, M.; Lu, S.J.; Tamir, A.; Kerbel, R.S.; Ben-David, Y. Tyrosinase-related protein 2 as a mediator of melanoma specific resistance to cis-diamminedichloroplatinum(II): Therapeutic implications. *Oncogene* **2000**, *19*, 395–402. [CrossRef]
24. Bloom, M.B.; Perry-Lalley, D.; Robbins, P.F.; Li, Y.; el-Gamil, M.; Rosenberg, S.A.; Yang, J.C. Identification of tyrosinase-related protein 2 as a tumor rejection antigen for the B16 melanoma. *J. Exp. Med.* **1997**, *185*, 453–459. [CrossRef] [PubMed]
25. Wallbaum, S.; Grau, N.; Schmid, A.; Frick, K.; Neeb, A.; Sleeman, J.P. Cell cycle quiescence can suppress transcription from an ecdysone receptor-based inducible promoter in mammalian cells. *Biotechniques* **2009**, *46*, 433–440. [CrossRef] [PubMed]
26. de Jel, M.M.; Schott, M.; Lamm, S.; Neuhuber, W.; Kuphal, S.; Bosserhoff, A.K. Loss of CYLD accelerates melanoma development and progression in the Tg(Grm1) melanoma mouse model. *Oncogenesis* **2019**, *8*, 56. [CrossRef]
27. Pollock, P.M.; Cohen-Solal, K.; Sood, R.; Namkoong, J.; Martino, J.J.; Koganti, A.; Zhu, H.; Robbins, C.; Makalowska, I.; Shin, S.S.; et al. Melanoma mouse model implicates metabotropic glutamate signaling in melanocytic neoplasia. *Nat. Genet.* **2003**, *34*, 108–112. [CrossRef]
28. Meyerholz, D.K.; Suarez, C.J.; Dintzis, S.M.; Frevert, C.W. 9-Respiratory System. In *Comparative Anatomy and Histology*, 2nd ed.; Treuting, P.M., Dintzis, S.M., Montine, K.S., Eds.; Academic Press: San Diego, CA, USA, 2018; pp. 147–162.
29. Schiffner, S.; Chen, S.; Becker, J.C.; Bosserhoff, A.K. Highly pigmented Tg(Grm1) mouse melanoma develops non-pigmented melanoma cells in distant metastases. *Exp. Dermatol.* **2012**, *21*, 786–788. [CrossRef]

30. Taus, L.J.; Flores, R.E.; Seyfried, T.N. Quantification of metastatic load in a syngeneic murine model of metastasis. *Cancer Lett.* **2017**, *405*, 56–62. [CrossRef]
31. Orlow, S.J.; Silvers, W.K.; Zhou, B.K.; Mintz, B. Comparative decreases in tyrosinase, TRP-1, TRP-2, and Pmel 17/silver antigenic proteins from melanotic to amelanotic stages of syngeneic mouse cutaneous melanomas and metastases. *Cancer Res.* **1998**, *58*, 1521–1523. [PubMed]
32. Meeth, K.; Wang, J.X.; Micevic, G.; Damsky, W.; Bosenberg, M.W. The YUMM lines: A series of congenic mouse melanoma cell lines with defined genetic alterations. *Pigment. Cell Melanoma Res.* **2016**, *29*, 590–597. [CrossRef]
33. Fang, D.; Hallman, J.; Sangha, N.; Kute, T.E.; Hammarback, J.A.; White, W.L.; Setaluri, V. Expression of microtubule-associated protein 2 in benign and malignant melanocytes: Implications for differentiation and progression of cutaneous melanoma. *Am. J. Pathol.* **2001**, *158*, 2107–2115. [CrossRef]
34. Lenggenhager, D.; Curioni-Fontecedro, A.; Storz, M.; Shakhova, O.; Sommer, L.; Widmer, D.S.; Seifert, B.; Moch, H.; Dummer, R.; Mihic-Probst, D. An Aggressive Hypoxia Related Subpopulation of Melanoma Cells is TRP-2 Negative. *Transl. Oncol.* **2014**, *7*, 206–212. [CrossRef]
35. Bolander, A.; Agnarsdottir, M.; Stromberg, S.; Ponten, F.; Hesselius, P.; Uhlen, M.; Bergqvist, M. The protein expression of TRP-1 and galectin-1 in cutaneous malignant melanomas. *Cancer Genom. Proteom.* **2008**, *5*, 293–300.
36. Journe, F.; Id Boufker, H.; Van Kempen, L.; Galibert, M.D.; Wiedig, M.; Sales, F.; Theunis, A.; Nonclercq, D.; Frau, A.; Laurent, G.; et al. TYRP1 mRNA expression in melanoma metastases correlates with clinical outcome. *Br. J. Cancer.* **2011**, *105*, 1726–1732. [CrossRef]
37. El Hajj, P.; Gilot, D.; Migault, M.; Theunis, A.; van Kempen, L.C.; Sales, F.; Fayyad-Kazan, H.; Badran, B.; Larsimont, D.; Awada, A.; et al. SNPs at miR-155 binding sites of TYRP1 explain discrepancy between mRNA and protein and refine TYRP1 prognostic value in melanoma. *Br. J. Cancer.* **2015**, *113*, 91–98. [CrossRef] [PubMed]
38. Tief, K.; Hahne, M.; Schmidt, A.; Beermann, F. Tyrosinase, the key enzyme in melanin synthesis, is expressed in murine brain. *Eur. J. Biochem.* **1996**, *241*, 12–16. [CrossRef] [PubMed]
39. Chi, D.D.; Merchant, R.E.; Rand, R.; Conrad, A.J.; Garrison, D.; Turner, R.; Morton, D.L.; Hoon, D.S. Molecular detection of tumor-associated antigens shared by human cutaneous melanomas and gliomas. *Am. J. Pathol.* **1997**, *150*, 2143–2152.
40. Gautron, A.; Migault, M.; Bachelot, L.; Corre, S.; Galibert, M.D.; Gilot, D. Human TYRP1: Two functions for a single gene? *Pigment Cell Melanoma Res.* **2021**, *34*, 836–852. [CrossRef] [PubMed]

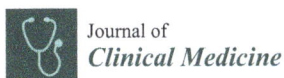

Article

Identification of microRNAs Targeting the Transporter Associated with Antigen Processing TAP1 in Melanoma

Maria-Filothei Lazaridou [1], Chiara Massa [1], Diana Handke [1], Anja Mueller [1], Michael Friedrich [1], Karthikeyan Subbarayan [1], Sandy Tretbar [1], Reinhard Dummer [2], Peter Koelblinger [3] and Barbara Seliger [1,*]

1 Institute of Medical Immunology, Martin Luther University Halle-Wittenberg, Magdeburger Str. 2, 06112 Halle, Germany; marifili.lazaridou@uk-halle.de (M.-F.L.); chiara.massa@uk-halle.de (C.M.); diana.handke@uk-halle.de (D.H.); anjamueller@uk-halle.de (A.M.); michael.friedrich@uk-halle.de (M.F.); karthik.subbarayan@uk-halle.de (K.S.); sandy.tretbar@uk-halle.de (S.T.)
2 Institute of Dermatology, University Hospital Zürich, 8091 Zürich, Switzerland; Reinhard.Dummer@usz.ch
3 Department of Dermatology and Allergology, University Hospital Salzburg, 5020 Salzburg, Austria; p.koelblinger@salk.at
* Correspondence: Barbara.Seliger@uk-halle.de; Tel.: +49-(0)-345-557-4054

Received: 29 June 2020; Accepted: 14 August 2020; Published: 20 August 2020

Abstract: The underlying molecular mechanisms of the aberrant expression of components of the HLA class I antigen processing and presentation machinery (APM) in tumors leading to evasion from T cell-mediated immune surveillance could be due to posttranscriptional regulation mediated by microRNAs (miRs). So far, some miRs controlling the expression of different APM components have been identified. Using in silico analysis and an miR enrichment protocol in combination with small RNA sequencing, miR-26b-5p and miR-21-3p were postulated to target the 3' untranslated region (UTR) of the peptide transporter TAP1, which was confirmed by high free binding energy and dual luciferase reporter assays. Overexpression of miR-26b-5p and miR-21-3p in melanoma cells downregulated the TAP1 protein and reduced expression of HLA class I cell surface antigens, which could be reverted by miR inhibitors. Moreover, miR-26b-5p overexpression induced a decreased T cell recognition. Furthermore, an inverse expression of miR-26b-5p and miR-21-3p with TAP1 was found in primary melanoma lesions, which was linked with the frequency of CD8+ T cell infiltration. Thus, miR-26-5p and miR-21-3p are involved in the HLA class I-mediated immune escape and might be used as biomarkers or therapeutic targets for HLA class I^{low} melanoma cells.

Keywords: immune escape; microRNA; melanoma; transporter associated with antigen processing

1. Introduction

Human solid tumors including melanoma develop different strategies to escape T cell-mediated immune surveillance such as loss or downregulation of human leukocyte antigens (HLA) class I molecules. This is frequently due to defects in the expression of various components of the antigen processing and presentation machinery (APM), which can be associated with disease progression and reduced patient survival [1–4]. Alterations in the HLA class I pathway may be a result of the selective pressure of the immune system and could occur in patients treated with immunotherapies [5,6]. During the last few decades, the underlying molecular mechanisms of HLA class I and APM component deficiencies have been characterized demonstrating a high diversity, ranging from deregulation to rather rare structural alterations [3,7–9]. The deregulation of HLA class I APM components in tumors could occur at the transcriptional, epigenetic, posttranscriptional and/or posttranslational level and depend on the tumor type analyzed [2,10–12]. Recently, the posttranscriptional regulation of HLA class I APM components has come into focus, which could be mediated by RNA binding proteins (RBP) or small non-coding microRNAs (miRs) [13–16].

MiRs with a length of approximately 20–23 nucleotides belong to the family of small non-coding RNAs [17] and play an important role in the posttranscriptional control of gene expression by binding to the 5′ UTR, 3′ UTR or coding sequence of the targeted mRNAs [18] either preventing translation or inducing degradation [17]. A broad spectrum of miRs have been identified to be abnormally expressed in hematologic malignancies and solid tumors including melanoma [19]. Dependent on their targets, miRs could influence tumor formation, metastasis, disease progression as well as the composition of the immune cell infiltration of the tumor microenvironment (TME) [20]. They function as oncogenes or tumor suppressor genes, but could also participate in immune escape or altered immune responses by targeting or affecting the expression of different immune modulatory molecules in tumor and immune cells [14].

The implementation of different strategies, such as in silico prediction, miR arrays, small RNA sequencing, RNA affinity approaches and luciferase (luc) reporter gene assays, resulted in the identification and functional characterization of a small number of miRs targeting the 3′UTR of the HLA class I heavy chain (HC), HLA-G, TAP1 or TAP2 [21–28]. Due to this limited information, the identification of novel miRs involved in HLA class I mediated immune escape mechanisms is urgently needed and might lead to a better understanding of tumor development and progression as well as response or resistance to immunotherapies such as checkpoint inhibitors or adoptive cell therapy [29–34]. To identify novel and specific miRs, the miRNA trapping by RNA in vitro affinity purification (miTRAP) assay has been shown to provide a rapid, reliable and easy-to-handle protocol for the enrichment of regulatory miRs for RNAs of choice in the cellular context of interest [35,36]. Apart from the 3′UTR, the target sequences can be the 5′UTR or the coding sequence (CDS) [35]. MiRs targeting immune modulatory molecules might serve as prognostic and/or predictive tumor markers or be used as therapeutic tools alone or in combination with immunotherapies [14,37].

Malignant melanoma represents the most common skin cancer with an incidence that has rapidly increased over the past few decades [38,39]. The interaction of melanoma cells with cells of the TME influences the biology of melanoma cells, such as proliferation, differentiation and progression [40]. Furthermore, melanoma cells are often highly immunogenic and have the capacity to induce an adaptive immune response [41]. This might be due to their high mutational burden leading to the expression of tumor-associated antigens (TAA) [42,43]. However, melanoma cells escape T cell recognition by different mechanisms, like inefficient antigen processing and presentation, modulation of immune stimulatory or immune suppressive molecules and alterations in the cellular composition of the TME [29,44–46]. This knowledge has led to the approval of therapeutic approaches aiming to overcome immune evasion, i.e., anti-CTLA-4 and anti-PD1 antibodies [39]. Another possibility might be to target immune modulatory miRs that have been demonstrated to be involved in innate and adaptive immune responses [47].

Therefore, in this study, miTRAP combined with small RNA sequencing was employed to identify novel miRs targeting TAP1 [35,36,48]. Two selected miRs were functionally analyzed in melanoma cell lines. In addition, their clinical relevance regarding survival outcome in melanoma patients and association with tumor immune cell infiltration was determined.

2. Experimental Section

2.1. Cell Lines and Cell Culture Conditions

The human embryonic kidney cell line HEK293T and the human TAP-negative T2 cell lines (ATCC® CRL-1992™) were obtained from the American Tissue Culture Collection (ATCC), the human melanoma cell lines FM3 (ESTDAB-007), FM81 (ESTDAB-026) and MZ-Mel2 (CVCL-1435) [49] from the European Searchable Tumour Cell Line and Data Bank (ESTDAB project; http://www.ebi.ac.uk/ipd/estdab) [50,51] and BUF1379 from Soldano Ferrone (Department of Surgery, Massachusetts General Hospital, Harvard Medical School, Boston, MA, USA). The HEK293T cells were cultured in Dulbecco's Modified Eagles Medium (DMEM, Invitrogen, Carlsbad, CA, USA), while all the other cell lines were maintained in Roswell Park Memorial Institute 1640 medium (RPMI 1640, Invitrogen) supplemented with 10% (v/v) fetal calf serum (FCS) (PAN, Aidenbach, Germany), 2 mM L-glutamine (Lonza, Basel, Switzerland) and 1% penicillin/streptomycin (v/v, Sigma-Aldrich, Saint Louis, MO, USA) at 37 °C in 5% (v/v) CO_2 humidified air. T2 cells negative for TAP1, TAP2, LMP2, LMP7 and MHC class II antigens served as a control for peptide pulsing [52]. T cells specific for the HLA-A2-restricted Melan A/Mart-1 epitope were kindly provided by Pedro Romero (Ludwig Institute for Cancer Research, Lausanne, Switzerland) and cultured in RPM 1640 supplemented with 8% human serum.

2.2. Human Melanoma Tissues

Tissue samples from cutaneous malignant melanoma used in this study ($n = 20$) were collected between 2008 and 2016 in the Department of Dermatology, University Hospital of Zurich, Zurich, Switzerland [53]. The study was performed according to the declaration of Helsinki and approved by the ethical committees of the University Hospital in Zurich (KEK-ZH-No. 647 and 800) as well as of the University Hospital in Salzburg (E-No. 2142). The clinical data from the melanoma patients as well as the PD-L1 expression and immune cell infiltration of the tumor lesions have recently been published [53].

2.3. Plasmids and Cloning

The recombinant vectors for luciferase reporter assays, oligonucleotide sequences used for PCR reactions and cloning strategies have recently been described [35,36,54] and are listed in Supplementary Table S1. The recombinant plasmid DNA pcDNA™ 3.1(+) (Invitrogen) with the two MS2 loops was kindly provided by Prof. Dr. Stefan Hüttelmaier (Institute of Molecular Medicine, Martin Luther University Halle-Wittenberg, Halle (Salle, Germany). All amplified inserts were sequenced for their identity prior to subcloning into the respective vectors.

2.4. MiRNA Trapping by RNA In Vitro Affinity Purification (miTRAP)

MiTRAP is a suitable method for the identification of miRs that specifically target immune relevant molecules. Detailed protocols for the different steps of this method have been recently published [35,36,48,55]. Briefly, the TAP1 3' UTR (NM_000593.5) was cloned upstream of the coding sequence for two MS2 stem loop structures, in vitro transcribed with RiboMAX large scale RNA production system (Promega, Mannheim, Germany) and used for the enrichment of TAP1-specific miRs from cell lysates of MZ-Mel2 (CVCL_1435) [49]. Then, amylose resin beads (NEB) were washed and incubated with the fusion protein maltose-binding protein (MBP) fused to the MS2-binding protein, blocked with yeast tRNA (Invitrogen) and bovine serum albumin (BSA; Invitrogen) and incubated with the bait RNAs (TAP1 3' UTR or the sequence encoding only the two MS2 loops (MS2) as a negative control) and the cell lysate. With the exception of cell lysis, all steps were performed at room temperature under constant agitation. For miR analysis, RNA complexes were eluted twice with 15 mM maltose and miR were purified from maltose solution by phenol–chloroform extraction. Untreated cell lysate was used for RNA extraction and applied as an input control. The miR enrichment in the eluates was further validated by RT-qPCR. For protein analysis, protein complexes were eluted once with Laemmli buffer and together with 1%, 0.5%, and 0.2% dilution series of the cell lysate, prepared as input controls, were subjected to Western blot analysis using 10% SDS-PAA gels.

2.5. Isolation of Plasmid DNA, Cellular RNA, miRNA and qPCR Analysis

Plasmid DNA was isolated either with NucleoSpin® Plasmid or the NucleoBond® Xtra Midi kits (Macherey-Nagel, Schkeuditz, Germany) for small or medium scale plasmid preparation, respectively. The NucleoSpin® Gel and PCR Clean-up kit (Macherey-Nagel) was employed for the DNA purification of the PCR products and the digested plasmids with the respective restriction enzymes as recently described [56].

Total cellular RNA from cell cultures was isolated using the NucleoSpin RNA kit (Macherey-Nagel, Schkeuditz, Germany) according to the manufacturer's instructions. Total cellular RNA and miR were extracted from cell cultures using the TRIzol reagent (Invitrogen) according to the manufacturer's instructions. For RNA isolation from paraffin-embedded tissue sections, total RNA was extracted using the NucleoSpin Tissue kit (Macherey-Nagel). The isolated RNA was treated with DNaseI (New England Biolabs (NEB), Ipswich, MA, USA) for 30 min at 37 °C, inactivated with 50 mM EDTA for 10 min at 75 °C and then used as template for cDNA synthesis.

RT-qPCR was performed as previously described [51,57]. Briefly, RNA was reverse transcribed into cDNA using RevertAid™ H Minus First Strand cDNA synthesis kit (Thermo Scientific, Waltham, MA, USA) together with oligo dT primers (Thermo Scientific) for mRNA and miR specific stem loop primers for the miR [57–59]. For qPCR reaction, the 2× SYBR Green qPCR Master Mix (Absource, Munich, Germany) was employed with target-specific primers (Supplementary Table S1). The reverse transcription reactions were carried out in a 96-well labcycler (Sensoquest, Göttingen, Germany) and the qPCR reactions in a BIO-RAD 96-well iCycler (BIO-RAD Laboratories, Inc., Hercules, CA, USA). For qPCR, the relative changes of RNA abundance were determined by the ΔCt method using the housekeeping genes glyceraldehyde-3-phosphate dehydrogenase (GAPDH) or β-actin (ACTB) for normalization, whereas the relative miR expression levels were normalized to the corresponding expression levels of the small non-coding RNA RNU6A. The reactions were performed at least in triplicates for each biological replicate.

2.6. Protein Extraction and Western Blot Analysis

For Western blot analysis, 50 µg protein/lane was separated in 10% SDS-PAGE gels, transferred onto nitrocellulose membranes (Schleicher & Schuell, Munich, Germany) and stained with Ponceau S performed as previously described [60]. Immunodetection was performed using the following specific primary antibodies (Ab): anti-TAP1 (ab13516, Abcam, Cambridge, UK), anti-TAP2, kindly provided by Soldano Ferrone, anti-AGO2 (ab156870, Abcam) and anti-MBP Abs (ab9084, Abcam). Staining with anti-GAPDH (#2118, Cell Signaling Technology, Danvers, MA, USA) or ACTB Ab (ab8227, Abcam) served as a loading control. The membranes were then stained with suitable horseradish peroxidase (HRP) conjugated secondary Abs (DAKO, Hamburg, Germany or Cell Signaling Technology, Danvers, MA, USA), before the signal was visualized with the Pierce Western Blot Signal Enhancer substrate (Thermo Scientific) and recorded with a LAS3000 camera system (Fuji LAS3000, Fuji GmbH, Düsseldorf, Germany) using the Image Reader LAS3000 software. The immunostaining signals were subsequently analyzed using the ImageJ software (NIH, Bethesda, Rockville, MD, USA). Relative protein expression levels are provided as arbitrary units by setting the peak values of the corresponding GAPDH signals to 1.

2.7. Luciferase Reporter Assay

The TAP1 3' UTR was cloned in the pmiR-Glo Dual-Luciferase miRNA target expression vector (Promega, Madison, Washington, DC, USA) with the restriction enzymes NheI and SalI (Thermo Scientific) as recently described [56]. For the deletion of the binding side of miR-26b-5p or miR-21-3p in the TAP1 3' UTR, specific primers were designed according to the NEBaseChanger software (https://nebasechanger.neb.com/, NEB) (Supplementary Table S1). The Q5® Site-Directed Mutagenesis kit (NEB) was employed according to manufacturer's instructions. On day zero, 1×10^4 HEK293T cells/well were seeded into 96-well plates. After 12–16 h, the cells were co-transfected with 30 nM mimics (Sigma-Aldrich) and 5 ng recombinant TAP1 3' UTR pmiR-Glo vector using Lipofectamin 2000 (Invitrogen). The cells were washed with phosphate-buffered saline (PBS) 48 h post-transfection and lysed in lysis buffer (Promega). The firefly and renilla luciferase (luc) activities were determined using the DualGlo reagent (Promega) with the GloMax 96-Microplate luminometer (Promega) kindly provided by Prof. Guido Posern (Institute of Biophysical Chemistry, Martin Luther University Halle-Wittenberg, Halle (Saale, Germany) with the Dual-Luciferase® Reporter Assay System (Promega) according to manufacturer's instructions. Firefly luc (FFL) activities were normalized to Renilla luc (RL) activities yielding relative light units (RLU). The empty pmiR-Glo vector only containing the multiple cloning site served as a negative control. RLU ratios were normalized to control populations. All experiments were performed at least three times in triplicates.

2.8. Transfection of miR

To determine the impact of miR on the expression of HLA class I APM components, 3×10^5 cells were seeded in 6-well plates and transiently transfected after 12–16 h with mimics (30 nM) or inhibitors (100 nM) (miR-26b-5p, miR-21-3p or the negative control (NC), Sigma-Aldrich) using 9 µL Lipofectamine RNAiMAX (Invitrogen) according to the manufacturer's instructions. The cells were harvested 48 h post-transfection for subsequent qPCR, Western blot, flow cytometric and functional analyses.

2.9. Flow Cytometry

The monoclonal antibodies (mAb) employed for flow cytometry were the PE-Cyanine7-labelled anti-HLA-ABC (BioLegend, San Diego, CA, USA), the APC-labelled anti-HLA-BC (BioLegend), the unconjugated anti-HLA-A2 (kindly provided by Soldano Ferrone) and the PE-labelled-secondary goat anti-mouse Ab (Jackson ImmunoResearch, Cambridgeshire, UK) at concentrations recommended by the manufacturers. Briefly, $1–5 \times 10^5$ cells were incubated with the appropriate amounts of respective Ab at 4 °C in darkness for 30 min. The stained cells were measured on a BD FACS LSRFortessa (Becton Dickinson (BD), New Jersey, NJ, USA) and subsequently analyzed with the FACS Diva analysis software (BD). The data are expressed as mean specific fluorescence intensities (MFI).

2.10. CD107a Degranulation Assay

Tumor cell susceptibility to HLA-A2 restricted MART1 specific CD8$^+$ T cells was evaluated by the CD107a degranulation assay [61,62]. Briefly, target cells were co-incubated with effector cells at a 1:1 ratio at 37 °C. After one hour of incubation, an anti-CD107a Ab (Biolegend, San Diego, CA, USA) was added and after an additional 3 h, the effector cells were stained with the anti-CD3 and anti-CD8Ab (Biolegend) and analyzed on a Navios flow cytometer (Beckman Coulter, Brea, CA, USA). Effector cells alone were used to determine the spontaneous degranulation that was removed from the specific one.

Incubation with peptide-pulsed versus unpulsed T2 cells was used as a positive control for the functionality of the clone.

2.11. Immunohistochemical Staining of the Paraffin-Embedded Tissue Sections of Melanoma Patients

Formalin-fixed paraffin-embedded (FFPE) tumor samples were processed and analyzed at collaborating institutions in Zurich and Salzburg. The studies were performed according to the declaration of Helsinki and approved by the ethical committees of the University Hospital in Zurich (KEK-ZH-No. 647 and 800) as well as of the University Hospital in Salzburg (E-No. 2142). Four µm thick sections were cut from each FFPE tissue block and stained using the Dako Autostainer Plus platform (Agilent Technologies Inc., Santa Clara, CA, USA) as recently described [53].

Immunohistochemical stains were independently evaluated by three independent dermatopathologists. A consensus-based score was derived for every single evaluation. Cell counts were estimated by averaging at least ten high-powered fields (HPF, 400× magnification) representative of the entire tumor. The expression of TAP1 in tumor cells was graded into four categories regarding their frequency (0%, 1–10%, 11–30%, >30%). For the present study, TAP1^{high} (>30%) and TAP1^{low} (0–10%) lesions were processed as published by Lazaridou et al. (Oncoimmunol.2020 9,1:1–14) [56].

2.12. Next-Generation Sequencing Analysis

As previously described in the miTRAP method [35,36], miR can be eluted from the beads for downstream analyses, such as small RNA sequencing. Small RNA sequencing and data analyses were provided for two biological replicates of the miTRAP eluates of TAP1 3′UTR, together with the background and input controls by Novogene Co., Ltd. (Hong Kong, China).

The reads were mapped with bowtie1 [63] against human rRNA and tRNA databases. MiRs were detected and quantified with mirdeep * [64] from mirBase (v21) [65] and were represented as counts per miR loci taking into account that an miR can be encoded by multiple loci.

2.13. Functional and Pathway Enrichment Analyses

Gene Ontology (GO) analysis was performed using the respective database (http://www.geneontology.org/) enrichment analysis. Predicted target gene candidates of miRs identified in this study [66] were categorized regarding their function into the biological process (BP), molecular function (MF), and cellular component (CC) [67]. It provides all GO terms significantly enriched in the predicted target gene candidates of the enriched known as well as novel identified miRs compared to the reference gene background (in this study the MS2 control) as well as the genes corresponding to certain biological functions. The corrected p-value (q-value) of <0.05 and the gene count of ≥2 was chosen as a significant threshold [67].

2.14. Bioinformatics—Survival Analysis

In silico analysis was performed using the starbase v2.0 web tool (http://starbase.sysu.edu.cn/) [68,69] in order to predict the association of the expression of TAP1 and HLA class I molecules with the survival of melanoma patients. The statistical differences in the gene expression values between the patients' groups with "high" and "low" mRNA expression levels were evaluated by ANOVA tests implemented in the web tool. The p-values were corrected for multiple testing according to the false discovery rate. All cut-off expression levels and their resulting groups were correlated with the patients' survival and used for the generation of the Kaplan–Meier curves, which allowed to discriminate patients into "good" and "bad" prognosis cohorts. Kaplan–Meier analysis was performed to estimate the disease specific survival probability and distant metastasis free survival probability according to mRNA expression status using this dataset.

For this purpose, the "TCGA Skin Cutaneous Melanoma (SKCM)" dataset [70–76] was chosen and 440 unique melanoma patients were included for the analysis. For determination of high and low expression levels of TAP1 and HLA class I, the cut-off modus "median" divided the patients into two groups containing the same number of patients. The raw p-value significance was calculated for every graph with the web database and Pearson's correlation with the transform 2log setting. The 2log expression ratio was compared and a linear regression was calculated. The expression pattern of TAP1 and HLA class I molecules were correlated to the clinical parameters. A p-value < 0.05 was considered as significant.

2.15. Statistical Analysis

Microsoft Excel 2010 (Microsoft Corporation, Redmond, WA, USA), SPSS version 15.0 and GraphPad Prism version 8 were used for analysis. A p-value < 0.05 was considered statistically significant using paired or unpaired t-tests respectively.

3. Results

3.1. Clinical Relevance of TAP1 and HLA Class I Molecules Regarding Survival of Tumor Patients

As already shown by our group and others, a decreased expression of several HLA class I APM components, such as TAP1, HLA-A, HLA-B and HLA-C, has been associated with poor patient survival in several types of cancer, including cutaneous melanoma [2,77–80]. Using the "starbase" web tool (http://starbase.sysu.edu.cn/) and several available datasets including the "TCGA Skin Cutaneous Melanoma (SKCM)" dataset [70,81], the correlation between the expression of TAP1 and HLA class I loci was re-evaluated in order to determine the prognostic relevance of TAP1 (Table 1a), HLA-A (Table 1b), HLA-B (Table 1c) and HLA-C (Table 1d) expression patterns in different cancer types including skin cutaneous melanoma. These data demonstrated a correlation of high levels of TAP1 and HLA class I loci with an increased overall survival (OS) of tumor patients including melanoma, with the exception of cancers in immune privileged organs (brain, eye, thymus). As shown in Figure 1, higher TAP1 (a), HLA-A (b), HLA-B (c) and HLA-C (d) mRNA transcript levels correlated with an increased OS of melanoma patients. Furthermore, the expression of TAP1 and HLA-A (Figure 1e), TAP1 and HLA-B (Figure 1f) as well as TAP1 and HLA-C (Figure 1g) were associated.

Table 1. Correlation of the expression pattern of TAP1 and HLA class I loci in different cancer types with the patients' survival.

Abbreviation	Type of Cancer	Number of Cases	Median Gene Expression	Correlation	p-Value
		a: TAP1			
OV	ovarian serous adenocarcinoma	374	18.68	positive	0.00053
LGG	brain lower grade glioma	523	11.19	negative	0.0032
SKCM	skin cutaneous melanoma	440	41.39	positive	0.0033
UVM	uveal melanoma	80	9.02	negative	0.0069
COAD	colon adenocarcinoma	447	44.99	positive	0.044
THYM	thymoma	118	24.35	negative	0.1
UCEC	uterine corpus endometrial carcinoma	537	21.75	positive	0.56
THCA	thyroid carcinoma	509	12.61	negative	0.8
		b: HLA-A			
LGG	brain lower grade glioma	523	133.35	negative	0.00012
SKCM	skin cutaneous melanoma	440	671.89	positive	0.00052
UCEC	uterine corpus endometrial carcinoma	537	523.84	positive	0.0074
UVM	uveal melanoma	80	502.23	negative	0.0081
THCA	thyroid carcinoma	509	468.03	positive	0.043
OV	ovarian serous adenocarcinoma	374	219.47	positive	0.059
THYM	thymoma	118	325.13	negative	0.063
COAD	colon adenocarcinoma	447	516.21	positive	0.26
		c: HLA-B			
SKCM	skin cutaneous melanoma	440	620.14	positive	5.7×10^{-6}
LGG	brain lower grade glioma	523	129.28	negative	0.00027
UVM	uveal melanoma	80	238.66	negative	0.0011
THYM	thymoma	118	390.69	negative	0.0026
OV	ovarian serous cystadenocarcinoma	374	300.77	positive	0.0069
UCEC	uterine corpus endometrial carcinoma	537	545.19	positive	0.053
COAD	colon adenocarcinoma	447	629.70	positive	0.18
THCA	thyroid carcinoma	509	503.74	positive	0.22
		d: HLA-C			
LGG	brain lower grade glioma	523	117.10	negative	2.0×10^{-7}
SKCM	skin cutaneous melanoma	440	458.38	positive	3.9×10^{-5}
THYM	thymoma	118	260.27	negative	0.0081
UVM	uveal melanoma	80	247.30	negative	0.011
UCEC	uterine corpus endometrial carcinoma	537	406.42	positive	0.2
OV	ovarian serous cystadenocarcinoma	374	270.08	positive	0.4
THCA	thyroid carcinoma	509	334.74	positive	0.36
COAD	colon adenocarcinoma	447	461.01	positive	0.85

Shown are the correlation of TAP1 (a), HLA-A (b), HLA-B (c) and HLA-C (d) expression levels with the overall survival of patients with different types of cancer. The expression levels and overall survival data were obtained by pan-cancer analysis using the TCGA data sets at the starbase v2.0 web tool (http://starbase.sysu.edu.cn/).

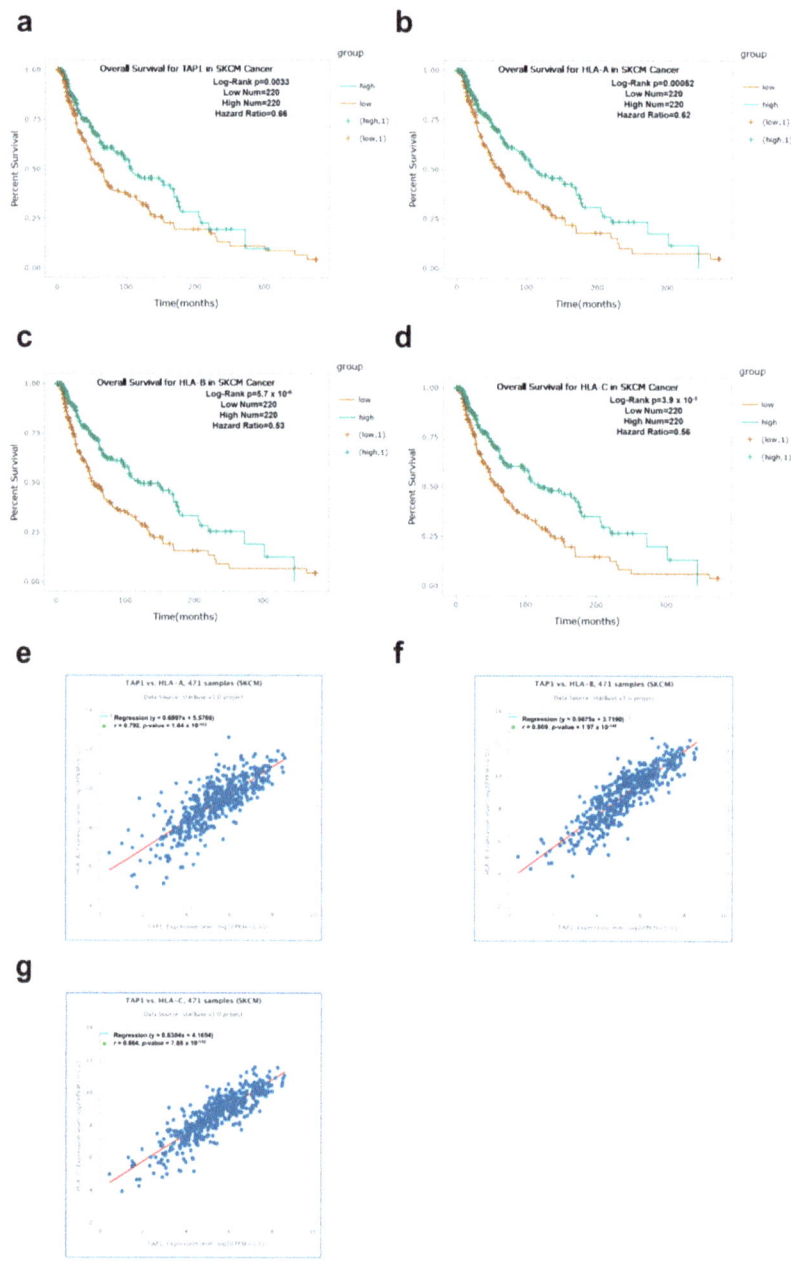

Figure 1. Correlation of TAP1 and HLA class I expression with the overall survival in melanoma patients. Kaplan–Meier estimation curves for overall survival (OS) probability of 440 individual melanoma patients based on the expression of TAP1 (**a**) HLA-A (**b**), HLA-B (**c**) and HLA-C (**d**) were generated by using the starbase v2.0 web tool and the "SKCM Cancer" dataset. The raw *p*-values were based on log-rank tests and were calculated for every graph with the web database (http://starbase.sysu.edu.cn/). In addition, TAP1 expression was correlated with HLA-A (**e**), HLA-B (**f**) or HLA-C (**g**) mRNA expression in the melanoma patients using the same dataset.

3.2. Identification of New Candidate miR Targeting TAP1 Using the miTRAP Assay

To identify miRs regulating TAP1 expression, the miTRAP method was employed [35,36,48,55]. Using a cell lysate of the melanoma cell line MZ-Mel2, the in vitro transcribed TAP1 3′ UTR, but not the MS2 control RNA nor the amylose resin beads loaded with MS2BP-MBP, specifically co-purified the RNA-induced silencing complex component argonaute 2 (AGO2) suggesting a putative posttranscriptional regulation of TAP1 expression by a binding of miRs (Figure 2a). The affinity purification of the bait RNA (TAP1 3′ UTR and MS2 control) was confirmed upon detection of the eluted TAP1 3′ UTR on a guanidinium thiocyanate denaturing agarose gel. The eluate-enriched miRs targeting the TAP1 3′ UTR from two biological replicates and the respective controls were subjected to small RNA sequencing.

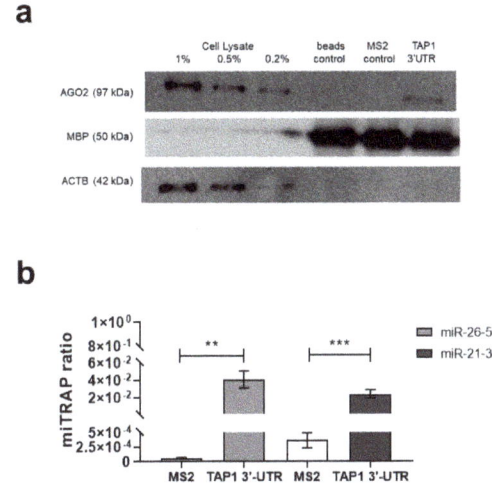

Figure 2. Detection of AGO2 at the 3′ UTR of TAP1 and presence of miRs in the miTRAP eluate. (**a**) Western blot-based detection of AGO2 was performed at the TAP1 3′ UTR in order to determine the presence of AGO2 in the cell lysate input control samples as well as on the target (TAP1 3′ UTR), control (MS2) RNA and in the amylose beads control (no RNA bait). Unspecific protein binding to RNA was excluded by the detection of ACTB, which lack in the beads control, MS2 control and target RNA. A signal for MBP of the MS2BP-MBP fusion protein is detected in the eluates, but not in the cell extract and served as control for equal loading of the MS2BP-MBP. (**b**) Enrichment of miRs in miTRAP eluates. Bar graph showing the miTRAP ratio of the two candidate miRs. The data were normalized to the input value, which was set to "1". The bars show the enrichment of each miR on the MS2 in comparison to the TAP1 3′ UTR. For miR-26b-5p, a 700-fold enrichment compared to the MS2 control RNA (MS2) is detected, while for miR-21-3p, only a 50-fold enrichment is observed. Shown are the normalized mean ± SE from a minimum of three different biological replicates, ** $p < 0.01$ and *** $p < 0.001$ in unpaired t-test.

The isolation of the miR fraction was based on size selection. Fractions of other RNA species, such as e.g., rRNA and tRNA, were excluded. The sequence length distribution demonstrated a major peak of 21–23 nt (Supplementary Figure S1). For analysis at the miR level, the transcripts per million (tpm) counts were used [36,53]. Selective binding of miRs to the TAP1 3′ UTR was determined relative to MS2 control by calculating the ratio of the respective tpm counts, indicating enrichment of the candidate miR as previously described [36,82]. In total, 352 of 2693 (13.07%) miRs determined by miRBase [65] were enriched in the TAP1 3′ UTR eluate when compared to the MS2 control (Supplementary Table S2). Among the enriched miRs, 2.27% (7 out of 352) were in silico predicted by 5 prediction tools, 3.98% (14/352) by 4 prediction tools, 3.98% (14/352) by 3 prediction tools, 13.64% (48/352) by 2 prediction tools, 49.72% (175/352) by 1 prediction tool and 26.42% (93/352) were not in silico predicted. These data suggest that the miTRAP allows a novel set of miR candidates to bind to the 3' UTR. In order to select the candidate miRs, several criteria were applied, such as (i) that a specific binding site for the respective candidate miRs within the TAP1 3'-UTR should be predicted by at least four out of the six selected bioinformatic tools, (ii) the tpm counts observed in the TAP1 3' UTR miTRAP eluate should be higher than 1000, while (iii) the tpm counts observed in the MS2 control miTRAP eluate should be less than 100 and (iv) the enrichment ratio should be higher than 50. Additionally, (v) a strong binding affinity of complementary structures between the putative miRs and the target TAP1 3' UTR calculated as a high free binding energy and (vi) a high "miTRAP ratio", defining the enrichment of miRs in the miTRAP eluate versus the input and determined by the ΔCt method were taken into consideration.

In silico analyses were performed for 21 of the candidate miRs identified by miTRAP and RNA-seq using the available prediction tools miRWalk 2.0 [83,84], microrna.org [85], miRDB [86], TargetScan [87], RNA22 [88] and RNAhybrid [89]. These include miR-21-3p, miR-22-3p, miR-140-3p, miR-590-3p, miR-26b-5p, miR-532-5p and miR-26a-5p (Table 2). Despite their in silico prediction, the enrichment ratios of miR-1273f, miR-1301-3p, miR-140-3p, miR-151a-5p, miR-151b, miR-24-1-5p, miR-24-2-5p, miR-28-5p, miR-330-3p, miR-504-3p, miR-508-5p, miR-512-3p, miR-548b-3p, miR-597-3p and miR-708-5p were less than 50. Moreover, miR-26a-5p, miR-532-5p and miR-590-3p had lower binding energy and/or enrichment ratios than miR-26b-5p or miR-21-3p, while the miTRAP ratio of miR-22-3p was lower than the miTRAP ratios of miR-26b-5p or miR-21-3p. Therefore, based on the in silico prediction by the selected bioinformatics tools, the RNA sequencing results, the free binding energy, the miTRAP ratio and current literature, miR-26b-5p and miR-21-3p were selected as novel candidate miRs targeting the TAP1 3' UTR for further analyses (Table 2). The enrichment of both candidate miRs was confirmed in the TAP1 3' UTR eluates by RT-qPCR. Candidate miRs are presented as a miTRAP ratio of miR abundance in the target TAP1 3' UTR or in the MS2 control eluates versus the input determined by the ΔCt method (Figure 2b).

Data from the GO analysis of the predicted target gene candidates from the enriched miRs of the miTRAP eluates are shown in Supplementary Figure S2, illustrating a categorization into biologic process, molecular function and cellular components. The molecular functions ATP binding and protein binding as well as the biologic process associated immune of genes located in the ER were highly enriched. Concerning the biologic processes, defense response and transmembrane/protein transport were also significantly enriched and are related to HLA class I APM components. The KEGG pathway analysis strengthens our assumption that miRs identified in the miTRAP eluate play a role in the regulation of antigen processing and presentation (Supplementary Table S3).

Table 2. In silico prediction of selected, enriched miRs in the TAP1 3′ UTR miTRAP eluates.

miRBase Accession Number	miR	RNA-Seq Enrichment Ratio	miRWalk	Microrna.org	miRDB	TargetScan	RNA22	RNAhybrid	In Silico Prediction Tools	Binding Energy (kcal/mol)
MIMAT0020601	hsa-miR-1273f	0.9	yes	Yes	no	yes	no	yes	4	−30.1
MIMAT0005797	hsa-miR-1301-3p	9.2	yes	Yes	no	yes	yes	yes	5	−29.0
MIMAT0004597	hsa-miR-140-3p	1.3	yes	Yes	no	yes	yes	yes	5	−24.0
MIMAT0004697	hsa-miR-151a-5p	19.1	yes	Yes	no	yes	yes	yes	5	−26.1
MIMAT0010214	hsa-miR-151b	6.3	yes	Yes	no	yes	no	yes	4	−24.8
MIMAT0004494	hsa-miR-21-3p	1036.0	yes	Yes	yes	yes	no	yes	5	−20.3
MIMAT0000077	hsa-miR-22-3p	102.9	yes	Yes	no	yes	yes	yes	5	−21.6
MIMAT0000079	hsa-miR-24-1-5p	5.0	yes	Yes	no	yes	no	yes	4	−25.8
MIMAT0004497	hsa-miR-24-2-5p	17.2	yes	Yes	no	yes	no	yes	4	−25.9
MIMAT0000082	hsa-miR-26a-5p	74.1	yes	Yes	no	yes	no	yes	4	−25.1
MIMAT0000083	hsa-miR-26b-5p	92.1	yes	Yes	no	yes	no	yes	4	−25.4
MIMAT0000085	hsa-miR-28-5p	16.1	yes	Yes	no	yes	no	yes	4	−20.9
MIMAT0000751	hsa-miR-330-3p	21.7	yes	Yes	no	yes	no	yes	4	−24.8
MIMAT0026612	hsa-miR-504-3p	16.2	yes	Yes	no	yes	no	yes	4	−27.2
MIMAT0004778	hsa-miR-508-5p	3.4	yes	Yes	no	yes	no	yes	4	−25.5
MIMAT0002823	hsa-miR-512-3p	4.0	yes	Yes	no	yes	no	yes	4	−27.0
MIMAT0002888	hsa-miR-532-5p	65.5	yes	Yes	no	yes	no	yes	4	−20.5
MIMAT0003254	hsa-miR-548b-3p	1.3	yes	Yes	yes	yes	no	yes	5	−22.4
MIMAT0004801	hsa-miR-590-3p	289.2	yes	Yes	yes	yes	no	yes	5	−12.8
MIMAT0026619	hsa-miR-597-3p	2.7	yes	Yes	no	yes	no	yes	4	−23.5
MIMAT0004926	hsa-miR-708-5p	13.8	yes	Yes	no	yes	no	yes	4	−24.3

Six different prediction tools were used to predict binding of miRs to the 3′ UTR of TAP1. Sum demonstrates how many of the six tools used predicted the binding.

3.3. Direct Interaction of miR-26b-5p and miR-21-3p with TAP1 3′ UTR

Using RNAhybrid [89], the binding affinity of complementary structures between the putative miRs and the target mRNA were calculated as a high free binding energy of −25.4 kcal/mol and −20.3 kcal/mol for miR-26b-5p or miR-21-3p and the TAP1 3′ UTR, respectively (Table 2 and Supplementary Figure S3a,b) indicating a high probability of interaction. Furthermore, the direct interaction between the two selected candidate miRs and the TAP1 3′ UTR was validated by the dual luc reporter assay. After transient transfection of HEK293T cells with the pMir-Glo vector containing the TAP1 3′ UTR in the presence of miR-26b-5p or miR-21-3p mimics, the luc activity significantly decreased upon overexpression of the miR in comparison to the miR mimic negative control (NC) (Figure 3a,b). As expected, the deletion of the binding sites of the candidate miR within the TAP1 3′ UTR altered neither the luc activity in the presence of the miR nor that of the NC (Figure 3a,b).

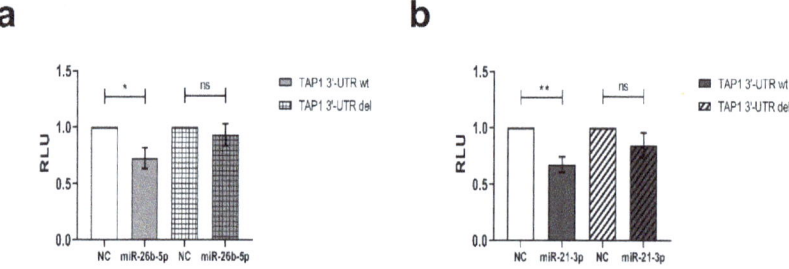

Figure 3. Identification of miR-26b-5p and miR-21-3p interaction with TAP1 3′ UTR. The dual luciferase reporter assay was performed with HEK293T cells using wt and del TAP1 3′ UTR as described in Materials and Methods together with miR-26b-5p (**a**) or miR-21-3p (**b**). Firefly luc (FFL) activities were internally normalized to Renilla luciferase activities yielding relative light units (RLU). Shown are the mean ± SE from 3 to 6 independent experiments upon normalization to the miR mimic NC. * $p < 0.05$, ** $p < 0.01$ in an unpaired *t*-test.

3.4. Downregulation of TAP1 Expression by miR-26b-5p and miR-21-3p

To determine whether miR-26b-5p and miR-21-3p, selectively co-purified with the TAP1 3′ UTR, regulate the TAP1 expression via binding to TAP1 3′ UTR, the respective miR mimics and NC were transiently transfected into the melanoma cell lines BUF1379, FM3 and FM81. Overexpression of both miRs was obtained in all three melanoma cell lines, but the level of overexpression varied among the three cell lines, based also on their constitutive miR expression level, with the highest levels for miR-21-3p in BUF1379 and FM3 cells. Cells transfected with the NC showed an miR expression pattern comparable to that of parental cells (Figure 4a,b). Overexpression of miR-26b-5p in BUF1379 and FM3 cells decreased the TAP1 mRNA and protein levels with approximately 30% when compared to controls (Figure 4c,g,h). In contrast, overexpression of miR-21-3p did not affect TAP1 mRNA levels (Figure 4d) in the melanoma cell lines analyzed, but interfered with TAP1 protein levels (Figure 4g,i) with a 25% decreased expression in melanoma transfectants compared to controls, potentially indicating a different type of action of miR-21-3p or miR-26-5p. As expected, the expression of other APM components, such as TAP2, was not affected by miR-26b-5p and miR-21-3p overexpression (Figure 4e–g). The miR-mediated downregulation of TAP1 was accompanied by decreased HLA class I surface antigen expression, but to a different extent among the melanoma cell lines. In contrast, HLA class I mRNA expression was not affected (Figure 5a,b) in the miR transfectants. As shown in Figure 5e, HLA-A2 surface expression was also significantly downregulated upon miR-26b-5p overexpression, whereas no effects were visible upon miR-21-3p overexpression. Interestingly, HLA-BC surface expression was upregulated upon overexpression of both miRs in BUF1379 cells (Figure 5g,h). Co-transfection of FM3 and FM81 cells with miR-26b-5p and miR-21-3p mimics was also performed and the expression levels of TAP1, TAP2 and HLA class I were evaluated by RT-qPCR, Western blot and/or flow cytometric analyses. Although both miRs were overexpressed during the co-transfection, no significant difference was observed compared to the single transfectants with miR-26b-5p or miR-21-3p, respectively.

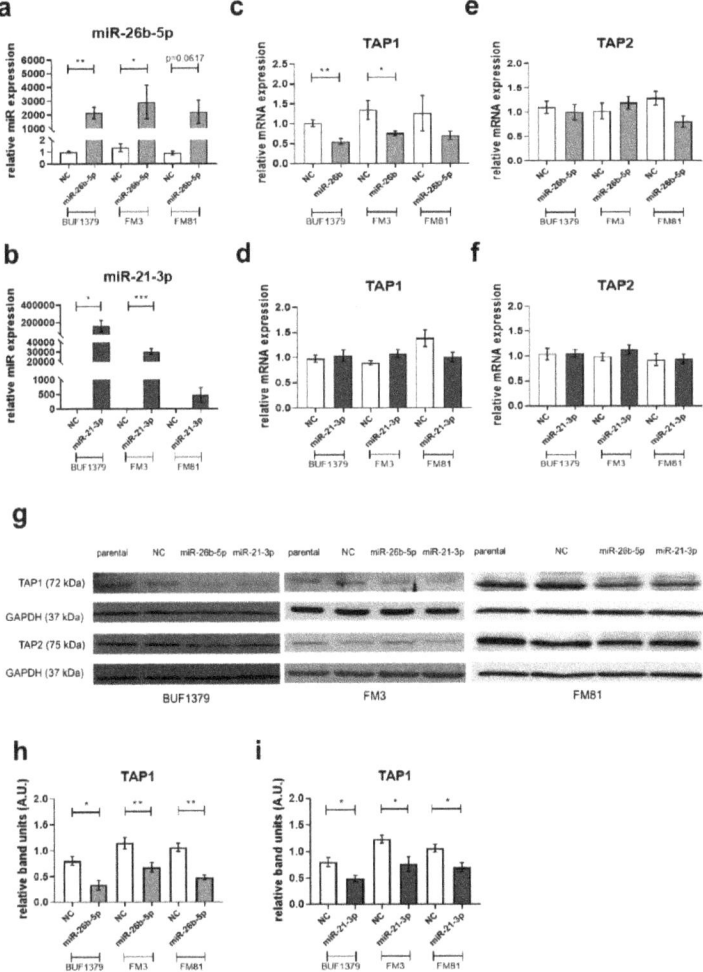

Figure 4. Effect of miRs overexpression on the expression of APM components in melanoma cell lines. BUF1379, FM3 and FM81 melanoma cells were left untreated (parental) or transiently transfected with miR mimics (miR-26b-5p or miR-21-3p) or miR mimic negative control (NC) as described in Materials and Methods. After 48 h of transfection, miR overexpression (**a**,**b**), as well as the mRNA expression levels of the indicated APM components, were determined by RT-qPCR (**c**–**f**). Protein expression was evaluated by Western blot (**g**–**i**). For quantification of Western blot results, the relative band density (A.U., arbitrary units) of transfectants was calculated to the respective parental melanoma cells and normalized to GAPDH expression. Shown are the normalized mean ± SE from a minimum of three different biological replicates and one representative Western blot, * $p < 0.05$, ** $p < 0.01$, *** $p < 0.001$ in an unpaired *t*-test.

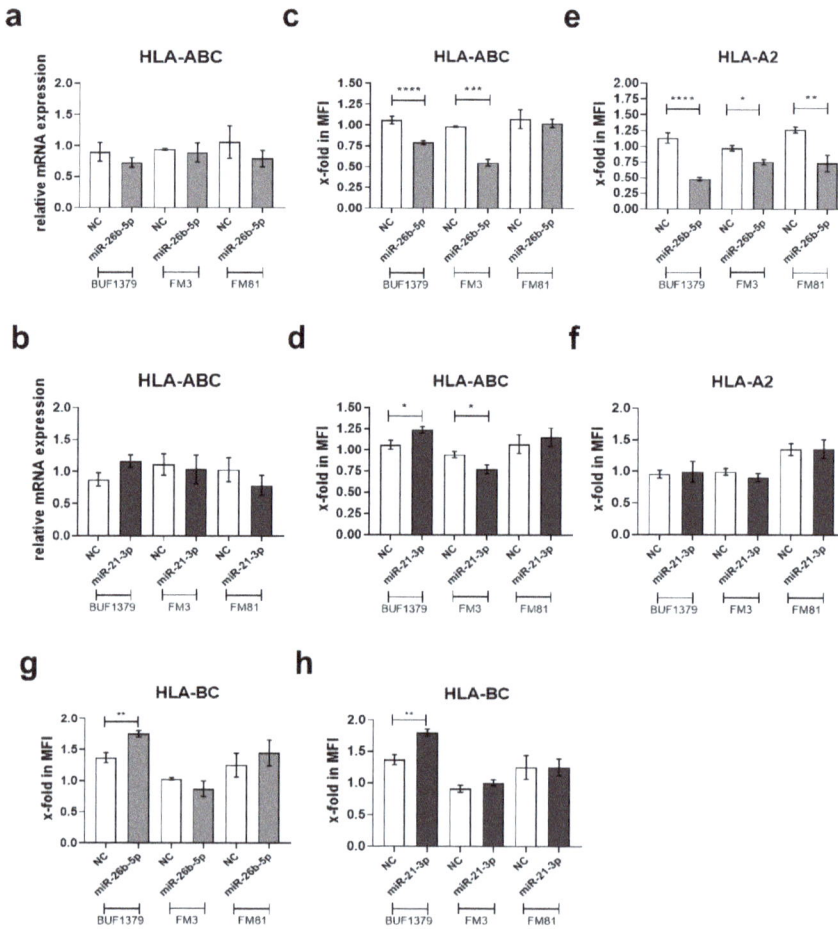

Figure 5. Effect of miRs overexpression on mRNA and surface expression of HLA class I in melanoma cell lines. BUF1379, FM3 and FM81 melanoma cells were transfected with 30 nM miR mimic negative control (NC) or miR mimics (miR-26b-5p or miR-21-3p) and after 48 h, the mRNA expression of HLA class I was determined by RT-qPCR (**a,b**) and the surface expression of HLA-ABC, HLA-A2 and HLA-BC was determined by flow cytometry (**c–h**). Shown are the normalized mean ± SE from a minimum of three different biological replicates, * $p < 0.05$, ** $p < 0.01$, *** $p < 0.001$ and **** $p < 0.0001$ in an unpaired t-test.

3.5. Reversion of the miR Effect by Inhibition of miR-26b-5p and miR-21-3p

To evaluate the specific effect of the candidate miRs on TAP1 expression, miR inhibitors and an inhibitor control were transiently transfected into BUF1379 and FM3 cells. MiR expression levels were significantly reduced (between 30–50%) both in the BUF1379 and FM3 transfectants when compared to cells transfected with NC inhibitors or parental cells (Figure 6a,b). Thus, miR inhibitors efficiently down-regulated the endogenous miR expression in BUF1379 and FM3 cells. This was accompanied by increased levels of TAP1 protein (Figure 6e,f) and at least partially of TAP1 mRNA (Figure 6c,d). HLA class I surface expression was upregulated in both melanoma cell lines (Figure 6g,h). Inhibition of miR-26b-5p or miR-21-3p in BUF1379 and FM3 cells increased HLA-A2 surface antigens (Figure 6i,j), while HLA-BC surface expression remained unchanged (Figure 6k,l).

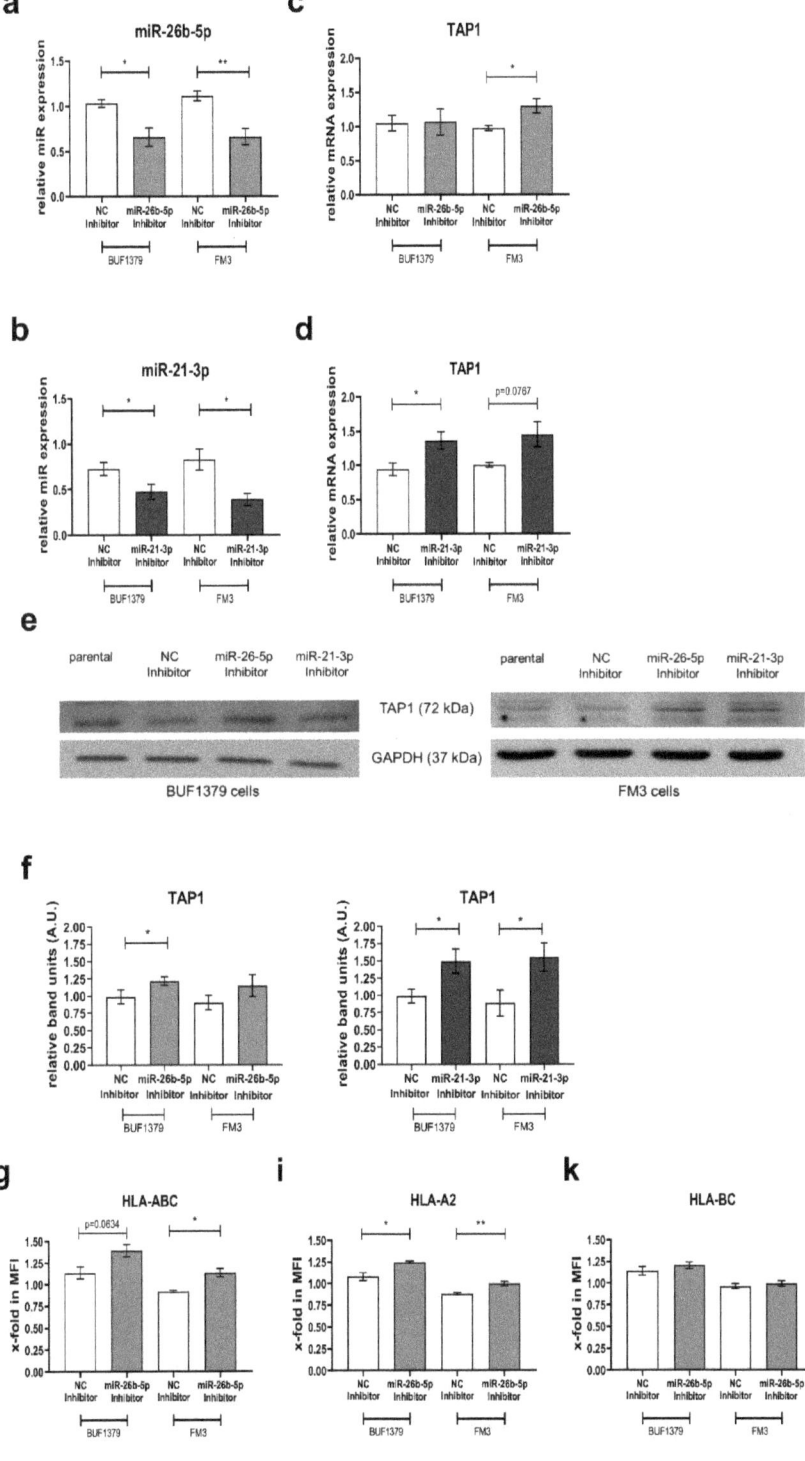

Figure 6. *Cont.*

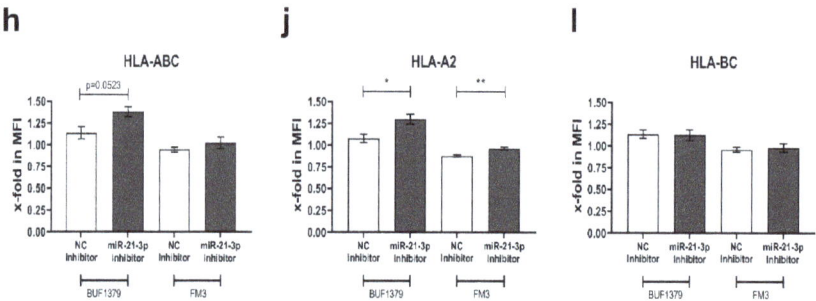

Figure 6. Effect of miRs inhibition on TAP1 and HLA class I expression in melanoma cell lines. BUF1379 and FM3 melanoma cells were left untreated (parental) or transiently transfected with the negative control inhibitor (NC Inhibitor) or the miR-26b-5p inhibitor or miR-21-3p inhibitor, respectively. After 48 h, miR inhibition (**a,b**) as well as TAP1 expression were determined on mRNA level by RT-qPCR (**c,d**). Protein expression was evaluated by Western blot (**e,f**) and flow cytometry (**g–l**). For quantification of Western blot results, the relative band density (A.U., arbitrary units) of transfectants was calculated to the respective parental melanoma cells and normalized to GAPDH expression. Shown are the normalized mean ± SE from a minimum of three different biological replicates and one representative Western blot, * $p < 0.05$, ** $p < 0.01$ in an un-paired t-test.

3.6. Correlation of the miR26b-5p-Mediated Downregulation of TAP1 with Decreased T Cell Recognition

To assess the functional relevance of the miR-induced suppression of TAP1 and consequently associated reduced HLA class I surface expression, the T cell-mediated recognition of miR transfectants was determined using a CD107a degranulation assay. Lower levels of CD107a positive T cells were found in response to BUF1379 cells overexpressing miR-26b-5p when compared to control transfectants (Figure 7).

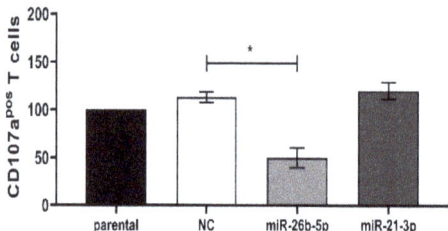

Figure 7. Effects of miR mimics on BUF1379 cell recognition by antigen-specific CD8$^+$ T cells. MelanA/MART1-specific CD8$^+$ T cells were incubated for 4 h with BUF1379 transfected with NC or miR mimics and evaluated for degranulation. Shown are the x-fold changes in CD107a positive cells from three independent experiments, * $p < 0.05$ in paired t-test.

3.7. Correlation between miR-26b-5p or miR-21-3p Expression with TAP1 and Immune Cell Infiltration in Melanoma Lesions

To determine the in vivo translatability of our data, miR-26b-5p and miR-21-3p expression levels were evaluated by RT-qPCR analysis in 20 FFPE sections of human primary melanoma scored as TAP1 low ($n = 10$) or TAP1 high ($n = 10$) based on the immunohistochemical staining of the lesions with anti-TAP1 specific mAb. While no difference was detected for miR-26b-5p (Figure 8a), a negative trend was found between miR-21-3p and TAP1 expression in the melanoma specimens (Figure 8b), thereby supporting our in vitro data. Since the immune cell infiltration of the same melanoma samples was previously analyzed for the presence of CD8$^+$ T cells by immunohistochemistry (IHC), it was possible to correlate TAP1 and miR expression to CD8 infiltration. As shown in Figure 8c,d, the TAP1 expression scores were directly correlated with the frequency of CD8$^+$ immune cells, with TAP1^{low} and TAP1^{high} melanoma lesions exhibiting the low and high frequency of CD8$^+$ T cells respectively. Furthermore, a direct link between TAP1^{low} and CD8^{low} infiltration with high miR-26b-5p and miR-21-3p expression and vice versa exists (Figure 8c,d).

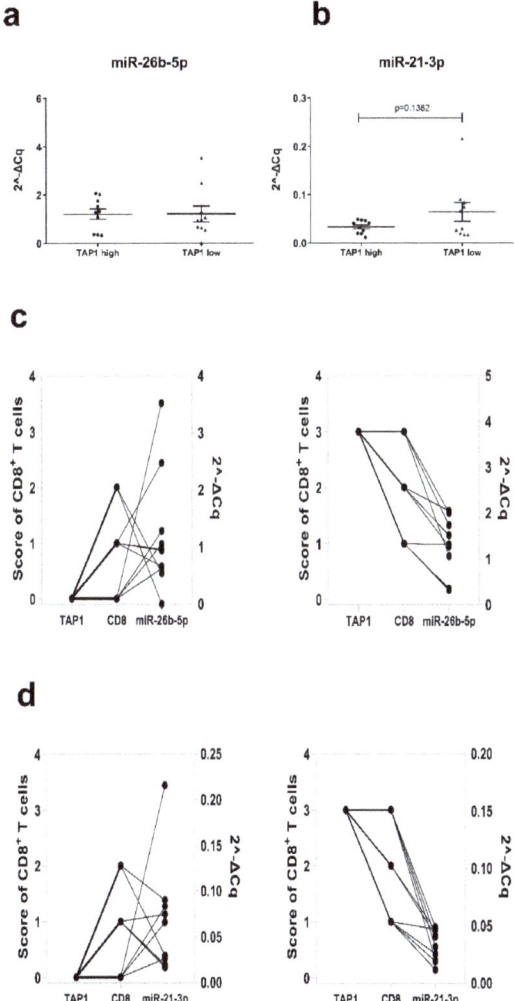

Figure 8. Inverse relation of miRs expression with TAP1 levels and CD8 infiltration in melanoma patients. Paraffin-embedded tissue sections from 20 primary melanoma patients were analyzed for miR-26b-5p or miR-21-3p expression levels by RT-qPCR and scored for TAP1 and CD8 expression as high or low by immunohistochemical staining. Comparison between TAP1 high ($n = 10$) and TAP1 low ($n = 10$) melanoma lesions is shown for miR-26b-5p (**a**) and miR-21-3p (**b**) expression. An overview of TAP1, CD8$^+$ T cells (left y-axis) and miR-26b-5p expression (right y-axis) for each individual patient among the TAP1 high (left) and TAP1 low (right) group is provided (**c**). Respective graphs are provided for miR-21-3p (**d**).

4. Discussion

During the last few years, the role of HLA class I APM components has gained rekindled interest, since this pathway has been shown to be involved in the process of resistance to immunotherapies, including checkpoint inhibitors and adoptive T cell therapy [37,90–92]. High expression levels of major APM components including TAP1 and HLA class I loci were directly associated with a better outcome for most cancer patients, including skin cutaneous melanoma, with the exception of brain tumors, uveal melanoma and thymoma (Table 1). Furthermore, TAP1 expression was associated with HLA class I expression (Figure 1). A deficient/reduced expression of HLA class I components frequently occurred and was linked to either structural alterations or an impaired expression of components of the APM and IFN signal transduction, which are controlled at distinct levels [31,37,92–95].

In this context, a number of miRs have been shown to act as critical regulators of anti-tumor immune responses, in particular in the context of solid tumors. The miR-mediated processes include (i) the regulation of the recruitment and activation of immune cells in the TME, (ii) the expression of immune modulatory molecules and (iii) the secretion of immune suppressive or immune stimulatory factors by tumor and immune cells [96,97]. Thus, miRs might have the potential to enhance or inhibit specific immune cell populations or immune modulatory molecules in tumor cells, hence influencing the anti-tumor immune response and possibly improving the efficacy of immunotherapy in cancer patients.

During the last few years, some miRs have been reported to target APM components and HLA class I molecules suggesting an important role of posttranscriptional control in the antigen processing and presentation process [98]. miR-9, miR-125a, miR-148 and miR-27a have been identified to modulate directly or indirectly the MHC class I surface expression of tumor cells [21,23,99]. Since TAP1 is a key component of the HLA class I APM pathway and is important for proper HLA class I surface expression, this study aimed to identify miRs targeting TAP1 using an miR enrichment protocol in combination with small RNA sequencing [36,48] instead of miR arrays, which identified miR-200a-5p and miR-346 as targets of the 3′ UTR of TAP1 [28]. Interestingly, GO analysis of enriched miRs by miTRAP, in combination with RNA sequencing, identified respective target genes involved in ATP and protein binding and was located in the ER. This is in line with the features of TAP1, (i) which transport peptides ATP-dependently from the cytosol into the ER and (ii) is located in the ER membrane [100,101].

Among the identified miRs, miR-21-3p and miR-26-5p were selected for further analysis and were demonstrated to directly target the 3′ UTR of TAP1. The binding was confirmed by several in silico prediction tools and the dual luc reporter assay. Moreover, the overexpression of miR-21-3p or miR-26b-5p resulted in a reduced TAP1 protein expression in melanoma cells. As a consequence of the reduced transport of cytosolically processed peptides into the ER, which are required for the assembly of the stable trimeric MHC-I/peptide complex [102,103], melanoma cells overexpressing the respective mimics had a reduced HLA class I surface expression. Particularly, upon miR-26b-5p overexpression, HLA-A2 surface expression was specifically downregulated, resulting in a decreased recognition of the transfected melanoma cells by HLA-A2-restricted CD8$^+$ T cells. Despite an overexpression of both miRs upon co-transfection in FM3 and FM81 cells with the respective miR mimics, the expression levels of TAP1 or the surface expression of HLA class I were not significantly different from that of the single transfectants with miR-26b-5p or miR-21-3p mimics respectively. Therefore, the results presented here provide an important mechanistic explanation for the reduced HLA class I expression on melanoma cells and its functional effect on immune cells.

The miR-21 family represents the prototype of oncomiRs and its expression is upregulated in various cancers, often correlating with tumor progression [104,105]. MiR-21-3p was among the top miRs isolated from invasive melanoma lesions and was differentially expressed between thin (0.75 mm) and thick (2.7 mm) melanoma, common melanocytic nevi and matched normal skin [106]. Its expression level correlated with the Breslow index, clinical stage and decreased survival of melanoma patients and increased from dysplastic nevi to melanoma and melanoma metastasis [107]. Since miR-21 has been shown to target cancer-relevant genes such as the phosphatase and tensin homolog

(PTEN), programmed cell death protein 4 (PCDP4), reversion-inducing cysteine-rich protein with Kazal motifs (RECK) and signal transducer activator of transcription 3 (STAT3), it is involved in carcinogenic processes and might serve as a diagnostic and prognostic biomarker or as a therapeutic target for several cancer types [105]. In melanoma, miR-21 expression is upregulated when compared to nevi [108] and affects genes associated with proliferation (PTEN, PI3K, Sprouty, PDCD4, FOXO1, TIPE2, p53, cyclin D1), evasion from apoptosis (FOXO1, FBXO11, APAF1, TIMP3, TIPE2), genetic instability (MSH2, FBXO11, hTERT), increased oxidative stress (FOXO1), angiogenesis (PTEN, HIF1α, TIMP3), invasion and metastasis (APAF1, PTEN, PDCD4, TIMP3) [109]. This was partially confirmed by functional analysis. For example, miR-21 and its target PTEN demonstrated an inverse expression in melanoma lesions, while anti-miR-21 altered PTEN expression in melanoma cell lines. MiR-21-3p was strongly enriched in miTRAP eluates of TAP1 and proved to directly bind to the 3′ UTR, thereby decreasing TAP1 protein expression, which supported its reported oncogenic role in melanoma, similar to what has been described in other types of cancers [108].

MiR-26b-5p also plays an important role in different malignancies, but in contrast to miR-21-3p it has been suggested to have a tumor-suppressive activity [110]. It is downregulated in various tumors including head and neck squamous cell carcinoma, bladder, prostate and liver cancer [111–115] and was correlated to the process of epithelial-mesenchymal transition in hepatocellular carcinoma [113,116]. Ectopic expression of miR-26b-5p can inhibit proliferation, induce apoptosis, suppress angiogenesis and/or decrease tumorigenicity and is therefore involved in controlling carcinogenesis and tumor progression in hepatocellular and bladder cancer [113,117–119]. So far, little information exists on the function of miR-26b-5p in melanoma. In melanoma, miR-26b-5p expression is decreased in primary tumors when compared to benign nevi [106]. Recently, miR-26b-5p has been shown to target the MAPK and AKT/mTOR signaling pathways by binding to the 3′ UTR of TRAF5 or TRIM44, respectively [120,121], which are involved in the malignant progression of melanoma cells. However, no direct effects of miR-26b-5p on the expression of immune modulatory molecules have been described neither in melanoma nor in other tumor types. In this context, it is noteworthy that miR-26a-5p bind to the 3′ UTR of CREB, which is a known regulator of MHC class I [122]. MiR-26b-5p was one of the strongly enriched miRs we identified in miTRAP eluates of TAP1, verified by small RNA sequencing. By directly targeting the 3′ UTR of TAP1, miR-26b-5p decreased TAP1 mRNA and protein expression and negatively interferes with the immunogenicity of tumor cells demonstrating that miR-26b-5p could have, instead of the published tumor suppressive activity, also a tumor-promoting activity by including an immune escape phenotype in melanoma cells. This is in line with a recent report demonstrating that miR-26b is a negative regulator of the NF-kB pathway, which is important for the expression of many immune modulatory molecules including cytokines and APM components [123]. These data suggest a dual role for miR-26b-5p in tumors.

5. Conclusions

Although further studies are required to provide more mechanistic insights into the link between miR-21-3p and miR-26b-5p high expression, HLA class I antigen presentation and CTL recognition, miR-21-3p/miR-26b-5p^{high} TAP1^{low} expression levels appear to be associated with a reduced CD8$^+$ T cell infiltrate and a more aggressive behavior of primary melanomas. Thus, both miRs are multifaceted by affecting different hallmarks of cancer including the tumor cell-host immunologic interactions, thereby extending their critical role in tumorigenesis. This opens a novel avenue for the development of strategies to improve patients' prognosis through enhancement of a response to (immuno)therapy and through avoidance of treatment resistance.

Supplementary Materials: The following are available online at http://www.mdpi.com/2077-0383/9/9/2690/s1, Figure S1: Sequence length distribution of miTRAP eluates, Figure S2: The GO terms of candidate targets of miRs enriched in the TAP1 3′ UTR miTRAP eluates vs the MS2 control, Figure S3: RNAhybrid figures, Table S1: List of primers, Table S2: List of the enriched miRs in TAP1 3′ UTR miTRAP eluates, Table S3: Significantly affected processes, components or functions by the enriched miRs in mi-TRAP eluates of the TAP1 3′ UTR.

Author Contributions: Conceptualization, B.S.; methodology, D.H., A.M. and S.T.; formal analysis and investigation, C.M., P.K., R.D., M.F., M.-F.L. and K.S.; writing—original draft preparation, B.S. and M.-F.L.; writing—B.S., M.-F.L. and C.M.; funding acquisition, B.S.; resources: R.D. and P.K.; supervision: B.S. All authors have read and agreed to the published version of the manuscript.

Funding: Deutsche Forschungsgemeinschaft DFG GRK1591 (105533105), SE-581.22-1, the German-Israeli foundation for scientific research and development GIF I-37-4145.II-2016 and Mildred Scheel Stiftung No. 70113861.

Acknowledgments: We would like to thank Maria Heise and Nicole Ott for excellent secretarial work.

Conflicts of Interest: The authors declare that they have no conflicts of interest.

Abbreviations

Ab: antibody; ACTB, β-actin; AGO2, argonaute 2; APM, antigen processing and presentation machinery; ATCC, American Tissue culture collection; BSA, bovine serum albumin; FCS, fetal calf serum; FFL, firefly luciferase; FFPE, formalin-fixed paraffin-embedded; GAPDH, glyceraldehyde-3-phosphate dehydrogenase; GO, gene ontology; HLA, human leukocyte antigen; HRP, horseradish peroxidase; HS, human serum; luc, luciferase; mAb, monoclonal antibody; MART, melanoma antigen recognized by T cells 1; MBP, maltose-binding protein; miR, microRNA; miTRAP, miRNA trapping by RNA in vitro affinity purification; NC, negative control; OS, overall survival; PBMC, peripheral blood mononuclear cell; RL, Renilla luc; RLU, relative light units; RTq-PCR, reverse transcribed quantitative PCR; TAA, tumor-associated antigen; TAP, transporter associated with antigen processing, tpn, tapasin; TCGA, The Cancer Genome Atlas; tpm, transcript per million; TME, tumor microenvironment; UTR, untranslated region.

References

1. Cai, L.; Michelakos, T.; Yamada, T.; Fan, S.; Wang, X.; Schwab, J.H.; Ferrone, C.R.; Ferrone, S. Defective HLA class I antigen processing machinery in cancer. *Cancer Immunol. Immunother.* **2018**, *67*, 999–1009. [CrossRef] [PubMed]
2. Seliger, B.; Ferrone, S. HLA Class I Antigen Processing Machinery Defects in Cancer Cells-Frequency, Functional Significance, and Clinical Relevance with Special Emphasis on Their Role in T Cell-Based Immunotherapy of Malignant Disease. *Methods Mol. Biol.* **2020**, *2055*, 325–350. [CrossRef] [PubMed]
3. Seliger, B. Molecular mechanisms of HLA class I-mediated immune evasion of human tumors and their role in resistance to immunotherapies. *HLA* **2016**, *88*, 213–220. [CrossRef] [PubMed]
4. Andersson, E.; Villabona, L.; Bergfeldt, K.; Carlson, J.W.; Ferrone, S.; Kiessling, R.; Seliger, B.; Masucci, G.V. Correlation of HLA-A02* genotype and HLA class I antigen down-regulation with the prognosis of epithelial ovarian cancer. *Cancer Immunol. Immunother.* **2012**, *61*, 1243–1253. [CrossRef] [PubMed]
5. Kalbasi, A.; Ribas, A. Tumour-intrinsic resistance to immune checkpoint blockade. *Nat. Rev. Immunol.* **2020**, *20*, 25–39. [CrossRef]
6. Mittal, D.; Gubin, M.M.; Schreiber, R.D.; Smyth, M.J. New insights into cancer immunoediting and its three component phases—Elimination, equilibrium and escape. *Curr. Opin. Immunol.* **2014**, *27*, 16–25. [CrossRef]
7. Jabrane-Ferrat, N.; Faille, A.; Loiseau, P.; Poirier, O.; Charron, D.; Calvo, F. Effect of gamma interferon on HLA class-I and -II transcription and protein expression in human breast adenocarcinoma cell lines. *Int. J. Cancer* **1990**, *45*, 1169–1176. [CrossRef]
8. Seliger, B. Novel insights into the molecular mechanisms of HLA class I abnormalities. *Cancer Immunol. Immunother.* **2012**, *61*, 249–254. [CrossRef]
9. Snyder, S.R.; Waring, J.F.; Zhu, S.Z.; Kaplan, S.; Schultz, J.; Ginder, G.D. A 3'-transcribed region of the HLA-A2 gene mediates posttranscriptional stimulation by IFN-gamma. *J. Immunol.* **2001**, *166*, 3966–3974. [CrossRef]
10. Campoli, M.; Ferrone, S. HLA antigen changes in malignant cells: Epigenetic mechanisms and biologic significance. *Oncogene* **2008**, *27*, 5869–5885. [CrossRef]
11. Rene, C.; Lozano, C.; Eliaou, J.F. Expression of classical HLA class I molecules: Regulation and clinical impacts: Julia Bodmer Award Review 2015. *HLA* **2016**, *87*, 338–349. [CrossRef]
12. Dovhey, S.E.; Ghosh, N.S.; Wright, K.L. Loss of interferon-gamma inducibility of TAP1 and LMP2 in a renal cell carcinoma cell line. *Cancer Res.* **2000**, *60*, 5789–5796. [PubMed]
13. Reches, A.; Nachmani, D.; Berhani, O.; Duev-Cohen, A.; Shreibman, D.; Ophir, Y.; Seliger, B.; Mandelboim, O. HNRNPR Regulates the Expression of Classical and Nonclassical MHC Class I Proteins. *J. Immunol.* **2016**, *196*, 4967–4976. [CrossRef] [PubMed]

14. Eichmuller, S.B.; Osen, W.; Mandelboim, O.; Seliger, B. Immune Modulatory microRNAs Involved in Tumor Attack and Tumor Immune Escape. *J. Natl. Cancer Inst.* **2017**, *109*. [CrossRef] [PubMed]
15. Yang, Q.; Cao, W.; Wang, Z.; Zhang, B.; Liu, J. Regulation of cancer immune escape: The roles of miRNAs in immune checkpoint proteins. *Cancer Lett.* **2018**, *431*, 73–84. [CrossRef] [PubMed]
16. Cano, F.; Rapiteanu, R.; Winkler, G.S.; Lehner, P.J. A non-proteolytic role for ubiquitin in deadenylation of MHC-I mRNA by the RNA-binding E3-ligase MEX-3C. *Nat. Commun.* **2015**, *6*, 8670. [CrossRef]
17. Bartel, D.P. MicroRNAs: Genomics, biogenesis, mechanism, and function. *Cell* **2004**, *116*, 281–297. [CrossRef]
18. Bartel, D.P. MicroRNAs: Target recognition and regulatory functions. *Cell* **2009**, *136*, 215–233. [CrossRef]
19. Jiang, C.; Chen, X.; Alattar, M.; Wei, J.; Liu, H. MicroRNAs in tumorigenesis, metastasis, diagnosis and prognosis of gastric cancer. *Cancer Gene Ther.* **2015**, *22*, 291–301. [CrossRef]
20. Nana-Sinkam, S.P.; Croce, C.M. MicroRNA regulation of tumorigenesis, cancer progression and interpatient heterogeneity: Towards clinical use. *Genome Biol.* **2014**, *15*, 445. [CrossRef]
21. Mari, L.; Hoefnagel, S.J.M.; Zito, D.; van de Meent, M.; van Endert, P.; Calpe, S.; Serra, M.D.C.S.; Heemskerk, M.H.M.; van Laarhoven, H.W.M.; Hulshof, M.; et al. microRNA 125a Regulates MHC-I Expression on Esophageal Adenocarcinoma Cells, Associated With Suppression of Antitumor Immune Response and Poor Outcomes of Patients. *Gastroenterology* **2018**, *155*, 784–798. [CrossRef] [PubMed]
22. Jasinski-Bergner, S.; Stoehr, C.; Bukur, J.; Massa, C.; Braun, J.; Huttelmaier, S.; Spath, V.; Wartenberg, R.; Legal, W.; Taubert, H.; et al. Clinical relevance of miR-mediated HLA-G regulation and the associated immune cell infiltration in renal cell carcinoma. *Oncoimmunology* **2015**, *4*, e1008805. [CrossRef] [PubMed]
23. Gao, F.; Zhao, Z.L.; Zhao, W.T.; Fan, Q.R.; Wang, S.C.; Li, J.; Zhang, Y.Q.; Shi, J.W.; Lin, X.L.; Yang, S.; et al. miR-9 modulates the expression of interferon-regulated genes and MHC class I molecules in human nasopharyngeal carcinoma cells. *Biochem. Biophys. Res. Commun.* **2013**, *431*, 610–616. [CrossRef] [PubMed]
24. Jasinski-Bergner, S.; Reches, A.; Stoehr, C.; Massa, C.; Gonschorek, E.; Huettelmaier, S.; Braun, J.; Wach, S.; Wullich, B.; Spath, V.; et al. Identification of novel microRNAs regulating HLA-G expression and investigating their clinical relevance in renal cell carcinoma. *Oncotarget* **2016**, *7*, 26866–26878. [CrossRef] [PubMed]
25. Manaster, I.; Goldman-Wohl, D.; Greenfield, C.; Nachmani, D.; Tsukerman, P.; Hamani, Y.; Yagel, S.; Mandelboim, O. MiRNA-mediated control of HLA-G expression and function. *PLoS ONE* **2012**, *7*, e33395. [CrossRef]
26. Albanese, M.; Tagawa, T.; Bouvet, M.; Maliqi, L.; Lutter, D.; Hoser, J.; Hastreiter, M.; Hayes, M.; Sugden, B.; Martin, L.; et al. Epstein-Barr virus microRNAs reduce immune surveillance by virus-specific CD8+ T cells. *Proc. Natl. Acad. Sci. USA* **2016**, *113*, E6467–E6475. [CrossRef]
27. Knox, B.; Wang, Y.; Rogers, L.J.; Xuan, J.; Yu, D.; Guan, H.; Chen, J.; Shi, T.; Ning, B.; Kadlubar, S.A. A functional SNP in the 3'-UTR of TAP2 gene interacts with microRNA hsa-miR-1270 to suppress the gene expression. *Environ. Mol. Mutagen.* **2018**, *59*, 134–143. [CrossRef]
28. Bartoszewski, R.; Brewer, J.W.; Rab, A.; Crossman, D.K.; Bartoszewska, S.; Kapoor, N.; Fuller, C.; Collawn, J.F.; Bebok, Z. The unfolded protein response (UPR)-activated transcription factor X-box-binding protein 1 (XBP1) induces microRNA-346 expression that targets the human antigen peptide transporter 1 (TAP1) mRNA and governs immune regulatory genes. *J. Biol. Chem.* **2011**, *286*, 41862–41870. [CrossRef]
29. Marzagalli, M.; Ebelt, N.D.; Manuel, E.R. Unraveling the crosstalk between melanoma and immune cells in the tumor microenvironment. *Semin. Cancer Biol.* **2019**, *59*, 236–250. [CrossRef]
30. Gettinger, S.; Choi, J.; Hastings, K.; Truini, A.; Datar, I.; Sowell, R.; Wurtz, A.; Dong, W.; Cai, G.; Melnick, M.A.; et al. Impaired HLA Class I Antigen Processing and Presentation as a Mechanism of Acquired Resistance to Immune Checkpoint Inhibitors in Lung Cancer. *Cancer Discov.* **2017**, *7*, 1420–1435. [CrossRef]
31. Kalbasi, A.; Ribas, A. Antigen Presentation Keeps Trending in Immunotherapy Resistance. *Clin. Cancer Res.* **2018**, *24*, 3239–3241. [CrossRef] [PubMed]
32. Cortez, M.A.; Anfossi, S.; Ramapriyan, R.; Menon, H.; Atalar, S.C.; Aliru, M.; Welsh, J.; Calin, G.A. Role of miRNAs in immune responses and immunotherapy in cancer. *Genes Chromosomes Cancer* **2019**, *58*, 244–253. [CrossRef] [PubMed]
33. Sharma, P.; Hu-Lieskovan, S.; Wargo, J.A.; Ribas, A. Primary, Adaptive, and Acquired Resistance to Cancer Immunotherapy. *Cell* **2017**, *168*, 707–723. [CrossRef] [PubMed]
34. Gide, T.N.; Wilmott, J.S.; Scolyer, R.A.; Long, G.V. Primary and Acquired Resistance to Immune Checkpoint Inhibitors in Metastatic Melanoma. *Clin. Cancer Res.* **2018**, *24*, 1260–1270. [CrossRef] [PubMed]

35. Tretbar, U.S.; Friedrich, M.; Lazaridou, M.F.; Seliger, B. Identification of Immune Modulatory miRNAs by miRNA Enrichment via RNA Affinity Purification. *Methods Mol. Biol.* **2019**, *1913*, 81–101. [CrossRef] [PubMed]
36. Braun, J.; Misiak, D.; Busch, B.; Krohn, K.; Huttelmaier, S. Rapid identification of regulatory microRNAs by miTRAP (miRNA trapping by RNA in vitro affinity purification). *Nucleic Acids Res.* **2014**, *42*, e66. [CrossRef]
37. Friedrich, M.; Jasinski-Bergner, S.; Lazaridou, M.F.; Subbarayan, K.; Massa, C.; Tretbar, S.; Mueller, A.; Handke, D.; Biehl, K.; Bukur, J.; et al. Tumor-induced escape mechanisms and their association with resistance to checkpoint inhibitor therapy. *Cancer Immunol. Immunother.* **2019**, *68*, 1689–1700. [CrossRef]
38. Pullen, A.M.; Kappler, J.W.; Marrack, P. Tolerance to self antigens shapes the T-cell repertoire. *Immunol. Rev.* **1989**, *107*, 125–139. [CrossRef]
39. Weiss, S.A.; Wolchok, J.D.; Sznol, M. Immunotherapy of Melanoma: Facts and Hopes. *Clin. Cancer Res.* **2019**, *25*, 5191–5201. [CrossRef]
40. Curtin, J.A.; Fridlyand, J.; Kageshita, T.; Patel, H.N.; Busam, K.J.; Kutzner, H.; Cho, K.H.; Aiba, S.; Brocker, E.B.; LeBoit, P.E.; et al. Distinct sets of genetic alterations in melanoma. *N. Engl. J. Med.* **2005**, *353*, 2135–2147. [CrossRef]
41. Shankaran, V.; Ikeda, H.; Bruce, A.T.; White, J.M.; Swanson, P.E.; Old, L.J.; Schreiber, R.D. IFNgamma and lymphocytes prevent primary tumour development and shape tumour immunogenicity. *Nature* **2001**, *410*, 1107–1111. [CrossRef] [PubMed]
42. Schumacher, T.N.; Schreiber, R.D. Neoantigens in cancer immunotherapy. *Science* **2015**, *348*, 69–74. [CrossRef] [PubMed]
43. Alexandrov, L.B.; Nik-Zainal, S.; Wedge, D.C.; Aparicio, S.A.; Behjati, S.; Biankin, A.V.; Bignell, G.R.; Bolli, N.; Borg, A.; Borresen-Dale, A.L.; et al. Signatures of mutational processes in human cancer. *Nature* **2013**, *500*, 415–421. [CrossRef]
44. Gajewski, T.F.; Schreiber, H.; Fu, Y.X. Innate and adaptive immune cells in the tumor microenvironment. *Nat. Immunol.* **2013**, *14*, 1014–1022. [CrossRef] [PubMed]
45. Maeurer, M.J.; Gollin, S.M.; Martin, D.; Swaney, W.; Bryant, J.; Castelli, C.; Robbins, P.; Parmiani, G.; Storkus, W.J.; Lotze, M.T. Tumor escape from immune recognition: Lethal recurrent melanoma in a patient associated with downregulation of the peptide transporter protein TAP-1 and loss of expression of the immunodominant MART-1/Melan-A antigen. *J. Clin. Investig.* **1996**, *98*, 1633–1641. [CrossRef]
46. Passarelli, A.; Mannavola, F.; Stucci, L.S.; Tucci, M.; Silvestris, F. Immune system and melanoma biology: A balance between immunosurveillance and immune escape. *Oncotarget* **2017**, *8*, 106132–106142. [CrossRef]
47. Cao, W.; Cheng, W.; Wu, W. MicroRNAs Reprogram Tumor Immune Response. *Methods Mol. Biol.* **2018**, *1699*, 67–74. [CrossRef]
48. Jasinski-Bergner, S.; Vaxevanis, C.; Heimer, N.; Lazaridou, M.F.; Friedrich, M.; Seliger, B. An altered miTRAP method for miRNA affinity purification with its pros and cons. *Methods Enzymol.* **2020**, *636*, 323–337. [CrossRef]
49. Bignell, G.R.; Greenman, C.D.; Davies, H.; Butler, A.P.; Edkins, S.; Andrews, J.M.; Buck, G.; Chen, L.; Beare, D.; Latimer, C.; et al. Signatures of mutation and selection in the cancer genome. *Nature* **2010**, *463*, 893–898. [CrossRef]
50. Pawelec, G.; Marsh, S.G. ESTDAB: A collection of immunologically characterised melanoma cell lines and searchable databank. *Cancer Immunol. Immunother.* **2006**, *55*, 623–627. [CrossRef]
51. Wulfanger, J.; Biehl, K.; Tetzner, A.; Wild, P.; Ikenberg, K.; Meyer, S.; Seliger, B. Heterogeneous expression and functional relevance of the ubiquitin carboxyl-terminal hydrolase L1 in melanoma. *Int. J. Cancer* **2013**, *133*, 2522–2532. [CrossRef] [PubMed]
52. Salter, R.D.; Cresswell, P. Impaired assembly and transport of HLA-A and -B antigens in a mutant TxB cell hybrid. *EMBO J.* **1986**, *5*, 943–949. [CrossRef] [PubMed]
53. Koelblinger, P.; Emberger, M.; Drach, M.; Cheng, P.F.; Lang, R.; Levesque, M.P.; Bauer, J.W.; Dummer, R. Increased tumour cell PD-L1 expression, macrophage and dendritic cell infiltration characterise the tumour microenvironment of ulcerated primary melanomas. *J. Eur. Acad. Dermatol. Venereol. JEADV* **2019**, *33*, 667–675. [CrossRef] [PubMed]
54. Fander, J.; Kielstein, H.; Buttner, M.; Koelblinger, P.; Dummer, R.; Bauer, M.; Handke, D.; Wickenhauser, C.; Seliger, B.; Jasinski-Bergner, S. Characterizing CD44 regulatory microRNAs as putative therapeutic agents in human melanoma. *Oncotarget* **2019**, *10*, 6509–6525. [CrossRef] [PubMed]

55. Yoon, J.H.; Srikantan, S.; Gorospe, M. MS2-TRAP (MS2-tagged RNA affinity purification): Tagging RNA to identify associated miRNAs. *Methods* **2012**, *58*, 81–87. [CrossRef] [PubMed]
56. Lazaridou, M.-F.; Gonschorek, E.; Massa, C.; Friedrich, M.; Handke, D.; Mueller, A.; Jasinski-Bergner, S.; Dummer, R.; Koelblinger, P.; Seliger, B. Identification of miR-200a-5p targeting the peptide transporter TAP1 and its association with the clinical outcome of melanoma patients. *Oncoimmunology* **2020**, *9*, 1774323. [CrossRef]
57. Chen, C.; Ridzon, D.A.; Broomer, A.J.; Zhou, Z.; Lee, D.H.; Nguyen, J.T.; Barbisin, M.; Xu, N.L.; Mahuvakar, V.R.; Andersen, M.R.; et al. Real-time quantification of microRNAs by stem-loop RT-PCR. *Nucleic Acids Res.* **2005**, *33*, e179. [CrossRef]
58. Varkonyi-Gasic, E.; Wu, R.; Wood, M.; Walton, E.F.; Hellens, R.P. Protocol: A highly sensitive RT-PCR method for detection and quantification of microRNAs. *Plant Methods* **2007**, *3*, 12. [CrossRef]
59. Kramer, M.F. Stem-loop RT-qPCR for miRNAs. *Curr. Protoc. Mol. Biol.* **2011**. [CrossRef]
60. Bukur, J.; Herrmann, F.; Handke, D.; Recktenwald, C.; Seliger, B. Identification of E2F1 as an important transcription factor for the regulation of tapasin expression. *J. Biol. Chem.* **2010**, *285*, 30419–30426. [CrossRef]
61. Alter, G.; Malenfant, J.M.; Altfeld, M. CD107a as a functional marker for the identification of natural killer cell activity. *J. Immunol. Methods* **2004**, *294*, 15–22. [CrossRef] [PubMed]
62. Lorenzo-Herrero, S.; Sordo-Bahamonde, C.; Gonzalez, S.; Lopez-Soto, A. CD107a Degranulation Assay to Evaluate Immune Cell Antitumor Activity. *Methods Mol. Biol.* **2019**, *1884*, 119–130. [CrossRef] [PubMed]
63. Langmead, B.; Trapnell, C.; Pop, M.; Salzberg, S.L. Ultrafast and memory-efficient alignment of short DNA sequences to the human genome. *Genome Biol.* **2009**, *10*, R25. [CrossRef] [PubMed]
64. An, J.; Lai, J.; Lehman, M.L.; Nelson, C.C. miRDeep*: An integrated application tool for miRNA identification from RNA sequencing data. *Nucleic Acids Res.* **2013**, *41*, 727–737. [CrossRef]
65. Kozomara, A.; Birgaoanu, M.; Griffiths-Jones, S. miRBase: From microRNA sequences to function. *Nucleic Acids Res.* **2019**, *47*, D155–D162. [CrossRef] [PubMed]
66. Young, M.D.; Wakefield, M.J.; Smyth, G.K.; Oshlack, A. Gene ontology analysis for RNA-seq: Accounting for selection bias. *Genome Biol.* **2010**, *11*, R14. [CrossRef]
67. Wei, L.; He, F.; Zhang, W.; Chen, W.; Yu, B. Bioinformatics analysis of microarray data to reveal the pathogenesis of diffuse intrinsic pontine glioma. *Biol. Res.* **2018**, *51*, 26. [CrossRef]
68. Li, J.H.; Liu, S.; Zhou, H.; Qu, L.H.; Yang, J.H. StarBase v2.0: Decoding miRNA-ceRNA, miRNA-ncRNA and protein-RNA interaction networks from large-scale CLIP-Seq data. *Nucleic Acids Res.* **2014**, *42*, D92–D97. [CrossRef]
69. Yang, J.H.; Li, J.H.; Shao, P.; Zhou, H.; Chen, Y.Q.; Qu, L.H. Starbase: A database for exploring microRNA-mRNA interaction maps from Argonaute CLIP-Seq and Degradome-Seq data. *Nucleic Acids Res.* **2011**, *39*, D202–D209. [CrossRef]
70. Guan, J.; Gupta, R.; Filipp, F.V. Cancer systems biology of TCGA SKCM: Efficient detection of genomic drivers in melanoma. *Sci. Rep.* **2015**, *5*, 7857. [CrossRef]
71. Ellrott, K.; Bailey, M.H.; Saksena, G.; Covington, K.R.; Kandoth, C.; Stewart, C.; Hess, J.; Ma, S.; Chiotti, K.E.; McLellan, M.; et al. Scalable Open Science Approach for Mutation Calling of Tumor Exomes Using Multiple Genomic Pipelines. *Cell Syst.* **2018**, *6*, 271–281. [CrossRef] [PubMed]
72. Gao, Q.; Liang, W.W.; Foltz, S.M.; Mutharasu, G.; Jayasinghe, R.G.; Cao, S.; Liao, W.W.; Reynolds, S.M.; Wyczalkowski, M.A.; Yao, L.; et al. Driver Fusions and Their Implications in the Development and Treatment of Human Cancers. *Cell Rep.* **2018**, *23*, 227–238. [CrossRef] [PubMed]
73. Hoadley, K.A.; Yau, C.; Hinoue, T.; Wolf, D.M.; Lazar, A.J.; Drill, E.; Shen, R.; Taylor, A.M.; Cherniack, A.D.; Thorsson, V.; et al. Cell-of-Origin Patterns Dominate the Molecular Classification of 10,000 Tumors from 33 Types of Cancer. *Cell* **2018**, *173*, 291–304. [CrossRef] [PubMed]
74. Liu, J.; Lichtenberg, T.; Hoadley, K.A.; Poisson, L.M.; Lazar, A.J.; Cherniack, A.D.; Kovatich, A.J.; Benz, C.C.; Levine, D.A.; Lee, A.V.; et al. An Integrated TCGA Pan-Cancer Clinical Data Resource to Drive High-Quality Survival Outcome Analytics. *Cell* **2018**, *173*, 400–416. [CrossRef]
75. Sanchez-Vega, F.; Mina, M.; Armenia, J.; Chatila, W.K.; Luna, A.; La, K.C.; Dimitriadoy, S.; Liu, D.L.; Kantheti, H.S.; Saghafinia, S.; et al. Oncogenic Signaling Pathways in The Cancer Genome Atlas. *Cell* **2018**, *173*, 321–337. [CrossRef]

76. Taylor, A.M.; Shih, J.; Ha, G.; Gao, G.F.; Zhang, X.; Berger, A.C.; Schumacher, S.E.; Wang, C.; Hu, H.; Liu, J.; et al. Genomic and Functional Approaches to Understanding Cancer Aneuploidy. *Cancer Cell* **2018**, *33*, 676–689. [CrossRef]
77. Sinn, B.V.; Weber, K.E.; Schmitt, W.D.; Fasching, P.A.; Symmans, W.F.; Blohmer, J.U.; Karn, T.; Taube, E.T.; Klauschen, F.; Marme, F.; et al. Human leucocyte antigen class I in hormone receptor-positive, HER2-negative breast cancer: Association with response and survival after neoadjuvant chemotherapy. *Breast Cancer Res.* **2019**, *21*, 142. [CrossRef]
78. Helgadottir, H.; Andersson, E.; Villabona, L.; Kanter, L.; van der Zanden, H.; Haasnoot, G.W.; Seliger, B.; Bergfeldt, K.; Hansson, J.; Ragnarsson-Olding, B.; et al. The common Scandinavian human leucocyte antigen ancestral haplotype 62.1 as prognostic factor in patients with advanced malignant melanoma. *Cancer Immunol. Immunother.* **2009**, *58*, 1599–1608. [CrossRef]
79. Seliger, B.; Ritz, U.; Abele, R.; Bock, M.; Tampe, R.; Sutter, G.; Drexler, I.; Huber, C.; Ferrone, S. Immune escape of melanoma: First evidence of structural alterations in two distinct components of the MHC class I antigen processing pathway. *Cancer Res.* **2001**, *61*, 8647–8650.
80. Garrido, F.; Aptsiauri, N. Cancer immune escape: MHC expression in primary tumours versus metastases. *Immunology* **2019**, *158*, 255–266. [CrossRef]
81. Luebker, S.A.; Zhang, W.; Koepsell, S.A. Comparing the genomes of cutaneous melanoma tumors to commercially available cell lines. *Oncotarget* **2017**, *8*, 114877–114893. [CrossRef] [PubMed]
82. Zhou, L.; Chen, J.; Li, Z.; Li, X.; Hu, X.; Huang, Y.; Zhao, X.; Liang, C.; Wang, Y.; Sun, L.; et al. Integrated profiling of microRNAs and mRNAs: microRNAs located on Xq27.3 associate with clear cell renal cell carcinoma. *PLoS ONE* **2010**, *5*, e15224. [CrossRef] [PubMed]
83. Dweep, H.; Gretz, N. miRWalk2.0: A comprehensive atlas of microRNA-target interactions. *Nat. Methods* **2015**, *12*, 697. [CrossRef] [PubMed]
84. Dweep, H.; Sticht, C.; Pandey, P.; Gretz, N. miRWalk—Database: Prediction of possible miRNA binding sites by "walking" the genes of three genomes. *J. Biomed. Inform.* **2011**, *44*, 839–847. [CrossRef]
85. Betel, D.; Wilson, M.; Gabow, A.; Marks, D.S.; Sander, C. The microRNA.org resource: Targets and expression. *Nucleic Acids Res.* **2008**, *36*, D149–D153. [CrossRef] [PubMed]
86. Wong, N.; Wang, X. miRDB: An online resource for microRNA target prediction and functional annotations. *Nucleic Acids Res.* **2015**, *43*, D146–D152. [CrossRef]
87. Agarwal, V.; Bell, G.W.; Nam, J.W.; Bartel, D.P. Predicting effective microRNA target sites in mammalian mRNAs. *eLife* **2015**, *4*. [CrossRef]
88. Miranda, K.C.; Huynh, T.; Tay, Y.; Ang, Y.S.; Tam, W.L.; Thomson, A.M.; Lim, B.; Rigoutsos, I. A pattern-based method for the identification of MicroRNA binding sites and their corresponding heteroduplexes. *Cell* **2006**, *126*, 1203–1217. [CrossRef]
89. Rehmsmeier, M.; Steffen, P.; Hochsmann, M.; Giegerich, R. Fast and effective prediction of microRNA/target duplexes. *RNA* **2004**, *10*, 1507–1517. [CrossRef]
90. Ribas, A.; Wolchok, J.D. Cancer immunotherapy using checkpoint blockade. *Science* **2018**, *359*, 1350–1355. [CrossRef]
91. O'Donnell, J.S.; Teng, M.W.L.; Smyth, M.J. Cancer immunoediting and resistance to T cell-based immunotherapy. *Nat. Rev. Clin. Oncol.* **2019**, *16*, 151–167. [CrossRef] [PubMed]
92. Andersen, R.; Westergaard, M.C.W.; Kjeldsen, J.W.; Muller, A.; Pedersen, N.W.; Hadrup, S.R.; Met, O.; Seliger, B.; Kromann-Andersen, B.; Hasselager, T.; et al. T-cell Responses in the Microenvironment of Primary Renal Cell Carcinoma-Implications for Adoptive Cell Therapy. *Cancer Immunol. Res.* **2018**, *6*, 222–235. [CrossRef] [PubMed]
93. Huang, L.; Malu, S.; McKenzie, J.A.; Andrews, M.C.; Talukder, A.H.; Tieu, T.; Karpinets, T.; Haymaker, C.; Forget, M.A.; Williams, L.J.; et al. The RNA-binding Protein MEX3B Mediates Resistance to Cancer Immunotherapy by Downregulating HLA-A Expression. *Clin. Cancer Res.* **2018**, *24*, 3366–3376. [CrossRef] [PubMed]
94. Grasso, C.S.; Giannakis, M.; Wells, D.K.; Hamada, T.; Mu, X.J.; Quist, M.; Nowak, J.A.; Nishihara, R.; Qian, Z.R.; Inamura, K.; et al. Genetic Mechanisms of Immune Evasion in Colorectal Cancer. *Cancer Discov.* **2018**, *8*, 730–749. [CrossRef]

95. Donia, M.; Harbst, K.; van Buuren, M.; Kvistborg, P.; Lindberg, M.F.; Andersen, R.; Idorn, M.; Ahmad, S.M.; Ellebaek, E.; Mueller, A.; et al. Acquired Immune Resistance Follows Complete Tumor Regression without Loss of Target Antigens or IFNgamma Signaling. *Cancer Res.* **2017**, *77*, 4562–4566. [CrossRef]
96. Gilles, M.E.; Slack, F.J. Let-7 microRNA as a potential therapeutic target with implications for immunotherapy. *Expert Opin. Ther. Targets* **2018**, *22*, 929–939. [CrossRef]
97. Paladini, L.; Fabris, L.; Bottai, G.; Raschioni, C.; Calin, G.A.; Santarpia, L. Targeting microRNAs as key modulators of tumor immune response. *J. Exp. Clin. Cancer Res.* **2016**, *35*, 103. [CrossRef]
98. Seliger, B. Immune modulatory microRNAs as a novel mechanism to revert immune escape of tumors. *Cytokine Growth Factor Rev.* **2017**, *36*, 49–56. [CrossRef]
99. Colangelo, T.; Polcaro, G.; Ziccardi, P.; Pucci, B.; Muccillo, L.; Galgani, M.; Fucci, A.; Milone, M.R.; Budillon, A.; Santopaolo, M.; et al. Proteomic screening identifies calreticulin as a miR-27a direct target repressing MHC class I cell surface exposure in colorectal cancer. *Cell Death Dis.* **2016**, *7*, e2120. [CrossRef]
100. Neefjes, J.; Gottfried, E.; Roelse, J.; Gromme, M.; Obst, R.; Hammerling, G.J.; Momburg, F. Analysis of the fine specificity of rat, mouse and human TAP peptide transporters. *Eur. J. Immunol.* **1995**, *25*, 1133–1136. [CrossRef]
101. Cresswell, P.; Bangia, N.; Dick, T.; Diedrich, G. The nature of the MHC class I peptide loading complex. *Immunol. Rev.* **1999**, *172*, 21–28. [CrossRef] [PubMed]
102. Heemels, M.T.; Ploegh, H. Generation, translocation, and presentation of MHC class I-restricted peptides. *Annu. Rev. Biochem.* **1995**, *64*, 463–491. [CrossRef] [PubMed]
103. Lankat-Buttgereit, B.; Tampe, R. The transporter associated with antigen processing: Function and implications in human diseases. *Physiol. Rev.* **2002**, *82*, 187–204. [CrossRef]
104. Pfeffer, S.R.; Yang, C.H.; Pfeffer, L.M. The Role of miR-21 in Cancer. *Drug Dev. Res.* **2015**, *76*, 270–277. [CrossRef] [PubMed]
105. Bautista-Sanchez, D.; Arriaga-Canon, C.; Pedroza-Torres, A.; De La Rosa-Velazquez, I.A.; Gonzalez-Barrios, R.; Contreras-Espinosa, L.; Montiel-Manriquez, R.; Castro-Hernandez, C.; Fragoso-Ontiveros, V.; Alvarez-Gomez, R.M.; et al. The Promising Role of miR-21 as a Cancer Biomarker and Its Importance in RNA-Based Therapeutics. *Mol. Ther. Nucleic Acids* **2020**, *20*, 409–420. [CrossRef] [PubMed]
106. Babapoor, S.; Wu, R.; Kozubek, J.; Auidi, D.; Grant-Kels, J.M.; Dadras, S.S. Identification of microRNAs associated with invasive and aggressive phenotype in cutaneous melanoma by next-generation sequencing. *Lab. Investig. A J. Tech. Methods Pathol.* **2017**, *97*, 636–648. [CrossRef]
107. Neagu, M.; Constantin, C.; Cretoiu, S.M.; Zurac, S. miRNAs in the Diagnosis and Prognosis of Skin Cancer. *Front. Cell Dev. Biol.* **2020**, *8*, 71. [CrossRef]
108. Saldanha, G.; Potter, L.; Lee, Y.S.; Watson, S.; Shendge, P.; Pringle, J.H. MicroRNA-21 expression and its pathogenetic significance in cutaneous melanoma. *Melanoma Res.* **2016**, *26*, 21–28. [CrossRef]
109. Melnik, B.C. MiR-21: An environmental driver of malignant melanoma? *J. Transl. Med.* **2015**, *13*, 202. [CrossRef]
110. Gao, J.; Liu, Q.G. The role of miR-26 in tumors and normal tissues (Review). *Oncol. Lett.* **2011**, *2*, 1019–1023. [CrossRef]
111. Jin, F.; Wang, Y.; Li, M.; Zhu, Y.; Liang, H.; Wang, C.; Wang, F.; Zhang, C.Y.; Zen, K.; Li, L. MiR-26 enhances chemosensitivity and promotes apoptosis of hepatocellular carcinoma cells through inhibiting autophagy. *Cell Death Dis.* **2017**, *8*, e2540. [CrossRef] [PubMed]
112. Cochetti, G.; Poli, G.; Guelfi, G.; Boni, A.; Egidi, M.G.; Mearini, E. Different levels of serum microRNAs in prostate cancer and benign prostatic hyperplasia: Evaluation of potential diagnostic and prognostic role. *Onco Targets Ther.* **2016**, *9*, 7545–7553. [CrossRef] [PubMed]
113. Wang, Y.; Sun, B.; Sun, H.; Zhao, X.; Wang, X.; Zhao, N.; Zhang, Y.; Li, Y.; Gu, Q.; Liu, F.; et al. Regulation of proliferation, angiogenesis and apoptosis in hepatocellular carcinoma by miR-26b-5p. *Tumour. Biol.* **2016**, *37*, 10965–10979. [CrossRef]
114. Shaikh, I.; Ansari, A.; Ayachit, G.; Gandhi, M.; Sharma, P.; Bhairappanavar, S.; Joshi, C.G.; Das, J. Differential gene expression analysis of HNSCC tumors deciphered tobacco dependent and independent molecular signatures. *Oncotarget* **2019**, *10*, 6168–6183. [CrossRef] [PubMed]

115. Lekchnov, E.A.; Amelina, E.V.; Bryzgunova, O.E.; Zaporozhchenko, I.A.; Konoshenko, M.Y.; Yarmoschuk, S.V.; Murashov, I.S.; Pashkovskaya, O.A.; Gorizkii, A.M.; Zheravin, A.A.; et al. Searching for the Novel Specific Predictors of Prostate Cancer in Urine: The Analysis of 84 miRNA Expression. *Int. J. Mol. Sci.* **2018**, *19*, 88. [CrossRef]
116. Shen, G.; Lin, Y.; Yang, X.; Zhang, J.; Xu, Z.; Jia, H. MicroRNA-26b inhibits epithelial-mesenchymal transition in hepatocellular carcinoma by targeting USP9X. *BMC Cancer* **2014**, *14*, 393. [CrossRef] [PubMed]
117. Miyamoto, K.; Seki, N.; Matsushita, R.; Yonemori, M.; Yoshino, H.; Nakagawa, M.; Enokida, H. Tumour-suppressive miRNA-26a-5p and miR-26b-5p inhibit cell aggressiveness by regulating PLOD2 in bladder cancer. *Br. J. Cancer* **2016**, *115*, 354–363. [CrossRef]
118. Lu, J.; He, M.L.; Wang, L.; Chen, Y.; Liu, X.; Dong, Q.; Chen, Y.C.; Peng, Y.; Yao, K.T.; Kung, H.F.; et al. MiR-26a inhibits cell growth and tumorigenesis of nasopharyngeal carcinoma through repression of EZH2. *Cancer Res.* **2011**, *71*, 225–233. [CrossRef]
119. Zhang, B.; Liu, X.X.; He, J.R.; Zhou, C.X.; Guo, M.; He, M.; Li, M.F.; Chen, G.Q.; Zhao, Q. Pathologically decreased miR-26a antagonizes apoptosis and facilitates carcinogenesis by targeting MTDH and EZH2 in breast cancer. *Carcinogenesis* **2011**, *32*, 2–9. [CrossRef]
120. Li, M.; Long, C.; Yang, G.; Luo, Y.; Du, H. MiR-26b inhibits melanoma cell proliferation and enhances apoptosis by suppressing TRAF5-mediated MAPK activation. *Biochem. Biophys. Res. Commun.* **2016**, *471*, 361–367. [CrossRef]
121. Wei, C.Y.; Wang, L.; Zhu, M.X.; Deng, X.Y.; Wang, D.H.; Zhang, S.M.; Ying, J.H.; Yuan, X.; Wang, Q.; Xuan, T.F.; et al. TRIM44 activates the AKT/mTOR signal pathway to induce melanoma progression by stabilizing TLR4. *J. Exp. Clin. Cancer Res.* **2019**, *38*, 137. [CrossRef] [PubMed]
122. Friedrich, M.; Heimer, N.; Stoehr, C.; Steven, A.; Wach, S.; Taubert, H.; Hartmann, A.; Seliger, B. CREB1 is affected by the microRNAs miR-22-3p, miR-26a-5p, miR-27a-3p, and miR-221-3p and correlates with adverse clinicopathological features in renal cell carcinoma. *Sci. Rep.* **2020**, *10*, 6499. [CrossRef] [PubMed]
123. Li, H.; Wang, Y.; Song, Y. MicroRNA-26b inhibits the immune response to Mycobacterium tuberculosis (M.tb) infection in THP-1 cells via targeting TGFbeta-activated kinase-1 (TAK1), a promoter of the NF-kappaB pathway. *Int. J. Clin. Exp. Pathol.* **2018**, *11*, 1218–1227. [PubMed]

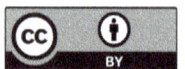

© 2020 by the authors. Licensee MDPI, Basel, Switzerland. This article is an open access article distributed under the terms and conditions of the Creative Commons Attribution (CC BY) license (http://creativecommons.org/licenses/by/4.0/).

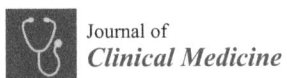

Article

Comparison of *BRAF* Mutation Screening Strategies in a Large Real-Life Series of Advanced Melanoma Patients

Maria Colombino [1,†], Carla Rozzo [2,†], Panagiotis Paliogiannis [3,†], Milena Casula [1], Antonella Manca [2], Valentina Doneddu [3], Maria Antonietta Fedeli [3], Maria Cristina Sini [1], Grazia Palomba [1], Marina Pisano [2], Paolo A. Ascierto [4], Corrado Caracò [4], Amelia Lissia [3], Antonio Cossu [3] and Giuseppe Palmieri [2,*]

1. Unit of Cancer Genetics, Institute of Biomolecular Chemistry (ICB), 07100 Sassari, Italy; colombinom@yahoo.it (M.C.); casulam@yahoo.it (M.C.); mariacristina.sini@cnr.it (M.C.S.); graziap68@yahoo.it (G.P.)
2. Unit of Cancer Genetics, Institute of Genetic and Biomedical Research (IRGB), National Research Council (CNR), Traversa La Crucca 3, 07100 Sassari, Italy; carlamaria.rozzo@cnr.it (C.R.); antonella.manca@cnr.it (A.M.); marina.pisano@cnr.it (M.P.)
3. Department of Medical, Surgical, and Experimental Sciences, University of Sassari, Viale San Pietro 43, 07100 Sassari, Italy; panospaliogiannis@gmail.com (P.P.); valentinadoneddu@gmail.com (V.D.); mariaant.fedeli@hotmail.it (M.A.F.); a_lissia@yahoo.it (A.L.); cossu@uniss.it (A.C.)
4. Unità Melanoma, Istituto Nazionale Tumori "Fondazione Pascale", Via Mariano Semmola 53, 80131 Naples; Italy; paolo.ascierto@gmail.com (P.A.A.); corrado.caraco@istitutotumori.na.it (C.C.)
* Correspondence: gpalmieri@yahoo.com; Tel.: +39-0792841303
† These authors contributed equally.

Received: 28 June 2020; Accepted: 27 July 2020; Published: 30 July 2020

Abstract: Malignant melanoma (MM) is one of the deadliest skin cancers. *BRAF* mutation status plays a predominant role in the management of MM patients. The aim of this study was to compare *BRAF* mutational testing performed by conventional nucleotide sequencing approaches with either real-time polymerase chain reaction (rtPCR) or next-generation sequencing (NGS) assays in a real-life, hospital-based series of advanced MM patients. Consecutive patients with AJCC (American Joint Committee on Cancer) stage IIIC and IV MM from Sardinia, Italy, who were referred for molecular testing, were enrolled into the study. Initial screening was performed to assess the mutational status of the *BRAF* and *NRAS* genes, using the conventional methodologies recognized by the nationwide guidelines, at the time of the molecular classification, required by clinicians: at the beginning, Sanger-based sequencing (SS) and, after, pyrosequencing. The present study was then focused on *BRAF* mutation detecting approaches only. *BRAF* wild-type cases with available tissue and adequate DNA were further tested with rtPCR (Idylla™) and NGS assays. Globally, 319 patients were included in the study; pathogenic *BRAF* mutations were found in 144 (45.1%) cases examined with initial screening. The rtPCR detected 11 (16.2%) and 3 (4.8%) additional *BRAF* mutations after SS and pyrosequencing, respectively. NGS detected one additional *BRAF*-mutated case (2.1%) among 48 wild-type cases previously tested with pyrosequencing and rtPCR. Our study evidenced that rtPCR and NGS were able to detect additional *BRAF* mutant cases in comparison with conventional sequencing methods; therefore, we argue for the preferential utilization of the aforementioned assays (NGS and rtPCR) in clinical practice, to eradicate false-negative cases and improve the accuracy of *BRAF* detection.

Keywords: melanoma; targeted therapies; BRAF; druggable mutations; real-time PCR; NGS assay

1. Introduction

Malignant melanoma (MM) is the deadliest form of skin cancer; it is estimated to affect more than 100,000 individuals, causing approximately 7000 deaths in the United States (US) in 2020 [1]. In Italy, an increase in MM incidence has been observed in the last decade, and approximately 12,300 new cases have been estimated (4% of all tumors) in 2019, representing the second and third most frequent neoplasia (9% and 7% of all tumors) in young men and women, respectively [2,3]. In the past, few effective therapeutic options were available for advanced MM patients, with response rates to conventional chemotherapy and immunomodulation therapy being limited to about 15–19% [4,5]. In the last few years, new therapeutic options have revolutionized the treatments of patients with III/IV American Joint Committee on Cancer (AJCC) stage melanomas. They include therapies targeted to specific genetic tumor mutations, as well as immunotherapy with immune checkpoint inhibitors (ICIs) [5,6].

Targeted therapies essentially consist of inhibitors of BRAF, a serine-threonine kinase that is constitutively activated in about one half of MMs carrying a mutation in the codon 600 of the *BRAF* oncogene [7]. Mutation at the codon V600 of the *BRAF* gene represents more than 97% of all *BRAF* mutations [8]. The most frequent alteration, occurring in about 75% of the cases, is a transversion of T to A at nucleotide 1799, which results in a substitution of a valine for glutamic acid at position 600 of the BRAF kinase (V600E) [8]. Less common substitutions are valine for lysine (V600K, up to 20%), arginine (V600R, 1%), leucine (V600M, 0,3%), and aspartic acid (V600D, 0,1%), as well as rarer mutations in other codons such as K601E or D594N [7,9]. The discovery and description of the crystal structure of the mutated BRAF protein [10] led to the development of several specific inhibitors, such as vemurafenib, dabrafenib, and encorafenib, which have been approved both in the US and Europe for the treatment of advanced (AJCC stage IIIC and stage IV) MM-harboring BRAF V600 mutations [11–14]. These BRAF inhibitors, administered in combination with MEK inhibitors, resulted in rapid therapeutic responses, with significant improvements in both progression-free and overall survival in large fractions of metastatic MM patients [2,15].

Molecular testing to determine *BRAF* mutation status has therefore become standard-of-care in the modern clinical management of patients with advanced MM, being currently the only available biomarker that can predict therapeutic responses to treatments with combined BRAF and MEK inhibitors. *BRAF* testing is currently recommended by both the National Comprehensive Cancer Network (NCCN) and the European Society for Medical Oncology (ESMO) guidelines for advanced melanoma patients [16,17]; the *BRAF* V600 mutation must be detected by using an FDA-approved (USA) or CE-IVD-certified (Europe) test [17–19].

More recently, several studies have demonstrated the impact of immune checkpoint inhibitors and targeted therapies on disease control in the adjuvant setting [20]. A long-term benefit of a 12-month adjuvant treatment with a combination of BRAF and MEK inhibitors (dabrafenib and trametinib, respectively) has been observed in patients with resected stage III *BRAF* V600 mutant melanoma [21,22]; in a recent update, median relapse-free survival was not reached in treated patients after a median follow-up of 60 months [23]. These findings highlight the significance of the assessment of the *BRAF* mutational status in all stage III MM patients for a more appropriate clinical decision. Overall, the detection of the *BRAF* V600 mutation plays a predictive role in the management of MM patients, identifying those with a potential sensitivity to combined treatments with BRAF and MEK inhibitors, either in advanced (stage IV or unresectable stage III) or resectable high-stage disease [24,25]. Identification of *NRAS* mutations may be also useful for a comprehensive molecular classification of the MM patients, as well as for their potential enrolment in clinical trials testing specific pharmacologic agents.

From a clinical perspective, it is therefore mandatory to identify the best technique to detect *BRAF* mutations with the highest sensitivity and specificity. Generally, formalin-fixed and paraffin-embedded (FFPE) tissues from MM patients are used for mutational analysis, after paraffin removal and genomic DNA purification with standardized protocols. The aim of this study was to compare *BRAF* mutational testing performed with conventional nucleotide sequencing approaches (Sanger-based sequencing and pyrosequencing) and either real-time polymerase chain reaction (rtPCR) or next-generation sequencing (NGS) assays, in order to assess the levels of concordance between different techniques in a real-life, hospital-based series of 319 FFPE tissue samples from advanced MM patients from Sardinia, Italy.

2. Materials and Methods

2.1. Patients and Samples

Patients with a histologically proven diagnosis of advanced MM (AJCC stages IIIC and IV), originating from Sardinia, Italy, were consecutively collected at clinics across the entire island and referred for molecular testing at the laboratory of the National Research Council (CNR), Sassari, Italy, from October 2012 through September 2019. All patients regularly participating in the diagnosis and treatment programs for melanoma at the Hospitals across Sardinia Island had tumor-tissue samples available for molecular analysis before inclusion in the study. To avoid bias, patients were included regardless of age of onset, family history of cancer, disease characteristics, and gene tested (*BRAF* with or without *NRAS*); their demographic, clinical, and pathological data were retrieved and stored in a digital database. FFPE tumor samples of primary melanomas or metastases from each patient were collected. Histological classification, including Breslow thickness and disease stage at diagnosis, according with the 8th versions of AJCC staging system, was performed in all cases. All histological specimens with an ascertained tumor cell content greater than 60% were selected for mutation analysis; in some cases, the tissue sections were macrodissected by removing surrounding healthy tissue in order to obtain tumor samples with at least 70% neoplastic cells. All samples included in the study were assessed for the quality of the purified DNA, in order to ensure that discrepant cases could not arise from technical problems due to the insufficient sample quality.

The patients were informed about the aims and methods of the study and, before the tissue sample was collected (thus, at the time of initial molecular testing), given a written informed consent for both mutational analyses with molecular diagnostic purposes on tissue samples and participation in the study. The study was conducted in accordance with the principles of the Declaration of Helsinki and approved by the Committee for the Ethics of the Research and Bioethics of the National Research Council.

2.2. Molecular Testing

2.2.1. DNA Isolation and Screening

Genomic DNA was isolated from tissue sections, using a standard protocol. In particular, paraffin was removed from FFPE samples with Bio-Clear (Bio-Optica, Milan, Italy), and DNA was purified by using the QIAamp DNA FFPE Tissue kit (Qiagen Inc., Valencia, CA, USA). DNA quantitation and quality assessment were carried out with both a Nanodrop 2000 spectrophotometer (Thermo Scientific, Wilmington, DE, USA) and Qubit® 2.0 Fluorometer (Invitrogen, Carlsbad, CA, USA). DNA fragmentation status was evaluated with the Agilent 2200 TapeStation, system using the Genomic DNA ScreenTape assay (Agilent Technologies, Santa Clara, CA, USA), which is able to produce a DNA Integrity Number (DIN).

2.2.2. Sanger Sequencing (SS)

Polymerase chain reaction (PCR) was performed on 20 ng of genomic DNA in a Veriti 96-Well Fast Thermal Cycler (Life Technologies-Thermo Fisher Scientific, Waltham, MA, USA); all PCR-amplified products were directly sequenced using an automated ABI3130 fluorescence-cycle sequencer (Life Technologies-Thermo Fisher Scientific, Waltham, MA, USA). Sequencing conditions, as well as primer sets and PCR assay protocols, were as previously described [26,27]. Sequencing analysis was conducted in all samples in duplicate and in both directions (forward and reverse).

A nucleotide sequence was considered as valid when the quality value (QV) was higher than 20 (<1/100 error probability); in this study, the QV average was 35 (range, 30–45; <1/1000–1/10,000 error probability). Starting from the purified DNA, the flat cost of the SS analysis was around €50, and the time required for performing it was about 6 h.

2.2.3. Pyrosequencing

Quantitative measurements of *BRAF* mutations were performed with the Therascreen™ BRAF Pyro Kit (Qiagen Inc., Valencia, CA, USA), for the quantitative detection of mutations in codons 600, 469, and 464 of the human *BRAF* gene in genomic DNA. In particular, the Therascreen™ BRAF Pyro Kit detected the following variants: V600E (c.1799T > A/c.1799_1800TG > AA), V600G (c.1799T > G), V600A (c.1799T > C), V600M (c.1798G > A), V600D (c.1799_1800TG > AT), V600K (c.1798_1799GT > AA), V600R (c.1798_1799GT > AG), G469E (c.1406G > A), G469A (c.1406G > C), G469V (c.1406G > T), G469S (c.1405_1406GG > TC), G466E (c.1397G > A), G466V (c.1397G > T), G464E (c.1391G > A), and G464V (c.1391G > T). Each pyrosequencing assay, which included a positive (*BRAF* mutated) and a negative (*BRAF* wild-type) DNA sample as control, was performed on a PyroMark Q24 system (Qiagen Inc., Valencia, CA, USA), following the manufacturer's instructions. Starting from the purified DNA, the flat cost of the pyrosequencing analysis was around €90, and the time required for performing was about 4 h.

2.2.4. Real-Time PCR (rtPCR) Test

The rtPCR test was based on the use of the Idylla™ *BRAF* mutation assay (Biocartis, Mechelen, Belgium), a fully automated rtPCR-based diagnostic mutation analysis method. The test consists of allele-specific PCR reactions that enable the qualitative detection of the wild-type sequence (c.1799T) and the main mutations at codon 600 in *BRAF* gene: V600E (c.1799T > A), V600E2 (c.1799_1800 delinsAA), V600D (c.1799_1800 delinsAT/c.1799_1800 delinsAC), V600K (c.1798_1799 delinsAA), V600M (c.1798G > A), and V600R (c.1798_1799 delinsAG). In each rtPCR assay, an internal control to test quality of amplification is included. A solution with at least 40 nanograms of isolated genomic DNA was loaded onto the cartridge in our experiments. Starting from the purified DNA, the flat cost of the Idylla™ test was around €170, and the time required for performing was about 2 h.

2.2.5. Next-Generation Sequencing

Next-generation sequencing (NGS) analysis was performed by using either the Ion Torrent PGM System either the Ion S5 GeneStudio platform with a multiple-gene panel or the Oncomine Focus Assay (Life Technologies-Thermo Fisher Scientific, Waltham, MA, USA), arranged in two primer pools, and designed to explore the mutational status of selected regions within the main 52 genes involved in tumorigenesis. Amplicon libraries were generated by starting from 20 ng of genomic DNA, using the Ion AmpliSeq Library Kit-2.0 (Life Technologies-Thermo Fisher Scientific), and barcoding each sample, following the manufacturer's instructions. Cycling conditions were performed according to the DNA type and primer pairs per pool. Libraries were purified with Agencourt Ampure-XT Beads (Beckman Coulter, Brea, CA, USA); purified DNA was diluted at a final concentration of 50 pM, placed into the Ion Chef for emulsion PCR and Chip loading, and sequenced on the Ion S5 GeneStudio (Life Technologies-Thermo Fisher Scientific) with the Ion Hi-Q™ View Sequencing Kit (Life Technologies-Thermo Fisher Scientific). Sequencing data were processed with the Ion Torrent Software Suite *v.*5.10.1 (Life Technologies-Thermo Fisher Scientific) platform-specific pipeline software. The plugin Variant Caller (VC) Ion Reporter v.5.10.1.20 and the Integrative Genome Viewer (http://www.broadinstitute.org/igv) were used for variant annotation and reads visualizations, respectively. To get a total amount of at least 10 mutated alleles for each candidate amplicon, the following mutation selection criteria were adopted: coverage of >200 reads and frequency of mutated alleles >5% for gene amplicon. Starting from the purified DNA, the flat cost of the NGS analysis with the Oncomine Focus Assay was up to €450, and the time required for performing was about two and half days.

2.3. Statistical Analysis

Results were expressed as median values (range) and percentages. Statistical differences between groups were evaluated by using the chi-squared test or the Fisher exact test, as appropriate. Statistical significance was set at 0.005. Statistical analyses were performed by using MedCalc for Windows, version 15.4 64 bit (MedCalc Software, Ostend, Belgium).

3. Results

Globally, 319 advanced melanoma patients undergoing molecular analysis for diagnostic classification of the *BRAF/NRAS* mutational status were consecutively collected in a hospital-based manner and enrolled into the study. The median age at diagnosis was 65 years, and 183 (57%) were males. The demographic, clinical, and pathological characteristics of the patients are reported in Table 1. Patients originated from different geographical areas across Sardinia: 241 (76%) were from Sassari province in North Sardinia, and 78 (24%) were from the remaining parts of the island. Almost the entire series was composed by patients with MM (89.4%, n = 285); four (1.3%) cases were affected by mucosal melanoma, and 30 (9.4%) patients presented with MM metastasis from an occult primary tumor; among them, 22 (73.3%) cases had lymph node metastasis, while the remaining patients had visceral metastasis. Most lesions were distributed on the trunk (53%, n = 152), followed by the limbs (32%, n = 93) and head/neck (15%, n = 44). Nodular and superficial spreading melanomas were the most frequent histological variants (50% and 39%, respectively), with vast preponderance of >1 mm thick melanomas (92%). Ulcerated and not-ulcerated melanomas were similarly represented, whereas 81% of patients showed ≥1 mitosis (Table 1).

Table 1. Patient demographics and melanoma characteristics in the study population.

Characteristics	Data
Age at diagnosis, median (range)	65 (21–92)
Male gender, n (%)	183 (57.4)
Primary melanoma localization (n = 319)	
Limbs, n (%)	93 (29.2)
Head and neck, n (%)	44 (13.8)
Trunk, n (%)	152 (47.6)
Occult, n (%)	30 (9.4)
Lymph node metastasis, n (%)	22 (6.9)
Visceral metastasis, n (%)	8 (2.5)
Histology (n = 289)	
SSM, n (%)	146 (50.5)
Nodular, n (%)	112 (38.7)
Acral, n (%)	19 (6.6)
Lentigo maligna, n (%)	8 (2.8)
Mucosal, n (%)	4 (1.4)

Table 1. *Cont.*

Characteristics	Data
Breslow class (*n* = 285)	
≤1 mm, *n* (%)	23 (8.1)
>1-≤2 mm, *n* (%)	78 (27.4)
>2-≤4 mm, *n* (%)	95 (33.3)
>4 mm, *n* (%)	89 (31.2)
Ulceration (*n* = 248)	
Present, *n* (%)	137 (55.2)
Absent, *n* (%)	111 (44.8)
Mitosis number (*n* = 243)	
<1, *n* (%)	47 (19.3)
≥1, *n* (%)	196 (80.7)
AJCC stage at diagnosis (*n* = 285)	
IA-IB, *n* (%)	26 (9.2)
IIA-IIB, *n* (%)	107 (37.5)
IIC, *n* (%)	28 (9.8)
III, *n* (%)	101 (35.4)
IV, *n* (%)	23 (8.1)
Lymph node metastasis at diagnosis (*n* = 289)	
pN0, *n* (%)	171 (59.2)
pN+, *n* (%)	118 (40.8)

SSM, superficial spreading melanoma; AJCC, American Joint Committee on Cancer.

The mutational status of the *BRAF* and *NRAS* genes was initially assessed with the screening methodology conventionally used at the time of the molecular diagnosis, required by clinician for patients' classification: Sanger-based sequencing (SS), from 2009 to 2014, and pyrosequencing, from 2015 to 2019 (Figure 1). Additional tests (Idylla^{TM} and NGS) were performed in accordance with the availability of tissue samples and adequate amount and quality of the DNA to use. *BRAF* mutations were documented in 45% (144/319) of the initial tests performed, while *NRAS* mutations were present in 15% (40/272) of the tumors tested (Table 2). No concomitant mutation in *BRAF* and *NRAS* genes was detected, further confirming that deleterious mutations in these driver oncogenes are mutually exclusive in melanoma [28,29]. Globally, about two-thirds (184 cases) of Sardinian melanoma patients were found to carry a *BRAF* or *NRAS* mutation, even considering that some cases were not analyzed for *NRAS* mutations. No statistically significant differences have been found between genders in the distribution of mutations in both genes; however, the amount of patients aged less than 55 years was significantly higher in patients with *BRAF* mutations than in those without, and the amount of patients older than 55 was significantly greater in patients with *NRAS* mutations than in those without (Table 2). Indeed, in patients with less than 55 years of age, mutation rates were significantly higher for the *BRAF* than for the *NRAS* gene (58/95, 61% vs. 4/77, 5.2%; $p < 0.0001$). Overall, no differences in distribution of *BRAF* and *NRAS* mutations between rural and urban areas, both globally and within the two (north vs. middle-south) geographical parts of the island, were observed.

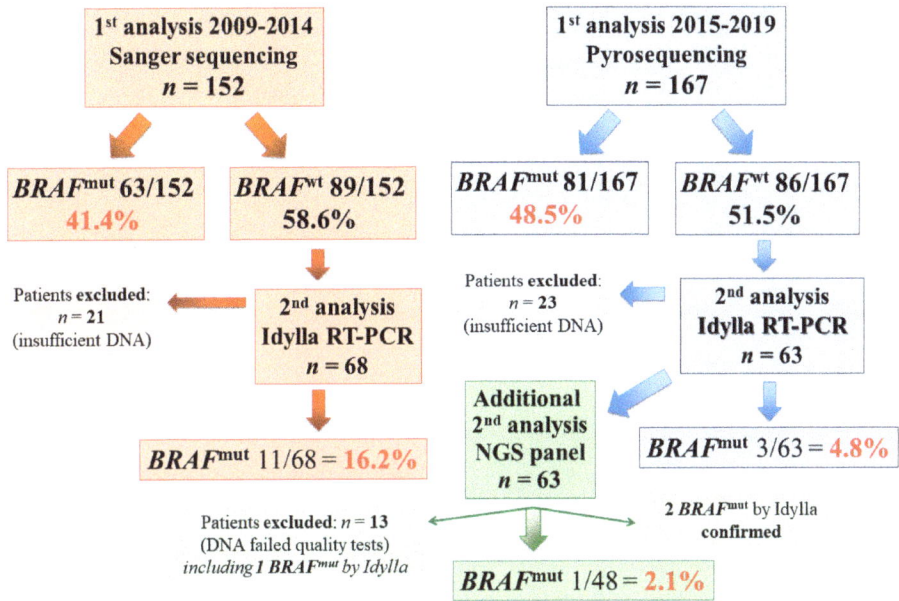

Figure 1. Tissue samples from advanced malignant melanoma (MM) patients analyzed for BRAF mutational status and screening methodologies used into the study. RT-PCR (written as rtPCR in the rest of the manuscript), real-time polymerase chain reaction; NGS, next-generation sequencing.

Table 2. Patient mutational status at first test screening by conventional analysis. In bold, significant p-value correlations.

Characteristics	Mutated	Wild-Type	p
BRAF (n = 319)			
Mutated, n (%)	144 (45.1)	175 (54.9)	
Gender, n (%)			
Male, n (%)	79 (54.9)	104 (59.4)	0.479
Female, n (%)	65 (45.1)	71 (40.6)	
Age at diagnosis, n (%)			
≤55 years, n (%)	58 (40.3)	37 (21.1)	**0.003**
>55 years, n (%)	86 (59.7)	138 (78.9)	
NRAS (n = 272)			
Mutated, n (%)	40 (14.7)	232 (85.3)	
Gender, n (%)			
Male, n (%)	25 (62.5)	129 (55.6)	0.522
Female, n (%)	15 (37.5)	103 (44.4)	
Age at diagnosis, n (%)			
≤55 years, n (%)	4 (10)	73 (31.5)	**0.004**
>55 years, n (%)	36 (90)	159 (68.5)	

The subtypes of the mutations found for each gene are summarized in Table 3. A very high proportion of *BRAF* mutations across samples was represented by the BRAF^{V600E} variant (120, 83.3%). All but one of the remaining *BRAF* variants were represented by other V600 subtypes: V600K (19, 13.2%),

V600D (3, 2.1%), and V600R (1, 0.7%) (Table 3). The K601E mutation was the only variant not affecting the codon 600 of *BRAF*, though it is a sequence variation still localized in the active kinase domain of the gene, which can respond to the targeted therapy. For *NRAS*, nearly all (35/40; 87.5%) mutations were found at the codon 61 of the gene: Q61R (n = 19), Q61K (n = 12), Q61L (n = 3), and Q61H (n = 1) (Table 3).

Table 3. *BRAF* and *NRAS* mutation spectrum. Frequencies are related to the total amount of mutated cases in *BRAF* (n = 144) and *NRAS* (n = 40) genes.

Exon	Mutation	Base Change	Amino Acid Change	Mutated Samples	%
BRAF					
15	V600D	1799–1800 TG>AT	Val to Asp	3	2.1
15	V600E	1799 T>A	Val to Glu	117	81.2
15	V600E	1799_1800TG>AA	Val to Glu	3	2.1
15	V600K	1798–99 GT>AA	Val to Lys	19	13.2
15	V600R	1798–99 GT>AG	Val to Arg	1	0.7
15	K601E	1790 T>G	Leu to Arg	1	0.7
NRAS					
2	G12A	35 G>C	Gly to Ala	1	2.5
2	G13D	38 G>A	Gly to Asp	2	5.0
2	G13R	37 G>C	Gly to Arg	2	5.0
3	Q61H	183 A>T	Gln to His	1	2.5
3	Q61K	181 C>A	Gln to Lys	12	30.0
3	Q61L	182 A>T	Gln to Leu	3	7.5
3	Q61R	182 A>G	Gln to Arg	19	47.5

All mutations detected in this study have been reported in the Human Gene Mutation Database (HGMD), at http://www.hgmd.cf.ac.uk/ac/index.php, and in the Catalogue of Somatic Mutations in Cancer (COSMIC), at http://www.sanger.ac.uk/genetics/CGP/cosmic/.

Successively, research was aimed at investigating differences in terms of sensitivity and specificity among the currently available molecular platforms for improving assessment of the mutational status. Given the high number of cases, we concentrate on *BRAF* mutations only in order to perform comparisons between the testing methods. Additional analyses with rtPCR/Idylla™ and NGS assays were performed on available FFPE tissue sections and/or DNA samples deriving from the same specimens used for first *BRAF* classification. Among the 144 patients carrying a *BRAF* mutated melanoma in our series (Figure 1), 61 DNA samples (30 cases evaluated by SS assay and 31 by pyrosequencing) were selected as adequate for further analyses. The Idylla™ test confirmed the presence of *BRAF* mutations in all 30 (100%) positive cases assessed by Sanger-based sequencing and in 30/31 (96.8%) mutated cases assessed by pyrosequencing. The latter discrepant case was further investigated with the NGS assay, which confirmed the presence of the *BRAF* mutation (thus confirming the result obtained by the pyrosequencing analysis).

Among the 175 *BRAF* wild-type cases, 42 of them were excluded, since the remaining available DNA was not sufficient or qualitatively adequate to perform further assays, and there was no availability of additional FFPE tissue sections (Figure 1). Overall, 131 *BRAF* wild-type samples (68 after SS and 63 after pyrosequencing) were re-analyzed by rtPCR/Idylla™ test; among the formers, 11 (16.2%) additional *BRAF* mutated cases were found, while among those initially tested with pyrosequencing, 3 (4.8%) additional *BRAF* mutated cases were detected (Figure 1). The difference was statistically significant (p = 0.047), even if the compared cases were not the same. Finally, 48 samples out of the

63 that underwent rtPCR/Idylla™ testing after pyrosequencing were also evaluated by NGS, and one additional mutation was detected; in this case, no statistically significant difference was found between the two methods ($p = 0.637$).

4. Discussion

BRAF molecular testing is currently imperative for the classification of stages III and IV MM patients, toward the selection of the appropriate therapeutic strategy. Several methods for *BRAF* testing are currently being used, including both companion diagnostic and laboratory-developed methods. The ideal method should be highly sensitive in detecting mutant alleles, and, at the same time, highly specific in detecting the correct mutation. Furthermore, it should be performable by using a small amount of biological material, considering that often the samples are small FFPE biopsies, and more than one analysis has to be carried out. In addition, the test should be inexpensive, easy, and quick to perform, with results that are easy to interpret. Currently, a unique test that contains all such features does not exist, and, often, more than one test is recommended.

The detection of *BRAF* mutations is commonly performed on DNA extracted from tumor tissue samples, using a molecular approach. In recent years, a *BRAF* mutation analysis conducted at protein level was introduced into the clinical practice, though its use remains controversial. The protein-based test is represented by an immunohistochemistry assay with a monoclonal antibody (VE1), which is specific for detecting the expression of $BRAF^{V600E}$ mutated protein in tumor tissue samples [30]. Nearly all tests currently in use are DNA-based. They include allele-specific PCR assays to selectively amplify the candidate *BRAF* codon and direct sequencing strategies (SS, pyrosequencing, or NGS) to determine the nucleotide sequence of the gene [31]. In Europe, at least three allele specific PCR tests have been CE-IVD certified for diagnostics: the PNAClamp™ BRAF Mutation detection kit (Panagene), the Cobas® 4800 BRAF V600 mutation kit (Roche Diagnostics), and the Idylla™ BRAF mutation kit (Biocartis). All rtPCR tests show higher sensitivity and specificity than those based on direct sequencing. Unfortunately, few studies have fully compared such different strategies for *BRAF* mutation screening. To date, no consensus on the best method to use in clinical practice exists.

The Idylla™ system, a fully automated rtPCR platform with several advantages over other techniques, has been recently introduced in clinical practice. Firstly, it is characterized by rapid turnaround times (approximately two hours), which is essential because it allows rapid decisions regarding the best treatment to adopt for the patient [32]. Furthermore, while the Cobas® test can detect the *BRAF* V600E mutation only, the Idylla™ test can detect all the actionable mutations at the codon V600 of the *BRAF* gene, including the less frequent V600D/K/R/M variants. In addition, cartridges that are able to detect the most relevant genetic alterations of both the *BRAF* and *NRAS* genes in a single assay are now available, and they can be also used in other tumors harboring such alterations (i.e., colorectal cancer) [33]. In their pivotal study, Barel et al. compared Idylla™ (NRAS-BRAF-EGFRS492R mutation assay—110 min per sample) with NGS and IHC for detection of *BRAF* and *NRAS* mutations in 36 patients with metastatic melanomas and found a global concordance between NGS and Idylla™ assays of 97.2% (35/36 cases) [34]. Interestingly, they noticed one difference in mutation genotyping, since NGS highlighted an NRAS G13C mutation, whereas the Idylla™ cartridges, which do not search the G13C alteration, reported an NRAS G12A [34].

Concordance with IHC was better evaluated in the study performed by Vallèe et al. [32]. When compared with their reference, the authors found an overall concordance of 89% for BRAF V600E mutation detection by IHC, while the Idylla™ system showed a concordance of 100% and 92.1% for *BRAF* and *NRAS* mutation detection, respectively. Furthermore, the Idylla™ showed a PPV and NPV of both 100% for *BRAF* mutation detection and a PPV and NPV of 100% and 87%, respectively, for *NRAS* mutation detection. They concluded that BRAF V600E immunohistochemistry is efficient for detecting the V600E mutation, but negative cases should be further evaluated by molecular approaches for other BRAF mutations.

In our study, we compared, for the first time, Idylla™ with all the available sequencing techniques (Sanger-based sequencing, pyrosequencing, and NGS sequencing) in a tissue-sample collection from MM patients undergoing mutational classification for clinical purposes in a real-life, hospital-based recruitment. NGS can provide information on a wider spectrum of genetic alterations, allowing for a better evaluation of the molecular landscape of the disease; in addition, it requires limited quantities of DNA and presents the highest diagnostic sensitivity (detection limit of 1–2%) [35]. Although it is able to identify all mutations present in the analyzed genomic regions (specificity of 100%; referred to as a comprehensive test), the interpretation of sequencing data may be somehow complex and requires a high level of expertise, making its application more difficult to be broadly introduced into the clinical practice [35]. In addition, it involves a longer turnaround time, it is more expensive, and it can be affected by DNA quality.

Our data showed that rtPCR is more accurate than both Sanger sequencing and pyrosequencing in detecting *BRAF* mutations. Firstly, we verified the existence of a quite absolute concordance among the three screening methods for the *BRAF* mutated cases analyzed in our series; overall, 60/61 (98.4%) Idylla™ tests confirmed the presence of the same *BRAF* mutation identified by the sequencing assay. One could speculate that the probability of detecting a false-positive *BRAF* mutated case is rare when using one of the three different approaches described above for mutation screening. Slightly more complex is the evaluation of the data among the *BRAF* wild-type cases from our series. As expected, the Idylla™ detection rates of missed *BRAF* mutations cases were significantly higher in wild-type cases assessed by SS, rather than in those by pyrosequencing. Indeed, Sanger-based direct DNA sequencing has the lowest diagnostic sensitivity (detection limit of 15–20%), though it is able to identify all the variants present in the analyzed genomic regions (specificity of 100%, again, referred to as a comprehensive test); pyrosequencing, instead, shows a higher sensitivity (detection limit of 5–8%) and a good mutation coverage (specificity of 90%; referred to as a near-comprehensive test). Finally, the ability of Idylla™ to detect such mutations was comparable with that of NGS, and both methods were more accurate than pyrosequencing. It has been reported that rtPCR techniques have a very high sensitivity (detection limit of 2–3%), but they can identify a limited number of mutations within specifically targeted genomic regions (specificity for each variant of up to 98%) [36–38]. In our study, we did not compare molecular techniques on DNA with IHC techniques on protein.

By summarizing pros and cons for each *BRAF* mutation testing strategy, we could infer the following:

NGS provides the maximum level of specificity (100%) and sensitivity (up to 98%) in detecting all gene variants (pros), but it requires skilled personnel and has several practical drawbacks (longer time for sample preparation and running, higher cost for reagents, and lack of guarantee of being able to complete the analysis in all FFPE samples due to DNA quality limitations) (cons);

Sanger-based direct sequencing achieves the highest specificity (100%) and can detect all sequence mutations in *BRAF* exons 11 and 15 (pros), but it presents the lowest diagnostic sensitivity (80–85%)—which requires a higher tumor cell representation into the tissue sample—and it is somehow time-consuming (cons).

Pyrosequencing is a simple-to-perform method and provides a good level of sensitivity (92–95%) (pros), but it does not achieve a complete mutation coverage specificity (up to 90%; in gene codons 600, 469, and 464 only; see Methods) (cons).

Real-time PCR is a rapid method which achieves the same maximum level of sensitivity of NGS (up to 98%), without requiring particular skills (pro), but it is able to identify a limited number of mutations (Idylla™ test: V600E/D/K/M/R, but not other V600 actionable variants, such as V600G/A—see Methods; Cobas® 4800 BRAF V600 mutation test: V600E/K mutations only) (con).

Our study has some limitations, mainly the retrospective design and the heterogeneity in the compared groups, dictated by its real-life nature. On the other hand, our work has several advantages, as it is the first study to compare four different DNA-based techniques, using the same specimen and same DNA per case, in order to avoid inter-tumoral heterogeneity. Finally, the study included patients from the same genetically homogeneous population from Sardinia, an island that experienced little immigration and genetic contamination in the past decades, due to its geographical location [39,40].

In conclusion, our findings provide support for both NGS and Idylla^{TM} assays to be adopted as the molecular method of choice for routine assessment of *BRAF* status in MM patients and to provide guidance toward the appropriate treatment strategy. These methods improved the diagnostic accuracy of *BRAF* testing via the detection of additional *BRAF* mutations in a subset of false-negative cases previously tested with Sanger sequencing or pyrosequencing. In attendance of further confirmations in larger prospectively designed studies, the use of two sensitive molecular methods may ensure the highest level of diagnostic accuracy.

Author Contributions: Conceptualization, M.C. (Maria Colombino) and G.P. (Giuseppe Palmieri); writing—original draft preparation, C.R. and G.P (Giuseppe Palmieri); writing—review and editing, P.P. and G.P. (Giuseppe Palmieri); investigation, M.C. (Maria Colombino), M.C. (Milena Casula), and A.M.; methodology, V.D. and M.A.F.; validation, M.C.S., G.P. (Grazia Palomba), and M.P.; visualization, P.A.A. and C.C.; data curation, A.L.; supervision, A.C. The members of MUS made substantial contributions in clinical data collection. The members of both AIRC and IMI contributed in data interpretation and critical discussion of the manuscript. All authors have read and agreed to the published version of the manuscript.

Funding: This work was partially founded by the Associazione Italiana per la Ricerca sul Cancro (AIRC) "Programma di ricerca 5 per Mille 2018—Id.21073".

Acknowledgments: The Melanoma Unit of Sassari (MUS) includes the following members who participated as investigators in this study and should be considered as co-authors: Roberto Dallocchio, Maria Serra (National Research Council-CNR, Sassari, Italy); Maria Filomena Dedola, Fabrizio Demaria, Maria Antonietta Montesu, Gildo Montroni, Stefano Profili, Corrado Rubino, Rosanna Satta, Tiziana Scotto, Germana Sini (Azienda Ospedaliero Universitaria-AOU, Sassari, Italy). The Italian Association for Cancer Research (AIRC) Study Group includes the following members who participated as investigators in this study and should be considered as co-authors: Michele Maio (Azienda Ospedaliera Universitaria Senese, Siena, Italy), Daniela Massi (Università di Firenze, Florence, Italy), Andrea Anichini (Istituto Nazionale dei Tumori, Milano, Italy), Ulrich Pfeffer (Azienda Ospedaliera Universitaria "San Martino", Genoa, Italy).The Italian Melanoma Intergroup (IMI) includes the following additional members who participated as investigators in this study and should be considered as co-authors: Antonio Maria Grimaldi (Istituto Nazionale Tumori Fondazione Pascale, Napoli, Italy); Mario Mandalà (Ospedale Papa Giovanni XXIII, Bergamo, Italy); Daniela Massi (Anatomia Patologica, Università di Firenze, Florence, Italy); Pietro Quaglino (Azienda Ospedaliera Universitaria Città della Salute e della Scienza, Torino, Italy); Paola Queirolo (Ospedale San Martino, Genova, Italy); and Ignazio Stanganelli (Università di Parma, Parma, Italy).

Conflicts of Interest: Paolo A. Ascierto has/had consultant and advisory role for Bristol Myers Squibb, Incyte, Merck Sharp & Dohme, Roche-Genentech, Novartis, Amgen, Array, Merck-Serono, and Pierre Fabre. He received research funds from Bristol Myers Squibb, Roche-Genetech, and Array. Giuseppe Palmieri has/had advisory role for Bristol Myers Squibb, Incyte, Merck Sharp & Dohme, Novartis, Pierre Fabre, and Roche-Genetech. All the remaining authors declare no conflict of interest.

References

1. Siegel, R.L.; Miller, K.D.; Jemal, A. Cancer statistics, 2020. *CA Cancer J. Clin.* **2020**, *70*, 7–30. [CrossRef] [PubMed]
2. Cossu, A.; Casula, M.; Cesaraccio, R.; Lissia, A.; Colombino, M.; Sini, M.C.; Budroni, M.; Tanda, F.; Paliogiannis, P.; Palmieri, G. Epidemiology and genetic susceptibility of malignant melanoma in North Sardinia, Italy. *Eur. J. Cancer Prev.* **2017**, *26*, 263–267. [CrossRef] [PubMed]
3. I Numeri del Cancro in Italia. Available online: https://www.aiom.it/wp-content/uploads/2019/09/2019_Numeri_Cancro-operatori-web.pdf (accessed on 11 May 2020).
4. Parker, B.S.; Rautela, J.; Hertzog, P.J. Antitumor actions of interferons: Implications for cancer therapy. *Nat. Rev. Cancer* **2016**, *16*, 131–144. [CrossRef] [PubMed]

5. Luke, J.J.; Flaherty, K.T.; Ribas, A.; Long, G.V. Targeted agents and immunotherapies: Optimizing outcomes in melanoma. *Nat. Rev. Clin. Oncol.* **2017**, *14*, 463–482. [CrossRef]
6. Su, M.Y.; Fisher, D.E. Immunotherapy in the precision medicine era: Melanoma and beyond. *PLoS Med.* **2016**, *13*, e1002196. [CrossRef]
7. Sini, M.C.; Doneddu, V.; Paliogiannis, P.; Casula, M.; Colombino, M.; Manca, A.; Botti, G.; Ascierto, P.A.; Lissia, A.; Cossu, A.; et al. Genetic alterations in main candidate genes during melanoma progression. *Oncotarget* **2018**, *9*, 8531–8541. [CrossRef]
8. Davies, H.; Bignell, G.R.; Cox, C.; Stephens, P.; Edkins, S.; Clegg, S.; Teague, J.; Woffendin, H.; Garnett, M.J.; Bottomley, W.; et al. Mutations of the BRAF gene in human cancer. *Nature* **2002**, *417*, 949–954. [CrossRef]
9. Greaves, W.O.; Verma, S.; Patel, K.P.; Davies, M.A.; Barkoh, B.A.; Galbincea, J.M.; Yao, H.; Lazar, A.J.; Aldape, K.D.; Medeiros, L.J.; et al. Frequency and spectrum of BRAF mutations in a retrospective, single institution study of 1112 cases of melanoma. *J. Mol. Diagn.* **2013**, *15*, 220–226. [CrossRef]
10. Wan, P.T.; Garnett, M.J.; Roe, S.M.; Lee, S.; Niculescu-Duvaz, D.; Good, V.M.; Project, C.G.; Jones, C.M.; Marshall, C.J.; Springer, C.J.; et al. Mechanism of activation of the RAF-ERK signaling pathway by oncogenic mutations of B-RAF. *Cell* **2004**, *116*, 855–867. [CrossRef]
11. Chapman, P.B.; Hauschild, A.; Robert, C.; Haanen, J.B.; Ascierto, P.; Larkin, J.; Dummer, R.; Garbe, C.; Testori, A.; Maio, M.; et al. BRIM-3 Study Group. Improved survival with vemurafenib in melanoma with BRAF V600E mutation. *N. Engl. J. Med.* **2011**, *364*, 2507–2516.
12. Hauschild, A.; Grob, J.J.; Demidov, L.V.; Jouary, T.; Gutzmer, R.; Millward, M.; Rutkowski, P.; Blank, C.U.; Miller, W.H., Jr.; Kaempgen, E.; et al. Dabrafenib in BRAF-mutated metastatic melanoma: A multicentre, open-label, phase 3 randomised controlled trial. *Lancet* **2012**, *380*, 358–365. [CrossRef]
13. Dummer, R.; Hauschild, A.; Lindenblatt, N.; Pentheroudakis, G.; Keilholz, U. Cutaneous melanoma: ESMO clinical practice guidelines for diagnosis, treatment, and follow-up. *Ann. Oncol.* **2016**, *26* (Suppl. 5), 126–132. [CrossRef] [PubMed]
14. Seth, R.; Messersmith, H.; Kaur, V.; Kirkwood, J.M.; Kudchadkar, R.; McQuade, J.L.; Provenzano, A.; Swami, U.; Weber, J.; Alluri, K.C.; et al. Systemic therapy for melanoma: ASCO Guideline. *J. Clin. Oncol.* **2020**, *31*, JCO2000198. [CrossRef] [PubMed]
15. Ascierto, P.A.; Agarwala, S.S.; Botti, G.; Budillon, A.; Davies, M.A.; Dummer, R.; Ernstoff, M.; Ferrone, S.; Formenti, S.; Gajewski, T.F.; et al. Perspectives in melanoma: Meeting report from the Melanoma Bridge (November 29th-1 December 1st, 2018, Naples, Italy). *J. Transl. Med.* **2019**, *17*, 234. [CrossRef] [PubMed]
16. National Comprehensive Cancer Network Guidelines. Available online: https://www.nccn.org/professionals/physician_gls/default.aspx (accessed on 11 May 2020).
17. Michielin, O.; van Akkooi, A.C.J.; Ascierto, P.A.; Dummer, R.; Keilholz, U.; ESMO Guidelines Committee. Electronic address: Clinicalguidelines@esmo.org. Cutaneous melanoma: ESMO Clinical Practice Guidelines for diagnosis, treatment and follow-up. *Ann. Oncol.* **2019**, *30*, 1884–1901. [CrossRef]
18. Coit, D.G.; Thompson, J.A.; Albertini, M.R.; Barker, C.; Carson, W.E.; Contreras, C.; Daniels, G.A.; DiMaio, D.; Fields, R.C.; Fleming, M.D.; et al. Cutaneous Melanoma, Version 2.2019, NCCN Clinical Practice Guidelines in Oncology. *J. Natl. Compr. Cancer Netw.* **2019**, *17*, 367–402. [CrossRef]
19. Garbe, C.; Amaral, T.; Peris, K.; Hauschild, A.; Arenberger, P.; Basholt, L.; Bataille, V.; Del Marmol, V.; Dréno, B.; Fargnoli, M.C.; et al. European consensus-based interdisciplinary guideline for melanoma. Part 2: Treatment—Update 2019. *Eur. J. Cancer* **2020**, *126*, 159–177.
20. Poklepovic, A.S.; Luke, J.J. Considering adjuvant therapy for stage II melanoma. *Cancer* **2020**, *126*, 1166–1174. [CrossRef]
21. Long, G.V.; Hauschild, A.; Santinami, M.; Atkinson, V.; Mandalà, M.; Chiarion-Sileni, V.; Larkin, J.; Nyakas, M.; Dutriaux, C.; Haydon, A.; et al. Adjuvant Dabrafenib plus Trametinib in Stage III BRAF-Mutated Melanoma. *N. Engl. J. Med.* **2017**, *377*, 1813–1823. [CrossRef]
22. Hauschild, A.; Dummer, R.; Schadendorf, D.; Santinami, M.; Atkinson, V.; Mandalà, M.; Chiarion-Sileni, V.; Larkin, J.; Nyakas, M.; Dutriaux, C.; et al. Longer Follow-Up Confirms Relapse-Free Survival Benefit with Adjuvant Dabrafenib Plus Trametinib in Patients with Resected BRAF V600-Mutant Stage III Melanoma. *J. Clin. Oncol.* **2018**, *36*, JCO1801219. [CrossRef]

23. Hauschild, A.; Dummer, R.; Santinami, M.; Atkinson, V.; Mandalà, M.; Kirkwood, J.M.; Chiarion Sileni, V.; Larkin, J.M.G.; Nyakas, M.; Dutriaux, C.; et al. Long-term benefit of adjuvant dabrafenib + trametinib (D+T) in patients (pts) with resected stage III BRAF V600–mutant melanoma: Five-year analysis of COMBI-AD. *J. Clin. Oncol.* **2020**, *38*, 10001. [CrossRef]
24. Dummer, R.; Ascierto, P.A.; Gogas, H.J.; Arance, A.; Mandala, M.; Liszkay, G.; Garbe, C.; Schadendorf, D.; Krajsova, I.; Gutzmer, R.; et al. Overall survival in patients with BRAF-mutant melanoma receiving encorafenib plus binimetinib versus vemurafenib or encorafenib (COLUMBUS): A multicentre, open-label, randomised, phase 3 trial. *Lancet Oncol.* **2018**, *19*, 1315–1327. [CrossRef]
25. Ascierto, P.A.; Lewis, K.D.; Di Giacomo, A.M.; Demidov, L.; Mandalà, M.; Bondarenko, I.; Herbert, C.; Mackiewicz, A.; Rutkowski, P.; Guminski, A.; et al. Prognostic impact of baseline tumour immune infiltrate on disease-free survival in patients with completely resected, BRAFv600 mutation-positive melanoma receiving adjuvant vemurafenib. *Ann. Oncol.* **2020**, *31*, 153–159. [CrossRef] [PubMed]
26. Colombino, M.; Capone, M.; Lissia, A.; Cossu, A.; Rubino, C.; De Giorgi, V.; Massi, D.; Fonsatti, E.; Staibano, S.; Nappi, O.; et al. BRAF/NRAS mutation frequencies among primary tumors and metastases in patients with melanoma. *J. Clin. Oncol.* **2012**, *30*, 2522–2529. [CrossRef] [PubMed]
27. Colombino, M.; Lissia, A.; Franco, R.; Botti, G.; Ascierto, P.A.; Manca, A.; Sini, M.C.; Pisano, M.; Paliogiannis, P.; Tanda, F.; et al. Unexpected distribution of cKIT and BRAF mutations among southern Italian patients with sinonasal melanoma. *Dermatology* **2013**, *226*, 279–284. [CrossRef] [PubMed]
28. The Cancer Genome Atlas Network. Genomic classification of cutaneous melanoma. *Cell* **2015**, *161*, 1681–1696.
29. Palmieri, G.; Ombra, M.; Colombino, M.; Casula, M.; Sini, M.; Manca, A.; Paliogiannis, P.; Ascierto, P.A.; Cossu, A. Multiple molecular pathways in melanomagenesis: Characterization of therapeutic targets. *Front. Oncol.* **2015**, *5*, 183. [CrossRef]
30. Feller, J.K.; Yang, S.; Mahalingam, M. Immunohistochemistry with a mutation-specific monoclonal antibody as a screening tool for the BRAFV600E mutational status in primary cutaneous malignant melanoma. *Mod. Pathol.* **2013**, *26*, 414–420. [CrossRef]
31. Sholl, L.M.; Andea, A.; Bridge, J.A.; Cheng, L.; Davies, M.A.; Ehteshami, M.; Gangadhar, T.C.; Kamel-Reid, S.; Lazar, A.; Raparia, K.; et al. Template for reporting results of biomarker testing of specimens from Patients with melanoma. *Arch. Pathol. Lab. Med.* **2016**, *140*, 355–357. [CrossRef]
32. Vallée, A.; Denis-Musquer, M.; Herbreteau, G.; Théoleyre, S.; Bossard, C.; Denis, M.G. Prospective evaluation of two screening methods for molecular testing of metastatic melanoma: Diagnostic performance of BRAF V600E immunohistochemistry and of a NRAS-BRAF fully automated real-time PCR-based assay. *PLoS ONE* **2019**, *14*, e0221123. [CrossRef]
33. Palomba, G.; Doneddu, V.; Cossu, A.; Paliogiannis, P.; Manca, A.; Casula, M.; Colombino, M.; Lanzillo, A.; Defraia, E.; Pazzola, A.; et al. Prognostic impact of KRAS, NRAS, BRAF, and PIK3CA mutations in primary colorectal carcinomas: A population-based study. *J. Transl. Med.* **2016**, *14*, 292. [CrossRef] [PubMed]
34. Barel, F.; Guibourg, B.; Lambros, L.; Le Flahec, G.; Marcorelles, P.; Uguen, A. Evaluation of a Rapid, Fully Automated Platform for Detection of BRAF and NRAS Mutations in Melanoma. *Acta Derm. Venereol.* **2018**, *98*, 44–49. [CrossRef] [PubMed]
35. Palmieri, G.; Colombino, M.; Casula, M.; Manca, A.; Mandalà, M.; Cossu, A.; Italian Melanoma Intergroup (IMI). Molecular pathways in melanomagenesis: What we learned from next-generation sequencing approaches. *Curr. Oncol. Rep.* **2018**, *20*, 86. [CrossRef]
36. Ihle, M.A.; Fassunke, J.; König, K.; Grünewald, I.; Schlaak, M.; Kreuzberg, N.; Tietze, L.; Schildhaus, H.U.; Büttner, R.; Merkelbach-Bruse, S. Comparison of high resolution melting analysis, pyrosequencing, next gene-ration sequencing and immunohistochemistry to conventional Sanger sequencing for the detection of p.V600E and non-p.V600E BRAF mutations. *BMC Cancer* **2014**, *14*, 13. [CrossRef] [PubMed]
37. Bruno, W.; Martinuzzi, C.; Andreotti, V.; Pastorino, L.; Spagnolo, F.; Dalmasso, B.; Cabiddu, F.; Gualco, M.; Ballestrero, A.; Bianchi-Scarrà, G.; et al. Heterogeneity and frequency of BRAF mutations in primary melanoma: Comparison between molecular methods and immunohistochemistry. *Oncotarget* **2017**, *8*, 8069–8082. [CrossRef] [PubMed]
38. Mosko, M.J.; Nakorchevsky, A.A.; Flores, E.; Metzler, H.; Ehrich, M.; van den Boom, D.J.; Sherwood, J.L.; Nygren, A.O. Ultrasensitive detection of multiplexed somatic mutations using MALDI-TOF Mass Spectrometry. *J. Mol. Diagn.* **2016**, *18*, 23–31. [CrossRef]

39. Casula, C.; Muggiano, A.; Cossu, A.; Budroni, M.; Caracò, C.; Ascierto, P.A.; Pagani, E.; Stanganelli, I.; Canzanella, S.; Sini, M.C.; et al. Role of key-regulator genes in melanoma susceptibility and pathogenesis among patients from South Italy. *BMC Cancer* **2009**, *9*, 352. [CrossRef]
40. Palomba, G.; Loi, A.; Porcu, E.; Cossu, A.; Zara, I.; Budroni, M.; Dei, M.; Lai, S.; Mulas, A.; Olmeo, N.; et al. Genome-wide association study of susceptibility loci for breast cancer in Sardinian population. *BMC Cancer* **2015**, *15*, 383. [CrossRef]

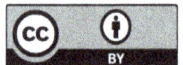

© 2020 by the authors. Licensee MDPI, Basel, Switzerland. This article is an open access article distributed under the terms and conditions of the Creative Commons Attribution (CC BY) license (http://creativecommons.org/licenses/by/4.0/).

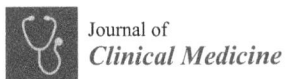

Article

Incidence of Melanoma in Catalonia, Spain, Is Rapidly Increasing in the Elderly Population. A Multicentric Cohort Study

Sebastian Podlipnik [1,2,*], Cristina Carrera [1,2,3], Aram Boada [4], Nina Richarz [4], Joaquim Marcoval [5], Josep Ramón Ferreres [5], Domingo Bodet [6], Rosa María Martí [7], Sonia Segura [8], Mireia Sabat [9], Joan Dalmau [10], Mònica Quintana [11], Antoni Azon [12], Neus Curcó [13], Manel Formigon [14], María Rosa Olivella-Garcés [15], Pedro Zaballos [16], Joaquim Sola [17], Loida Galvany [18], Carola Baliu-Piqué [19], Marta Alegre [20], Paola Pasquali [21], Josep Malvehy [1,2,3], Susana Puig [1,2,3] and on behalf of the Network of Melanoma Centres of Catalonia [†]

1. Hospital Clinic de Barcelona, University of Barcelona, 08036 Barcelona, Spain; criscarrer@yahoo.es (C.C.); jmalvehy@gmail.com (J.M.); susipuig@gmail.com (S.P.)
2. Institut d'Investigacions Biomediques August Pi I Sunyer (IDIBAPS), 08036 Barcelona, Spain
3. Biomedical Research Networking Center on Rare Diseases (CIBERER), ISCIII, 28029 Barcelona, Spain
4. Hospital Universitari Germans Trias i Pujol, Badalona, Universitat Autònoma de Barcelona, 08193 Barcelona, Spain; aramboada@gmail.com (A.B.); ninaricharz@hotmail.com (N.R.)
5. Hospital Universitari de Bellvitge, L'Hospital de Llobregat, 08907 Barcelona, Spain; jmarcoval@bellvitgehospital.cat (J.M.); joseramonferreresriera@yahoo.es (J.R.F.)
6. Hospital Vall d'Hebron, 08035 Barcelona, Spain; dombodet@hotmail.com
7. Hospital Universitari Arnau de Vilanova, 25198 Lleida, Spain; marti@medicina.udl.cat
8. Hospital del Mar, IMIM, 08003 Barcelona, Spain; ssegura@parcdesalutmar.cat
9. Hospital Parc Taulí, 08208 Sabadell, Spain; msabat@tauli.cat
10. Hospital Santa Creu i Sant Pau, 08041 Barcelona, Spain; jdalmau@santpau.es
11. Hospital Universitari Sagrat Cor, 08029 Barcelona, Spain; mquintanacodina@gmail.com
12. Hospital Sant Joan de Reus, 43204 Reus, Spain; azon3030@gmail.com
13. Hospital Universitari Mútua de Terrassa, 08221 Terrassa, Spain; ncurco@mutuaterrassa.cat
14. Consorci Sanitari de Terrassa, 08224 Terrassa, Spain; mformigon@cst.cat
15. Hospital de Sant Joan Despí Moisès Broggi, 08970 Barcelona, Spain; MariaRosa.OlivellaGarces@sanitatintegral.org
16. Hospital Sant Pau i Santa Tecla, 43003 Tarragona, Spain; pzaballos@aedv.es
17. Hospital General de Granollers, 08402 Barcelona, Spain; quimsola@yahoo.com
18. Hospital Dos de Maig, 08025 Barcelona, Spain; Loida.GalvanyRossell@sanitatintegral.org
19. Hospital d'Igualada, Consorci Sanitari de l'Anoia, 08700 Igualada, Spain; carola.baliu.pique@gmail.com
20. Hospital Plató, 08006 Barcelona, Spain; marta.alegre@hospitalplato.com
21. Pius Hospital de Valls, 43800 Valls, Spain; pasqualipaola@gmail.com
* Correspondence: podlipnik@clinic.cat; Tel.: +34-932279867
† Colaborators of the Network of Melanoma Centres of Catalonia: Marc Sagristà (Hospital de Calella), Oriol Yélamos (Hospital de la Santa Creu i Sant Pau), Sara Martín-Sala (Hospital Moisès Broggi. Consorci Sanitari Integral), Clara Matas-Nadal, Joan Angel, Xavier Soria and Sonia Gatius (Hospital Universitari Arnau de Vilanova, Lleida), Montserrat Bonfill-Ortí (Hospital Universitari de Bellvitge), Ane Jaka and Ariadna Quer (Hospital Universitari Germans Trias i Pujol, Badalona), Inés Zarzoso Muñoz, Emili Masferrer (Hospital Universitari Mututa Terrassa), Fani Martínez (Hospital Universitari Sant Joan de Reus).

Received: 18 September 2020; Accepted: 20 October 2020; Published: 23 October 2020

Abstract: The incidence of melanoma has been increasing worldwide during recent decades. The objective of the study was to analyse the trends in incidence for in situ and invasive melanoma in the Spanish region of Catalonia during the period of 2008–2017. We designed a cross-sectional study with an age-period-cohort analysis of melanoma patient data from the Network of Melanoma Centres in Catalonia. Our database covered a population of over seven million and included a total of

8626 patients with incident melanoma. The main outcome measures were crude and age-standardised incidence rates to the European 2013 standard population. Joinpoint regression models were used to evaluate the population trends. We observed an increase in the age-standardised incidence rate (per 100,000 population) of all melanoma subtypes from 11.56 in 2008 to 13.78 in 2017 with an average annual percent change (AAPC) of 3.5%. This incidence increase was seen exclusively in the older population. Moreover, the stratified analysis showed a statistically significant increase in the age-standardised incidence rate for invasive (AAPC 2.1%) and in situ melanoma (AAPC 6.5%). In conclusion, the incidence of melanoma has continued to increase in the elderly population over recent decades, with a rapidly increasing trend of in situ melanomas and the lentigo maligna subtype.

Keywords: melanoma; incidence; population-based study; epidemiology; Spain; skin cancer

1. Introduction

Melanoma is responsible for 1%–2% of all cancers worldwide and accounts for only 5% of all malignant skin tumours. However, it is one of the most aggressive forms of cancer and causes 75–90% of skin cancer-related deaths [1]. In addition, melanoma is one of the cancers that presents earlier in life and is one of the solid neoplasms that produces the greatest number of potential life years lost [2–4].

Despite the fact that major primary prevention campaigns have been implemented in recent decades [5–9], the number of melanoma cases continues to rise every year [10,11]. Recent data from the Surveillance, Epidemiology, and End Results (SEER) registry indicate that the incidence of melanoma is rapidly increasing, especially in older patients [10]. However, what it is even more worrying is the fact that there has been an increase in the incidence of melanoma in young adults, especially women between 25 and 39 years of age, often with high associated mortality [12].

In addition, incidence and mortality vary widely among different geographical areas, due to diverse ethnicities and social conditions, with the white race being the most affected in raw numbers [4]. WHO estimates of age-standardised incidence rates worldwide vary widely and show higher incidences in Australia and New Zealand with 33.6 cases per 100,000 population/year, followed by Europe with rates between 9 and 18.8 cases per 100,000 population and the United States with 12.6 cases per 100,000 population [11]. Specifically in Spain there is an incidence rate of 6.4 cases per 100,000 inhabitants per year and a prevalence of skin melanoma in the last five years of 18,181 cases [11]. Although the incidence of melanoma has been increasing globally over recent decades, SEER data has shown that for the first time, the mortality rate decreased by 17.9% in the period 2013–2016 [11,13]. These data may suggest that new drugs, introduced during the last decade for the management of metastatic and locally advanced melanoma, appear to improve survival [13,14].

In the present study, we analysed the population-based age-specific data for cutaneous melanoma in the Catalan population. A thorough knowledge of the incidence of melanoma in Spain is necessary to improve public health policies.

2. Material and Methods

This is a descriptive study with an age-period-cohort analysis of melanoma in the region of Catalonia, located in north-east Spain. We obtained the data on the Catalonian population from the Statistical Institute of Catalonia (IDESCAT) [15], and totals 16.23% of the Spanish population with 7,496,276 inhabitants in 2017, and corresponds to a predominantly white population. The melanoma incidence data was obtained from the Catalan registry of melanoma (Xarxa-melanoma) for the period of 2008–2017. The Xarxa-melanoma is a collaborative prospective database in which a total of 19 hospitals participate, covering most of the population of Catalonia. Cases diagnosed and monitored exclusively in private centres were not included in the database. These cases are a minority in Catalonia since most melanoma patients are seen in public hospitals, especially in the case of invasive tumours.

The research protocol received approval from the Research Ethics Committee of the Hospital Clinic of Barcelona (IRB number: HCB/2015/0298). All data were collected prospectively during the time period. This study followed the "strengthening the reporting of observational studies in epidemiology" (STROBE) statement [16].

We analysed all cases of invasive and in situ cutaneous melanoma, including all ages. To evaluate age periods, we used equally spaced two-year calendar periods to analyse differences in time. Category variables were compared using Pearson's x^2 test, or Fisher's exact test, when the expected observations were fewer than five. For continuous variables, we used the mean and standard deviation and linear model ANOVA test.

Annual incidence rates were age-standardised to the European standardised population [17] by the direct method to remove the confounding effect of age and to make valid comparisons between the incidence rates from different countries and 95% confidence intervals for age-adjusted rates were calculated using the Fay and Feuer method [18].

To examine the population trends in age-standardised incidence rate according to sex and histological subtype (invasive vs in situ), joinpoint regression models were used. We calculated the average annual percent change (AAPC) for each variable independently using a fixed period between 2008 and 2017 for an easier comparison of the subgroups. Moreover, we calculated the average annual percentage change (APC) with a maximum number of possible joinpoints set to one, based on the number of data points in the series [19]. A permutation test was used to determine the location of the joinpoints, when the change in trend was statistically significant. The resulting slope was recorded as the APC.

Statistical analyses were performed using the computing environment R and RStudio [20,21], and the Joinpoint Regression Software, version 4.8.0.1 (National Cancer Institute) [22]. All statistical analyses were two sided and assessed for statistical significance at $P < 0.05$.

3. Results

During the study period of 2008 to 2017, we identified a total of 8753 new cases of melanoma in the Catalonian region, of which 2896 were in situ and 5857 invasive. The analysis stratified by two-year groups revealed that there were no differences between the proportion of men and women over that time; however, the age of presentation of melanoma increased from a mean of 58.2 (SD 17.3) years in 2008 to 63.3 (SD 17.1) in 2017 ($P < 0.001$). Table 1 Moreover, there was a clear trend to diagnose a higher proportion of in situ than invasive melanomas, and the proportion of the lentigo maligna subtype also increased from 13.9% to 22.6%. (Table 1 and Figure 1).

Age-standardised incidence rate of melanoma data is summarised in Table 2. Between 2008 and 2017, there was a significant increase in the age-standardised incidence rate of melanoma per 100,000 population/year from 11.56 (95% CI, 11.38–11.75) in 2008 to 13.78 (95% CI, 13.57–13.98) in 2017. This means a 19% global increase with an average annual percentage change (AAPC) of 3.5% (95% CI, 2.1%, 5.0%) and an annual percentage change (APC) of 4.9% (95% CI, 2.7%, 7.0%). Moreover, the stratified curves for age-standardised incidence for subtypes of melanoma showed an increased trend for both groups. However the magnitude was greater for in situ melanomas (AAPC of 6.5%; 95% CI, 4.4%, 8.6%) than invasive melanomas (AAPC of 2.1%; 95% CI, 0.1%, 4.1%). The stratified analysis by sex showed a higher age-adjusted incidence of melanoma in men over the whole study period, and also showed a similar upward trend in both groups with an AAPC of 3.9% (95% CI, 2.2%, 5.6%) and 3.2% (95% CI, 1.6%, 4.9%) for men and women respectively (Figures 2 and 3).

Age-specific crude incidence rates by 10-year age bands for 2008 to 2017 showed a stable incidence rate during the follow-up period in patients under 60 years; however, from the 60–70 year age group, a rapid increase in incidence is seen as the age of presentation increases. Additionally, in 2017, the crude incidence rate for patients over the age of 80 years was 50.25 cases per 100,000 population (Figure 2).

Moreover, a pyramid plot stratified by sex showed that in women there is a double peak of incidence of melanoma in the 45–49 year bracket and then between 60 and 64 years, while men present a single peak of incidence later in life, between 65 and 69 years (Figure 4A). Moreover, the mean age at presentation of melanoma was 59.1 years in women (SD 17.7) and 62.8 years (16.6) in men ($P < 0.001$). A ridgeline plot shows the distribution of cases represented as density over the years in the study, clearly showing a bimodal distribution of cases in women and only one peak of incidence in men which is maintained during the study period (Figure 4B).

Table 1. Basal characteristics of the tumours.

	2008–2009 (N = 1543)	2010–2011 (N = 1500)	2012–2013 (N = 1696)	2014–2015 (N = 1906)	2016–2017 (N = 2108)	Total (N = 8753)	P Value
Gender							0.496
Female	789 (51.1%)	751 (50.1%)	897 (52.9%)	971 (50.9%)	1060 (50.3%)	4468 (51.0%)	
Male	754 (48.9%)	749 (49.9%)	799 (47.1%)	935 (49.1%)	1048 (49.7%)	4285 (49.0%)	
Age							<0.001
Mean (SD)	58.2 (17.3)	59.6 (17.3)	60.4 (17.3)	61.9 (17.0)	63.3 (17.1)	60.9 (17.3)	
Staging							<0.001
In situ	466 (30.2%)	476 (31.7%)	524 (30.9%)	638 (33.5%)	792 (37.6%)	2896 (33.1%)	
invasive	1077 (69.8%)	1024 (68.3%)	1172 (69.1%)	1268 (66.5%)	1316 (62.4%)	5857 (66.9%)	
Breslow index							0.219
Mean (SD)	2.2 (6.0)	2.4 (4.5)	2.4 (3.6)	2.2 (4.1)	2.1 (3.2)	2.3 (4.3)	
Tumour Location							0.001
Trunk	551 (41.4%)	527 (40.2%)	573 (38.8%)	740 (43.1%)	888 (45.1%)	3279 (42.0%)	
Head and neck	278 (20.9%)	302 (23.1%)	310 (21.0%)	371 (21.6%)	412 (20.9%)	1673 (21.4%)	
Lower limbs	254 (19.1%)	231 (17.6%)	280 (18.9%)	268 (15.6%)	298 (15.1%)	1331 (17.1%)	
Upper limbs	145 (10.9%)	148 (11.3%)	190 (12.9%)	219 (12.8%)	237 (12.0%)	939 (12.0%)	
Acral	97 (7.3%)	85 (6.5%)	107 (7.2%)	92 (5.4%)	107 (5.4%)	488 (6.3%)	
Mucosa	7 (0.5%)	17 (1.3%)	18 (1.2%)	27 (1.6%)	27 (1.4%)	96 (1.2%)	
Missing values	211	190	218	189	139	947	
Histological subtype							<0.001
SSM	871 (63.9%)	806 (61.7%)	884 (60.2%)	965 (59.5%)	1011 (55.1%)	4537 (59.7%)	
LMM	190 (13.9%)	183 (14.0%)	227 (15.5%)	306 (18.9%)	414 (22.6%)	1320 (17.4%)	
Nodular	180 (13.2%)	176 (13.5%)	193 (13.1%)	180 (11.1%)	189 (10.3%)	918 (12.1%)	
Acral lentiginous	65 (4.8%)	51 (3.9%)	85 (5.8%)	73 (4.5%)	74 (4.0%)	348 (4.6%)	
Mucosal	4 (0.3%)	13 (1.0%)	11 (0.7%)	16 (1.0%)	20 (1.1%)	64 (0.8%)	
Desmoplastic	10 (0.7%)	14 (1.1%)	10 (0.7%)	8 (0.5%)	15 (0.8%)	57 (0.8%)	
Spitzoid	3 (0.2%)	1 (0.1%)	8 (0.5%)	11 (0.7%)	21 (1.1%)	44 (0.6%)	
Nevoid	3 (0.2%)	1 (0.1%)	1 (0.1%)	4 (0.2%)	8 (0.4%)	17 (0.2%)	
Other	37 (2.7%)	62 (4.7%)	50 (3.4%)	60 (3.7%)	82 (4.5%)	291 (3.8%)	
Missing values	180	193	227	283	274	1157	

Only includes the evaluation of invasive melanomas.

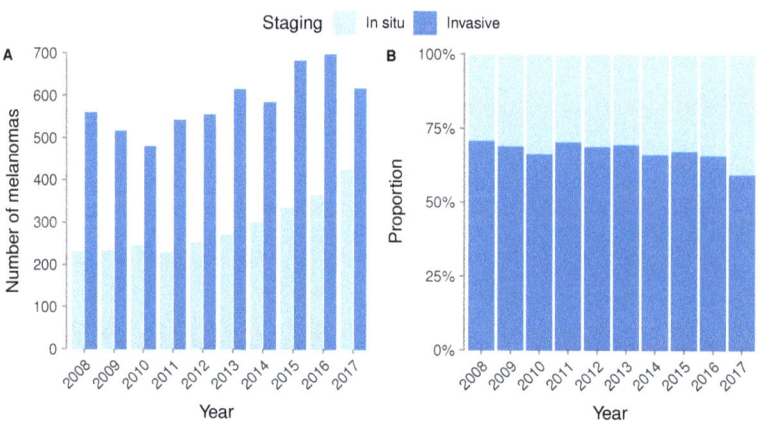

Figure 1. Distribution of invasive and in situ melanomas.

Finally, the analysis of melanoma subtypes showed that the age-standardised incidence rate of superficial spreading melanoma and lentigo maligna melanoma is increasing, while the proportion of patients with nodular, acral lentiginous and other subtypes of melanoma remains constant (Figure 2).

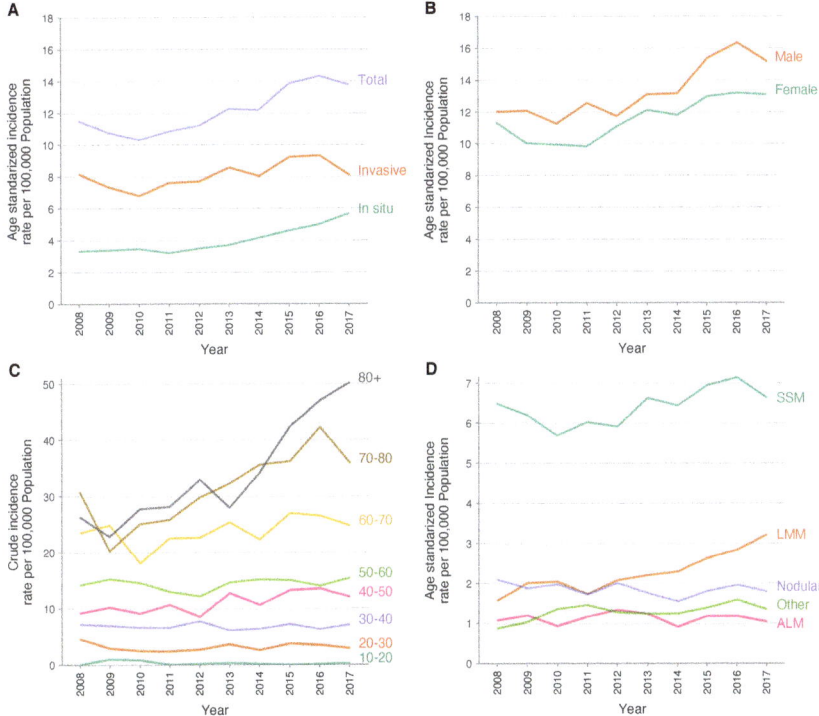

Figure 2. Trends in the incidence of melanoma in Catalunya. Abbreviations: ALM, acral lentiginous melanoma, LMM, lentiginous malignant melanoma; SSM, superficial spreading melanoma.

Table 2. Incidence of melanoma in Catalonia.

Year	Population	Cases	Crude Rate	ASIR	95% CI
Melanoma (Including In Situ Melanoma)					
2008	7,298,313	792	10.85	11.56	[11.38–11.75]
2009	7,416,605	751	10.13	10.80	[10.62–10.97]
2010	7,462,044	727	9.74	10.35	[10.18–10.52]
2011	7,501,853	773	10.30	10.88	[10.7–11.06]
2012	7,515,398	809	10.76	11.25	[11.07–11.43]
2013	7,478,968	887	11.86	12.30	[12.11–12.49]
2014	7,433,894	887	11.93	12.23	[12.05–12.43]
2015	7,424,754	1019	13.72	13.86	[13.65–14.06]
2016	7,448,332	1064	14.29	14.34	[14.14–14.55]
2017	7,496,276	1044	13.93	13.78	[13.57–13.98]

Table 2. *Cont.*

Year	Population	Cases	Crude Rate	ASIR	95% CI
Invasive melanoma					
2008	7,298,313	560	7.67	8.19	[8.04–8.35]
2009	7,416,605	517	6.97	7.38	[7.23–7.52]
2010	7,462,044	481	6.45	6.83	[6.7–6.98]
2011	7,501,853	543	7.24	7.64	[7.49–7.79]
2012	7,515,398	556	7.40	7.73	[7.58–7.88]
2013	7,478,968	616	8.24	8.57	[8.41–8.73]
2014	7,433,894	585	7.87	8.04	[7.89–8.2]
2015	7,424,754	683	9.20	9.23	[9.06–9.4]
2016	7,448,332	698	9.37	9.32	[9.16–9.49]
2017	7,496,276	618	8.24	8.08	[7.92–8.24]

Abbreviations: ASIR, age-standardised incidence rate.

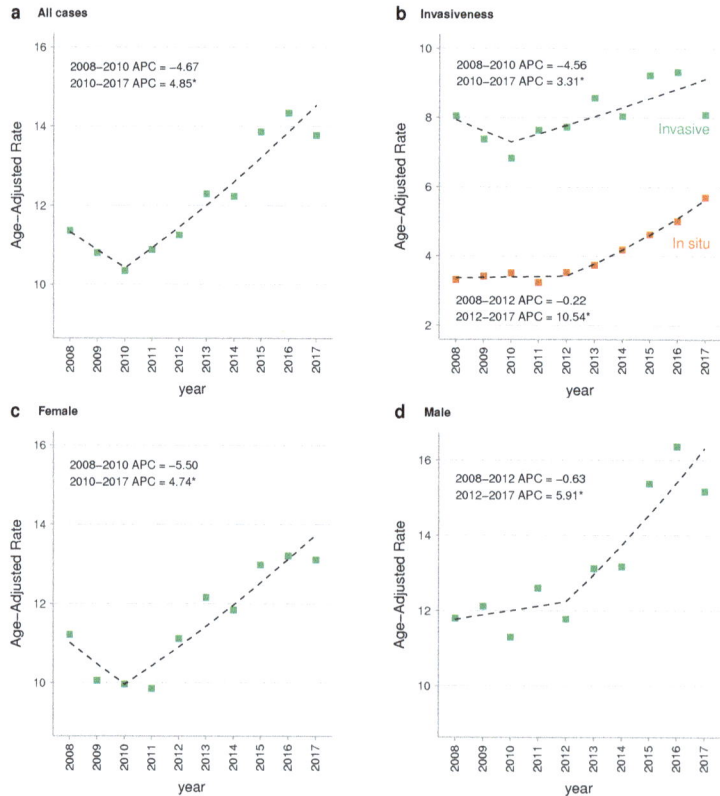

Figure 3. Joinpoint regression analysis of melanoma age-standardised incidence rate. European age-standardised incidence rate trends for melanoma lesions in Catalonia in the period 2008–2017. Squares shapes represent the observed values and dashed lines represent the joinpoint models. (*) APCs were significantly different from zero at alpha = 0.05. Abbreviations: APC, annual percent change.

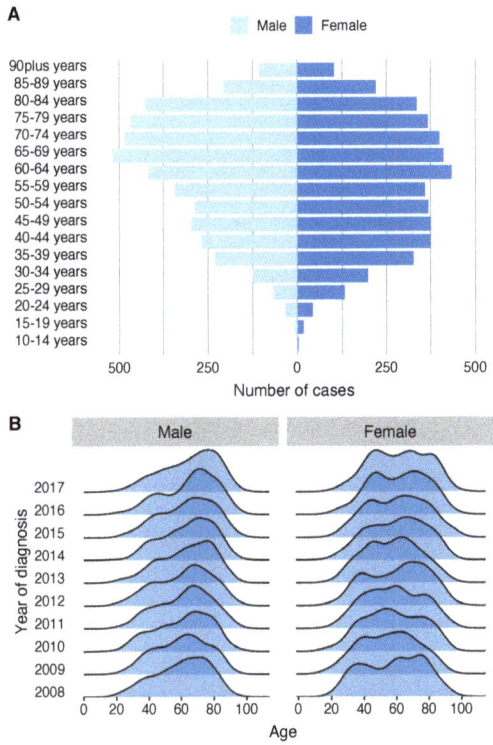

Figure 4. Pyramid plot in (**A**) shows that cases occur at younger ages in women showing a double peak of incidence; however, in men they present in a single peak of incidence at older ages. (**B**) shows a ridgeline with the distribution trend across the years of the study.

4. Discussion

Our study demonstrates that the incidence of melanoma in Catalonia continued to increase during the 2008 to 2017 period with a rising trend which mainly affected elderly patients. This increase has been consistently observed in other countries with predominantly Caucasian populations [23–25] and this rising trend is consisted with a previous period studied in Catalonia [26]. Despite this increase in incidence, the age-standardised incidence rate (ASIR) of invasive melanoma in Spain is relatively low (ASIR 6.4) in the GLOBOCAN registry in comparison with other European Mediterranean countries such as France (ASIR 13.6), Italy (ASIR 12.4), Greece (ASIR 8.7) and Malta (ASIR 8.0) [23]. This could be explained in part by an underestimation due to the lack of a comprehensive national Spanish melanoma registry. Another explanation could be the patient's phenotype (e.g., skin type, red hair) [27] and genotype (e.g., MC1R polymorphisms status), sunlight incidence during the year [28], sun-exposure behavior [29] and the Mediterranean diet which has also been reported as a favorable modifying factor of melanoma incidence [30]. A further possible explanation is the large foreign population living in Catalonia mainly coming from countries with a pigmented skin population and/or low melanoma incidence. In 2017, there were 1,041,362 immigrants which corresponds to 13.9% of the Catalan population: 27.7% were from Africa and 17.4% from South America which could dilute the cases of melanoma and lower the incidence rate [15].

Recent epidemiological data have shown a steady increase in the incidence of melanoma of 3% per year and it is expected that by 2030 the number of melanoma cases will double that of 2016 [25]. Our data showed an AAPC of 3.5% and APC of 4.9% during the last period which is consistent with what has been reported in the literature. If these predictions are accurate, the expected increase in melanoma prevalence will be associated with higher treatment costs, as some of these patients will require new target treatments and immunotherapy [25].

The analysis by melanoma subtype showed that the age-standardised incidence rate of invasive melanomas increased slightly with an AAPC of 2.1% while in situ melanomas almost doubled their incidence with an AAPC of 6.5%. These results are consistent with the findings of a large European study by Sacchetto et al. [31], who observed a significant incidence increase in both invasive (AAPC 4.0%) and more markedly for in situ melanoma (AAPC 7.7%). An increase in incidence of these proportions could mean a lifetime risk of developing in situ melanoma of 1 in 58 people [32]. Although the incidence of invasive melanoma is not as marked as in situ melanoma, the absolute number of thick melanomas continues to rise, which could have an serious impact in the mortality of the patients and costs related to the new treatments [32].

We have observed in this cohort that the proportion of invasive melanomas is higher than in situ melanomas with a ratio of approximately 2:1. This ratio is in line with other European cohorts [31]. On the other hand, in the SEER registry the ratio of invasive versus in-situ melanoma is close to 1:1 [10,33]. One possible explanation is that many low-risk patients are normally seen in private clinics and some of them are not entered in the regional registries.

The increasing trend in incidence during the study decade was observed in the 60–70 age group and above, while the younger age groups remained fairly stable. Moreover, the histological subtype that increased notably during this period is the lentigo maligna subtype. This trend was observed in the study by Swetter et al. who reported a significant increase in melanoma in-situ in the older population. They also found that lentigo maligna accounted for 79–83% of the total diagnoses of the in-situ subtype [34]. All these findings could be explained by accumulated harm from UV (ultraviolet) radiation since childhood as UV exposure and resulting from occupations with high sun exposure (>20 years) leading to the development of melanoma [27]. Large public initiatives to decrease sun exposure have been carried out for many years [5–9,35], but unfortunately, these campaigns will not benefit older people today who could have already had intense sun exposure during childhood. This could explain the significant increase in incidence from age 50 years onwards which we have seen in our study and the important increase in the lentigo maligna melanoma subtype. Another possible explanation for the increase in incidence has partially been attributed to the development of highly sensitive diagnostic techniques during the last decade, principally the use of dermatoscopy which has allowed the detection of clinically unidentifiable tumors [36].

In the stratified analysis by sex, we observed that in both sexes the age-standardised incidence rate showed a rising trend with an AAPC of 3.9% for men and 3.2% in women; moreover, the age-standardised incidence rate was higher in men throughout the study period. Different authors have described that melanoma incidence differs between men and women by age, with women having higher rates of melanoma early in life and men at later stages of life [37–39]. One biological explanation for this difference could be related to the hormonal profile. It has been seen that high levels of oestrogen during a woman's fertile period can promote the formation of reactive oxygen species which seem to favour the development of melanoma seen in younger women [40].

Strengths and Limitations

A strength of this study was the ability to collect all data prospectively from the main reference hospitals in Catalonia. As a limitation of the study, private centres are not included, resulting in a possible underestimation of a proportion of early melanomas as well as possible differences in melanoma subtypes. Furthermore, this study does not include mortality data.

- **Author Contributions:** Conceptualisation, all authors; formal analysis, S.P. (Sebastian Podlipnik) and S.P. (Susana Puig); funding acquisition—supporting, S.P. (Susana Puig), C.C. and J.M. (Josep Malvehy); investigation, S.P. (Sebastian Podlipnik); methodology S.P. (Sebastian Podlipnik), S.P. (Susana Puig), C.C. and J.M. (Josep Malvehy); data curation, all authors; software, S.P. (Sebastian Podlipnik); supervision, S.P. (Susana Puig) and

J.M. (Josep Malvehy); validation, S.P. (Sebastian Podlipnik) and S.P. (Susana Puig); visualisation, S.P. (Sebastian Podlipnik); writing—original, S.P. (Sebastian Podlipnik); writing—review and editing all authors. All authors have read and agreed to the published version of the manuscript.

Funding: The study in the Melanoma Unit, Hospital Clínic, Barcelona was supported in part by grants from Fondo de Investigaciones Sanitarias P.I. 12/00840, PI 15/00956, and PI 15/00716 Spain; by the CIBER de Enfermedades Raras of the Instituto de Salud Carlos III, Spain, co-funded by "Fondo Europeo de Desarrollo Regional (FEDER). Unión Europea. Una manera de hacer Europa"; by the AGAUR 2014_SGR_603 and 2017_SGR_1134 of the Catalan Government, Spain; by a grant from "Fundació La Marató de TV3, 201331-30", Catalonia, Spain; by the European Commission under the 6th Framework Programme, Contract n°: LSHC-CT-2006-018702 (GenoMEL); by CERCA Programme/Generalitat de Catalunya; by a Research Grant from "Fundación Científica de la Asociación Española Contra el Cáncer" GCB15152978SOEN, Spain; by a grant from the European Academy of Dermatology and Venereology (EADV) (PPRC-2017/19). Part of the work was developed at the building Centro Esther Koplowitz. Melanoma research at the Department of Dermatology of Hospital Universitari Arnau de Vilanova de Lleida is supported by grants from ISCIII (PI15/00711 to RMM, cofinanced by FEDER "Una manera de hacer Europa" and CIBERONC- CB16/12/00231) and from Fundació la Marató de TV3 (FMTV 201331-31 to RMM).

Acknowledgments: Thanks to our patients and their families who are the main reason for our studies. To Paul Hetherington for his help with English editing and correction of the manuscript in English.

Conflicts of Interest: The authors have no conflict of interest to declare. The sponsors had no role in the design and conduct of the study; in the collection, analysis, and interpretation of data, nor in the preparation, review, or approval of the manuscript.

References

1. Miller, A.J.; Mihm, M.C. Melanoma. *N. Engl. J. Med.* **2006**, *355*, 51–65. [CrossRef] [PubMed]
2. Guy, G.P.; Ekwueme, D.U. Years of Potential Life Lost and Indirect Costs of Melanoma and Non-Melanoma Skin Cancer. *PharmacoEconomics* **2011**, *29*, 863–874. [CrossRef] [PubMed]
3. Burnet, N.G.; Jefferies, S.J.; Benson, R.J.; Hunt, D.P.; Treasure, F.P. Years of life lost (YLL) from cancer is an important measure of population burden—And should be considered when allocating research funds. *Br. J. Cancer* **2005**, *92*, 241–245. [CrossRef] [PubMed]
4. Schadendorf, D.; van Akkooi, A.C.J.; Berking, C.; Griewank, K.G.; Gutzmer, R.; Hauschild, A.; Stang, A.; Roesch, A.; Ugurel, S. Melanoma. *Lancet* **2018**, *392*, 971–984. [CrossRef]
5. Stratigos, A.J.; Forsea, A.M.; van der Leest, R.J.T.; de Vries, E.; Nagore, E.; Bulliard, J.L.; Trakatelli, M.; Paoli, J.; Peris, K.; Hercogova, J.; et al. Euromelanoma: A dermatology-led European campaign against nonmelanoma skin cancer and cutaneous melanoma. Past, present and future. *Br. J. Dermatol.* **2012**, *167*, 99–104. [CrossRef]
6. Melia, J.; Cooper, E.J.; Frost, T.; Graham-Brown, R.; Hunter, J.; Marsden, A.; Du Vivier, A.; White, J.; Whitehead, S.; Warin, A.P. Cancer Research Campaign health education programme to promote the early detection of cutaneous malignant melanoma. II. Characteristics and incidence of melanoma. *Br. J. Dermatol.* **1995**, *132*, 414–21. [CrossRef]
7. Stang, A.; Jöckel, K.H.; Heidinger, O. Skin cancer rates in North Rhine-Westphalia, Germany before and after the introduction of the nationwide skin cancer screening program (2000–2015). *Eur. J. Epidemiol.* **2018**, *33*, 303–312. [CrossRef]
8. Katalinic, A.; Waldmann, A.; Weinstock, M.A.; Geller, A.C.; Eisemann, N.; Greinert, R.; Volkmer, B.; Breitbart, E. Does skin cancer screening save lives? *Cancer* **2012**, *118*, 5395–5402. [CrossRef] [PubMed]
9. Berwick, M.; Buller, D.B.; Cust, A.; Gallagher, R.; Lee, T.K.; Meyskens, F.; Pandey, S.; Thomas, N.E.; Veierød, M.B.; Ward, S. Melanoma Epidemiology and Prevention. In *Melanoma. Cancer Treatment and Research*; Kaufman, H., Mehnert, J., Eds.; Springer: Cham, Switzerland, 2016; pp. 17–49._2. [CrossRef]
10. National Cancer Institute. *SEER Cancer Stat Facts: Melanoma of the Skin;* National Cancer Institute: Bethesda, MD, USA. Available online: https://seer.cancer.gov/statfacts/html/melan.html (accessed on 22 October 2020).
11. International Agency for Research on Cancer; WHO. *GLOBOCAN 2012: Estimated Cancer Incidence, Mortality, and Prevalence Worldwide in 2018*; International Agency for Research on Cancer: Lyon, France, 2018.
12. Wong, D.J.L.; Ribas, A. Melanoma. In *Cancer Treatment and Research*; Springer International Publishing: Cham, Switzerland, 2016; Volume 167, pp. 251–262. [CrossRef]
13. Berk-Krauss, J.; Stein, J.A.; Weber, J.; Polsky, D.; Geller, A.C. New Systematic Therapies and Trends in Cutaneous Melanoma Deaths Among US Whites, 1986–2016. *Am. J. Public Health* **2020**, *110*, 731–733. [CrossRef] [PubMed]

14. Poizeau, F.; Kerbrat, S.; Happe, A.; Rault, C.; Drezen, E.; Balusson, F.; Tuppin, P.; Guillot, B.; Thuret, A.; Boussemart, L.; et al. Patients with metastatic melanoma receiving anticancer drugs: Changes in overall survival, 2010–2017. *J. Investig. Dermatol.* **2020**. [CrossRef] [PubMed]
15. Idescat. Tema. Población. Cifras de población. Available online: https://www.idescat.cat/ (accessed on 22 October 2012).
16. Von Elm, E.; Altman, D.G.; Egger, M.; Pocock, S.J.; Gøtzsche, P.C.; Vandenbroucke, J.P. The Strengthening the Reporting of Observational Studies in Epidemiology (STROBE) statement: Guidelines for reporting observational studies. *Lancet* **2007**, *370*, 1453–1457. [CrossRef]
17. Eurostat. *Revision of the European Standard Population. Report of Eurostat's Task Force*; Number 1346; Publications Office of the European Union: Luxembourg, 2013; p. 121. [CrossRef]
18. Fay, M.P.; Feuer, E.J. Confidence intervals for directly standardized rates: A method based on the gamma distribution. *Stat. Med.* **1997**, *16*, 791–801.:7<791::aid-sim500>3.0.co;2-%23. [CrossRef]
19. Number of Joinpoints—Joinpoint Help System. Available online: https://surveillance.cancer.gov/help/joinpoint/setting-parameters/method-and-parameters-tab/number-of-joinpoints (accessed on 22 October 2012).
20. RStudio Team. *RStudio: Integrated Development Environment for R*; RStudio Team: Boston, MA, USA, 2018. Available online: http://www.rstudio.com/ (accessed on 22 October 2012).
21. R Core Team. *R: A Language and Environment for Statistical Computing*; R Core Team: Vienna, Austria, 2020.
22. Joinpoint Regression Program, Version 4.8.0.1–April 2020; Statistical Methodology and Applications Branch, Surveillance Research Program, National Cancer Institute. Available online: https://surveillance.cancer.gov/joinpoint/ (accessed on 22 October 2020).
23. Bray, F.; Ferlay, J.; Soerjomataram, I.; Siegel, R.L.; Torre, L.A.; Jemal, A. Global cancer statistics 2018: GLOBOCAN estimates of incidence and mortality worldwide for 36 cancers in 185 countries. *CA Cancer J. Clin.* **2018**, *68*, 394–424. [CrossRef]
24. Clarke, C.A.; McKinley, M.; Hurley, S.; Haile, R.W.; Glaser, S.L.; Keegan, T.H.; Swetter, S.M. Continued Increase in Melanoma Incidence across all Socioeconomic Status Groups in California, 1998–2012. *J. Investig. Dermatol.* **2017**, *137*, 2282–2290. [CrossRef]
25. Gershenwald, J.E.; Guy, G.P. Stemming the Rising Incidence of Melanoma: Calling Prevention to Action. *J. Natl. Cancer Inst.* **2016**, *108*, djv381–djv381. [CrossRef] [PubMed]
26. Puig, S.; Marcoval, J.; Paradelo, C.; Azon, A.; Bartralot, R.; Bel, S.; Bigata, X.; Boada, A.; Campoy, A.; Carrera, C.; et al. Melanoma incidence increases in the elderly of Catalonia but not in the younger population: Effect of prevention or consequence of immigration? *Acta Derm. Venereol.* **2015**, *95*, 422–426. [CrossRef]
27. Carr, S.; Smith, C.; Wernberg, J. Epidemiology and Risk Factors of Melanoma. *Surg. Clin. N. Am.* **2020**, *100*, 1–12. [CrossRef]
28. Moan, J.; Baturaite, Z.; Porojnicu, A.C.; Dahlback, A.; Juzeniene, A. UVA, UVB and incidence of cutaneous malignant melanoma in Norway and Sweden. *Photochem. Photobiol. Sci.* **2012**, *11*, 191–198. [CrossRef]
29. Bataille, V.; Winnett, A.; Sasieni, P.; Newton Bishop, J.; Cuzick, J. Exposure to the sun and sunbeds and the risk of cutaneous melanoma in the UK: A case—Control study. *Eur. J. Cancer* **2004**, *40*, 429–435. [CrossRef]
30. Fortes, C.; Mastroeni, S.; Melchi, F.; Pilla, M.A.; Antonelli, G.; Camaioni, D.; Alotto, M.; Pasquini, P. A protective effect of the Mediterranean diet for cutaneous melanoma. *Int. J. Epidemiol.* **2008**, *37*, 1018–1029. [CrossRef]
31. Sacchetto, L.; Zanetti, R.; Comber, H.; Bouchardy, C.; Brewster, D.; Broganelli, P.; Chirlaque, M.; Coza, D.; Galceran, J.; Gavin, A.; et al. Trends in incidence of thick, thin and in situ melanoma in Europe. *Eur. J. Cancer* **2018**, *92*, 108–118. [CrossRef]
32. Glazer, A.M.; Winkelmann, R.R.; Farberg, A.S.; Rigel, D.S. Analysis of Trends in US Melanoma Incidence and Mortality. *JAMA Dermatol.* **2017**, *153*, 225. [CrossRef]
33. Siegel, R.L.; Miller, K.D.; Jemal, A. Cancer statistics, 2020. *CA Cancer J. Clin.* **2020**, *70*, 7–30. [CrossRef] [PubMed]
34. Swetter, S.M.; Boldrick, J.C.; Jung, S.Y.; Egbert, B.M.; Harvell, J.D. Increasing incidence of lentigo maligna melanoma subtypes: Northern California and national trends 1990–2000. *J. Investig. Dermatol.* **2005**, *125*, 685–691. [CrossRef]
35. Olsen, C.M.; Whiteman, D.C. Clinical Epidemiology of Melanoma. In *Cutaneous Melanoma*; Springer International Publishing: Cham, Switzerland, 2020; pp. 425–449._47. [CrossRef]

36. Lallas, A.; Apalla, Z.; Chaidemenos, G. New Trends in Dermoscopy to Minimize the Risk of Missing Melanoma. *J. Skin Cancer* **2012**, *2012*, 1–5. [CrossRef] [PubMed]
37. Olsen, C.M.; Thompson, J.F.; Pandeya, N.; Whiteman, D.C. Evaluation of Sex-Specific Incidence of Melanoma. *JAMA Dermatol.* **2020**, *156*, 553. [CrossRef]
38. Rastrelli, M.; Tropea, S.; Rossi, C.R.; Alaibac, M. Melanoma: Epidemiology, risk factors, pathogenesis, diagnosis and classification. *In Vivo* **2014**, *28*, 1005–1011.
39. Najita, J.S.; Swetter, S.M.; Geller, A.C.; Gershenwald, J.E.; Zelen, M.; Lee, S.J. Sex Differences in Age at Primary Melanoma Diagnosis in a Population-Based Analysis (US Surveillance, Epidemiology, and End Results, 2005–2011). *J. Investig. Dermatol.* **2016**, *136*, 1894–1897. [CrossRef]
40. Lira, F.; Podlipnik, S.; Potrony, M.; Tell-Martí, G.; Calbet-Llopart, N.; Barreiro, A.; Carrera, C.; Malvehy, J.; Puig, S. Inherited MC 1R variants in patients with melanoma are associated with better survival in women. *Br. J. Dermatol.* **2019**. [CrossRef] [PubMed]

Publisher's Note: MDPI stays neutral with regard to jurisdictional claims in published maps and institutional affiliations.

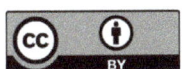

© 2020 by the authors. Licensee MDPI, Basel, Switzerland. This article is an open access article distributed under the terms and conditions of the Creative Commons Attribution (CC BY) license (http://creativecommons.org/licenses/by/4.0/).

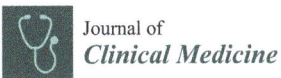

Journal of
Clinical Medicine

Review

An Update on the Role of Ubiquitination in Melanoma Development and Therapies

Frédéric Soysouvanh [1,†], Serena Giuliano [1,†], Nadia Habel [1,†], Najla El-Hachem [2], Céline Pisibon [1], Corine Bertolotto [1,3,‡] and Robert Ballotti [1,4,*,‡]

1. Inserm U1065, C3M, Team 1, Biology, and Pathologies of Melanocytes, University of Nice Côte d'Azur, 06200 Nice, France; frederic.soysouvanh@unice.fr (F.S.); serena.giuliano@univ-cotedazur.fr (S.G.); nadia.habel20@gmail.com (N.H.); celine.pisibon@etu.univ-cotedazur.fr (C.P.); corine.bertolotto@univ-cotedazur.fr (C.B.)
2. Laboratory of Cancer Signaling, University of Liège, 4020 Liège, Belgium; nelhachem@uliege.be
3. Equipe labellisée Fondation ARC 2019, 06200 Nice, France
4. Equipe labellisée Ligue Contre le Cancer 2020, 06200 Nice, France
* Correspondence: ballotti@unice.fr; Tel.: +33-4-89-06-43-32
† Equal contribution.
‡ Equal contribution.

Citation: Soysouvanh, F.; Giuliano, S.; Habel, N.; El-Hachem, N.; Pisibon, C.; Bertolotto, C.; Ballotti, R. An Update on the Role of Ubiquitination in Melanoma Development and Therapies. *J. Clin. Med.* **2021**, *10*, 1133. https://doi.org/10.3390/jcm10051133

Academic Editor: Lionel Larribère

Received: 8 January 2021
Accepted: 25 February 2021
Published: 8 March 2021

Publisher's Note: MDPI stays neutral with regard to jurisdictional claims in published maps and institutional affiliations.

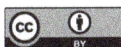

Copyright: © 2021 by the authors. Licensee MDPI, Basel, Switzerland. This article is an open access article distributed under the terms and conditions of the Creative Commons Attribution (CC BY) license (https://creativecommons.org/licenses/by/4.0/).

Abstract: The ubiquitination system plays a critical role in regulation of large array of biological processes and its alteration has been involved in the pathogenesis of cancers, among them cutaneous melanoma, which is responsible for the most deaths from skin cancers. Over the last decades, targeted therapies and immunotherapies became the standard therapeutic strategies for advanced melanomas. However, despite these breakthroughs, the prognosis of metastatic melanoma patients remains unoptimistic, mainly due to intrinsic or acquired resistances. Many avenues of research have been investigated to find new therapeutic targets for improving patient outcomes. Because of the pleiotropic functions of ubiquitination, and because each step of ubiquitination is amenable to pharmacological targeting, much attention has been paid to the role of this process in melanoma development and resistance to therapies. In this review, we summarize the latest data on ubiquitination and discuss the possible impacts on melanoma treatments.

Keywords: melanoma; treatment; ubiquitination

1. Introduction

Ubiquitination, one of the most conserved protein post-translational modifications, is controlled by the ubiquitin system, a dynamic multifaceted network involved in nearly all aspects of eukaryotic biology. Ubiquitination refers to the covalent attachment of a highly conserved 76-amino acid protein, the ubiquitin, to lysine residues on target proteins. The addition of a single ubiquitin protein or ubiquitin chain is mediated by a cascade of enzymatic reactions carried out by activating, conjugating, and ligating enzymes. The ubiquitination process is well-known to play a key role in protein homeostasis through the control of 26S-mediated proteasome degradation, but also includes nonproteolytic roles, such as receptor internalization, assembly of multiprotein complexes, inflammatory signaling, DNA damage repair, cell death, autophagy, or metabolism [1].

Many proteins, regulated by ubiquitination, control cellular processes relevant to tumorigenesis, such as the modulation of the activity of tumor promoters and suppressors. One of the best-known examples is the RING-type E3 ubiquitin ligase MDM2, a negative regulator of the p53 tumor suppressor [2]. Therefore, ubiquitination enzymes are considered potential therapeutic targets for cancers [3,4]. After the successful clinical application and the approval of proteasomal inhibitors for the treatment of multiple myeloma, substantial progress has been made in understanding the molecular mechanisms of ubiquitin in cancer-relevant processes, and shed light on the therapeutic potential of the ubiquitin system [5].

Even though defects in ubiquitination are not among the most frequent alterations in melanoma, this process has gained more and more attention in the field, as demonstrated by the nearly 300 publications on melanoma and ubiquitination since the last review of Ma et al. in 2017.

2. Brief Overview of Melanoma and Its Treatments

Historically, melanoma was a rare cancer, but its incidence has risen rapidly in the last decades. Melanomas represent about 5% of skin cancers, but they are responsible for 90% of deaths from skin cancers. Significant advances in the understanding of melanoma physiopathology have led to the development of new effective treatments for advanced melanomas. Indeed, the identification of BRAF^{V600} mutations in about 50% of melanomas has led to the development of the first targeted therapies (TTs) for patients harboring these mutations. Now, a combination of the BRAF inhibitor (BRAFi) and the MEK inhibitor (MEKi) has shown an overall response rate of up to 70% and has become the standard targeted treatment for BRAF^{V600}-mutated melanomas [6]. However, even though long-term responses have been reported, most patients develop resistance and relapse [7,8].

The other breakthrough in melanoma treatment came from immune checkpoint therapies (ICTs), using anti-CTLA4 (Cytotoxic T-Lymphocyte-associated antigen 4) or anti-PD-1 (Programmed cell death protein 1) antibodies. ICTs also showed a dramatic response rate of 44% for anti-PD-1, 20% for anti-CTLA4, and up to 58% when combining both treatments. More interestingly, up to 30% of patients showed a complete and durable response [6,7,9–12]. Now, the combination of CTLA-4, and PD-1 checkpoint blockades has been proven as a highly efficient treatment for patients with advanced melanomas [13,14]. However, more than half of the patients do not respond to ICT [8,15].

Despite treatment breakthroughs that for the first time improved the survival of patients, the prognosis of metastatic melanoma patients remains unoptimistic. Because of intrinsic or acquired resistance, approximately 50% of patients find themselves in a therapeutic dead-end, which has prompted further research of adjuvant therapies that can improve the efficiency of current standard treatments and patients' outcomes.

From this perspective, attention has been paid to the regulation of ubiquitination and its consequences on melanoma development and treatments. In this review, we focus on the latest data on ubiquitination in melanoma and discuss the possible impact on melanoma treatments.

3. A Glimpse of Ubiquitination Processes

Ubiquitination is catalyzed by three distinct biochemical steps: activation, conjugation, and ligation, performed by ubiquitin-activating enzymes (E1s), ubiquitin-conjugating enzymes (E2s), and ubiquitin ligases (E3s), respectively [16]. The first enzyme, E1, catalyzes ubiquitin activation by adenylation of the ubiquitin C-terminus. Subsequently, the mature ubiquitin (Ub) is transferred to the E2-conjugating enzymes. In the final step, the covalent linking of the ubiquitin on the target protein is catalyzed by the E3 ligase, acting as an adapter that recognizes the substrate and mediates the interaction with the Ub-E2. Different combinations of E2 and E3 are possible, providing a wide variability in signal integration and conveying [16] (Figure 1).

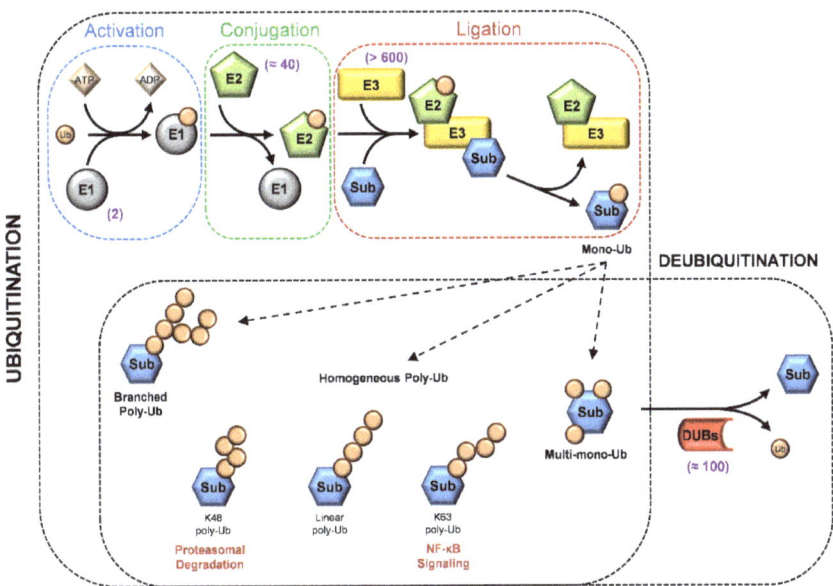

Figure 1. The ubiquitination and deubiquitination process. In the upper panel, three distinct biochemical steps are required for substrate (Sub) ubiquitination: activation performed by activating enzymes (E1s), conjugation by conjugating enzymes (E2s), and ligation by ubiquitin ligases (E3s). In the lower panel, there are different ubiquitin (Ub) modifications and a schematic representation of deubiquitination performed by deubiquitinating enzymes (DUBs). The number of members of each type of enzymes in mammals are highlighted in purple.

E3s are classified into two general classes on the basis of specific protein motifs, the HECT and the RING domain. The HECT domain family is endowed with an intrinsic E3 ligase activity, while the RING-E3 ligases are devoid of enzymatic activity and use the RING domain to bring the E2 ligase to the substrate. The RING domain E3 ligases are divided in single-subunit or multi-subunit proteins, in which the substrate-binding site and RING domain are in the same protein or in a different subunit of the complex [16,17].

The regulation of the various cellular processes is also mediated by different types of ubiquitination. The ubiquitin forms a peptide bond between the ε-NH2 group on the substrate lysyl residues and the C-terminus carboxyl group of Ub (monoubiquitination). It is also possible that multiple lysines in the same substrate are ubiquitinated (multi-monoubiquitination). Ubiquitin, once linked to the target protein, can itself be ubiquitinated on any of its lysine residues (K6, K11, K27, K29, K33, K48, and K63) or its N-terminus methionine (M1), generating poly-Ub chains (polyubiquitination) by the sequential addition of Ub. Poly-Ub chains are homogenous when, during elongation, each ubiquitin is attached to the previous one by the same lysine or methionine or is branched when ubiquitin is linked to a different residue than the previous one. Mixes of homogenous and branched chains also exist [16,18]. These different chain topologies trigger distinct outcomes indicating that the different types of ubiquitin chains can operate as a code, transferring various information to the target proteins [18].

For instance, canonical K48-linked poly-Ub chains are usually the principal signal to target substrates for 26S proteasome proteolysis [19,20]. In contrast, K63-linked chains can act as non-proteolytic signals in several intracellular pathways [21,22]. Ubiquitination can affect protein activity and/or degradation, influencing the regulation of numerous signal pathways. For instance, the NF-κB pathway activation occurs with the degradation of the inhibitor of the NF-κB transcription factor (IκBα). The proteolytic process is initiated by SCFβ-TrCP, a multi-subunit E3 ubiquitin ligase complex [23,24]. In addition, activation of the NF-κB pathway involves the E3 ligase tumor necrosis factor receptor-associated factor 6, TRAF6, which governs the K63-linked polyubiquitination on IKKg (NEMO). This process leads to the release of NF-κB from its inhibitor, and ultimately induces the expression of specific genes [21,22,25].

As ubiquitination is a reversible process, the removal of ubiquitin adducts also plays a key role in cellular biological functions. The deconjugation reactions are catalyzed by deubiquitinating enzymes (DUBs) that precisely cleave the peptide bond between ubiquitin and the target protein after the Gly76 C-terminus of ubiquitin, or between ubiquitins (Figure 1). On the basis of the sequence and domain conservation, DUBs can also be divided into distinct subfamilies, among which ubiquitin-specific proteases (USPs) represent the largest class [26].

Therefore, DUBs, as well as E1, E2, and E3 enzymes, contribute to modulating activation/deactivation, recycling and localizing regulatory proteins, and play important roles in diverse cellular processes, such as DNA repair, apoptosis, cell proliferation, and kinase activation [27].

Compelling evidence established the critical role of ubiquitination in melanoma progression. Indeed, mutations in the deubiquitinating enzyme BRCA1-associated protein 1 (BAP1), in the E3 ligase (or E3 ligase complex) Parkinson protein 2 (PARK2), and in the F-box and WD repeat-containing 7 protein (FBXW7), were shown to favor melanoma development [3]. Moreover, ubiquitination plays an instrumental role in key signaling pathways for melanoma pathogenesis, such as the NF-κB and Wnt/β-catenin pathways [3,28–31]. In the last three years, numerous studies have increased our knowledge on the involvement of ubiquitination processes in melanoma progression. In the following sections, we focus on the most recent reports dealing with the role of E2, E3, and DUB proteins in melanoma biology.

4. E2 Enzyme Involvement in Melanoma Progression

The E2 enzyme family is comprised of nearly 40 members that are involved in the conjugation of Ub or Ub-like molecules to target proteins. The E2 enzymes have been classified into 17 families according to a comprehensive phylogenetic analysis, but broadly fall into 4 different classes: class I contains only the Ub-conjugating (UBC) domain, classes II and III have N- or C-terminus extensions, respectively, and class IV has both N- and C-terminus extensions [32,33]. E2 enzymes are involved in cell cycle progression, DNA repair, apoptosis, and the stimulation of oncogenic signaling pathways (Table 1). In the following section, we describe the roles of E2 enzymes in melanoma progression.

Members of the E2 family were reported to be dysregulated in many cancer types, including melanoma [34]. Indeed, gene expression studies in primary cutaneous melanomas have shown that Ub-conjugating enzyme E2-T (UBE2T) gene expression positively correlates with cell proliferation, tumor progression, and poor prognosis outcome [35]. UBE2T has been involved in the development of various cancers, such as breast cancer through the inhibition of the expression of BRCA1, nasopharyngeal carcinoma by triggering the AKT/Glycogen Synthase Kinase (GSK)-3β/β-catenin pathway, or multiple myeloma as a poor prognosis marker [36–38]. A recent study from Dikshit et al. showed that Ub-conjugating enzyme E2-N (UBE2N/Ubc13), a class I E2 enzyme involved in DNA repair, was overexpressed in melanoma cells and played a critical role in melanoma growth and progression both in vitro and in vivo [39]. The systemic inhibition of UBE2N by a selective small molecule, NSC697923, impaired melanoma xenograft growth. In addition to its role in melanoma progression, the authors showed that UBE2N positively regulated and maintained the MEK/FRA1 (Fos-Related Antigen 1)/SOX10 (SRY-related HMG box-containing factor 10) signaling cascade that plays a key role in melanomas [39]. Another E2 enzyme was recently demonstrated to participate in melanoma progression. The Ub-conjugating enzyme E2-C (UBE2C), a key regulator of cell progression, is upregulated in melanomas compared to Spitz nevus [40]. Furthermore, the high mRNA expression level of UBE2C is associated with poor overall survival of patients with melanoma, according to the cancer genome atlas (TCGA) database [41]. The downregulation of UBE2C suppressed melanoma cell growth via the inactivation of the ERK and AKT signaling pathways and the induction of apoptosis. Finally, it was also shown that the knockdown of UBE2C inhibited the growth of xenografted melanoma [41].

Among the E2 family, some members can conjugate small molecules, called Ub-like proteins (UBL), such as small Ub-related modifier (SUMO), neural precursor cell expressed developmentally down-regulated protein 8 (NEDD8), autophagy-related protein 8 (ATG8), autophagy-related protein 12 (ATG12), Ub-related modifier 1 (URM1), Ub-fold modifier 1 (UFM1), human leukocyte antigen F locus adjacent transcript 10 (FAT10), and interferon-stimulated gene 15 (ISG15) [42]. Like ubiquitin, when conjugated to target proteins, UBLs can regulate their activity, stability, subcellular localization, or macromolecular interactions. Furthermore, a crosstalk between ubiquitylation and another post-translational modification, called SUMOylation, has been demonstrated. SUMOylation targets proteins involved in cell cycle regulation, proliferation, apoptosis, and DNA repair. Thus, SUMOylation could impact cancer progression and/or drug responsiveness. As Ub-conjugating enzyme E2-I (UBE2I), also known as Ubc9, is absolutely required for SUMOylation, it has been the subject of numerous studies as a potential target for cancer therapy [43,44]. In melanoma, Ubc9 seems to be upregulated, involved in proliferation, and could play a role in apoptosis evasion in response to chemotherapy treatments [43,45]. Interestingly, it was also demonstrated that Ubc9 interacted with the microphthalmia-associated transcription factor (MITF) [46]. The MITF plays a critical role in melanocyte differentiation, but also melanomagenesis, allowing the transition of melanoma cells between a differentiated-proliferative phenotype and a stem cell-like phenotype [47]. It was described that Ubc9 targets the MITF to the proteasome for degradation, and may favor the transition toward a dedifferentiated and metastatic melanoma phenotype [46]. Whether this regulation involved SUMOylation of ubiquitination remains to be clarified. Nevertheless, SUMOylation of the MITF is paramount for melanoma pathogenesis, as patients with a germline mutation that prevents K316 SUMOylation have an increased risk of developing melanoma [48]. Thus, Ubc9 appears to be a potential target to limit melanoma development.

The ubiquitin-conjugating enzyme E2S (UBE2S) could also play a role in melanoma and be an appealing target. Depletion of UBE2S using short hairpin RNA in melanoma cells resulted in an inhibition of proliferation, a cell cycle arrest, and an increase in apoptosis [49]. In vivo, UBE2S depletion resulted in tumor growth inhibition and the suppression of epithelial-to-mesenchymal transition (EMT)-related markers [49].

RAD6, a ubiquitin-conjugating E2 enzyme, was found to be overexpressed in primary and metastatic melanomas. RAD6 is encoded by two genes, UBE2A (RAD6A) and UBE2B (RAD6B), so Gajan et al. investigated their expression levels in normal melanocytes and melanomas. They demonstrated a selective upregulation of RAD6B in melanoma cells [50]. RAD6B was also linked to Wnt/β-catenin signaling during melanoma progression [51]. RAD6B depletion in metastatic melanoma decreased cell migration, tumor growth, and lung metastasis. The loss of RAD6B also inhibited protein steady-state levels of β-catenin and its transcriptional targets, such as MITF, SOX10, and vimentin. A pathway analysis of transcriptomic data highlighted the implication of various networks, amongst them protein ubiquitination and Wnt signaling [51]. Overall, these findings demonstrate a clear connection between RAD6B and Wnt/β-catenin signaling in melanoma cells and suggest the possibility of targeting RAD6B as a new strategy to treat melanoma.

The involvement of E2 enzymes in many cancer types suggests that specific small chemical inhibitors of E2 enzymes might be valuable in the treatment of cancers, including melanoma. Until now, few E2 enzyme inhibitors have been described [4]. For instance, Leucettamol A and Manadosterols A and B can inhibit Ubc13–UEV1A interaction and block the formation of their complex [4]. CC0651, a small-molecule selective allosteric site inhibitor of the E2 enzyme hCdc34, can block the ubiquitination and degradation of p27 and then inhibit tumor cell proliferation [4]. To date, none of these small molecules have been assessed in the context of melanoma.

Table 1. Summary table of identified E2 enzymes and their functional roles in melanoma.

E2 Class		E2s	Roles in Melanoma	Refs
I	UBC domain	UBE2N UBE2I UBE2B	Overexpressed, proliferation and malignancy Proliferation, apoptosis evasion, sumoylation of MITF	[39] [44–47] [50,51]
II	N-ter — UBC domain	UBE2C	Overexpressed, progression and pathogenesis Overexpressed, associated with poor prognosis	[40,41]
III	UBC domain — C-ter	UBE2T UBE2S	Overexpressed, biological role to be determined Proliferation, cell survival, tumor growth, EMT	[35] [49]
IV	N-ter — UBC domain — C-ter			

5. E3 Enzyme Involvement in Melanoma

The E3 ubiquitin ligases are considered the most important and specific enzymes in the ubiquitin conjugation machinery. In recent years, E3 ligases received interest as drug targets for their ability to regulate protein stability. Indeed, compared to inhibitors that block the protein degradation through the proteasome, drugs that target E3 ligase are expected to have better selectivity and less toxicity.

Generally, the E3 ligases are classified into four families based on the substrate binding domain: HECT-type, RING-finger-type, U-box-type, and PHD (plant homeodomain)-finger-type ligases. The largest family of E3 ligases is the RING-type SCF (Skp1, Cullins, F-box proteins) E3 family of ligases. SCF complexes consist of four proteins: RING box protein 1 (RBX1) Cullin Protein (CUL), S-phase Kinase-associated Protein 1 (SKP1), which are invariant among SCF complexes, and an F-box protein that varies [52]. Several recent studies have highlighted the critical role of E3 ligase on cancer progression. In line with this, E3 ligase alterations were shown to affect the BRAF and mitogen-activated protein kinase (MAPK) pathways, melanoma migration, and differentiation (Figure 2).

5.1. BRAF Pathway

Among the E3 ligase proteins, the F-box and WD repeat-containing 7 protein (FBXW7) was particularly well-studied in cancer progression [53–55]. In melanoma, an inactivating mutation of FBXW7 was reported to occur in 8% of melanoma patients [56]. FBXW7 was described as a negative regulator of the mitogen-activated protein kinase (MAPK) pathway by targeting BRAF for degradation. It was demonstrated that FBXW7 loss of function enhanced MAPK activity and promoted resistance to BRAF inhibitors in vitro and in vivo [57]. In parallel, another E3 ligase-targeting BRAF was identified. Wan et al. demonstrated that the APC/C E3 ligase complex and its activator fizzy-related protein 1 (FZR1) both negatively regulated BRAF activity through two distinct mechanisms involving proteolysis and the disruption of BRAF dimerization [58]. Importantly, the authors showed that a loss of FZR1 contributed to Vemurafenib resistance in melanoma cells [58]. These studies showed that E3 ligases can act as tumor suppressors, but some of them are considered as oncogenic players in melanoma progression. That is the case, for instance, of the itchy E3 ubiquitin-protein ligase, or ITCH, which was initially identified as a key enzyme in maintaining a balanced immune response and is strongly associated with autoimmune disease. The role of ITCH in malignancies was unveiled by its ability to tag different substrates for ubiquitination [59]. In melanoma, it was described that ITCH can directly interact with BRAF and promotes its lysine 27-linked polyubiquitination [60]. This atypical non-degradative polyubiquitination of BRAF allows for the recruitment of PP2A that dephosphorylates S365 and disrupts the interaction with the inhibitory scaffold protein 14.3.3, resulting in the sustained activation of BRAF and of its downstream signaling cascade [60].

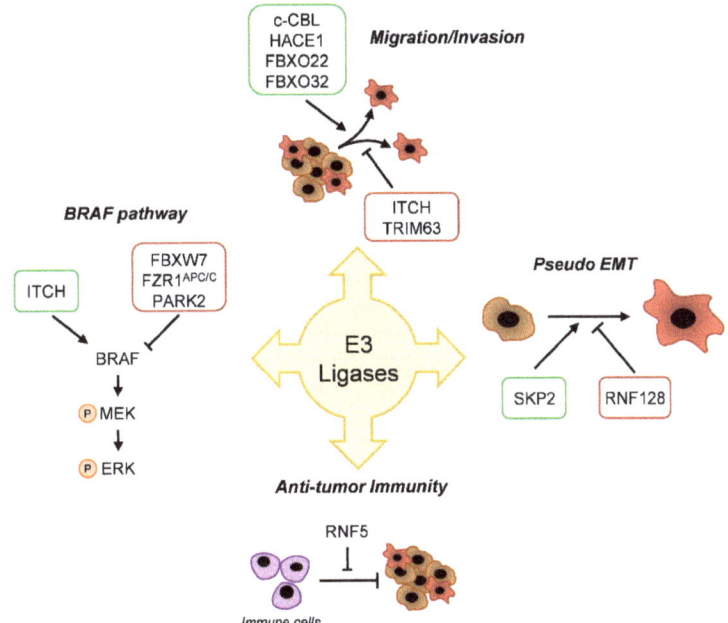

Figure 2. E3-conjugating enzymes implications in melanoma. E3-conjugating enzymes families have been described as players in melanoma progression; for instance, in the BRAF pathway, in the migration and invasion in epithelial-to-mesenchymal transition (EMT) or antitumor immunity. Green boxes are overexpressed in melanoma. Red boxes are underexpressed in melanoma.

The E3 ubiquitin ligase PARK2 was defined by Montagnani et al. as a tumor suppressor in malignant melanomas, by uncovering a new mechanism of PARK2 regulation. ELK1 (Ets-like protein 1), a known transcriptional effector of MAPK signaling, represses PARK2, leading to increased melanoma cell proliferation and tumor growth. Moreover, the inhibition of the BRAF-ERK1/2 axis increases PARK2 expression. The authors showed that overexpression of PARK2 in melanoma cells was associated with an antiproliferative effect and cell death in vitro and in vivo [61]. Thus, the reactivation of PARK2 may be an effective approach to counteract melanoma progression.

5.2. Migration/Invasion

As previously mentioned, ITCH can tag more than 50 substrates. Thus, it is not surprising that this E3 ligase is involved in several cellular processes like migration and invasion [59,60]. In a recent study, Wang et al. demonstrated that miR-10b, a microRNA targeting ITCH, promoted melanoma progression [62]. The downregulation of miR-10b significantly inhibited cell proliferation, migration, and invasion of melanoma cells in vitro. This work suggests the tumor-suppressing role of ITCH. Of note, FBXW7 was also reported to play a critical role in melanoma cell migration and metastasis [63].

By studying the molecular signature of melanoma, Rambow et al. identified the tripartite motif-containing protein 63 (TRIM63) E3 ligase as a new MITF target gene, and a core gene implicated in cell migration and invasion [64]. In addition, the casitas B-lineage lymphoma (c-CBL), an E3 ubiquitin ligase that was previously associated with acute myeloid leukemia, was found to be strongly expressed in human melanoma compared to benign melanocytic nevi [65]. The knockdown of c-CBL in melanoma cells resulted in decreased proliferation, migration, and spheroid formation. The authors also showed that the knockdown of c-CBL downregulated the FAK-GRB2-SRC signaling pathway, a system known to promote cell growth, proliferation, and motility of normal and neoplastic cells [65].

Recently, our group identified a new player in melanoma biology, the HECT domain and the ankyrin repeat-containing E3 ubiquitin-protein ligase 1 (HACE1). HACE1 is described as a tumor suppressor that catalyzes the degradative ubiquitination of active Rac1 (Ras-related C3 botulinum toxin substrate 1) GTPase [66]. The loss of HACE1 has promoted the progression of numerous cancers, such as breast cancer, hepatocellular carcinoma, or colorectal cancer [67–69]. In melanoma, even though expression levels of HACE1 are unchanged between nevi, primary, and metastatic melanoma, the loss of this E3 ligase impairs the migration of melanoma cells [70]. We demonstrated that HACE1 promoted the K27 ubiquitination of fibronectin and favored its secretion. Secreted fibronectin regulates ITGAV (Integrin subunit alpha V) and ITGB1 (Integrin beta-1) expression, globally promoting melanoma cell adhesion and migration. Thus, HACE1 plays a role in melanoma biology [70].

As a part of the SCF complexes, F-box proteins can critically affect cellular processes. A recent study on F-box only protein 22 (FBXO22) by Zheng et al. showed its role as an oncogene and as a potential target in malignant melanoma [71]. The F-box protein FBXO22 is known to specifically interact and induce degradative polyubiquitination of intracellular CD147, also known as basigin [72]. The authors showed a higher expression of FBXO22 in metastatic melanomas compared to normal skin tissue. Moreover, the downregulation of FBXO22 did not impair melanoma cell proliferation in vitro, but affected their migration in vitro and in vivo [71].

Very recently, our group identified FBXO32, a key component of the SCF ubiquitin-protein ligase complexes, as a MITF target, regulating melanoma cell migration and proliferation. Using loss of function approaches, we demonstrated that FBXO32 silencing in melanoma cell lines induced a downregulation of CDK6, a cell cycle protein promoting proliferation, and an upregulation of SMAD7, an inhibitor of the TGF-β pathway linked to cell migration. At the molecular level, FBOX32 seemed to interact with BRG1 (Brahma-related gene-1), a chromatin-remodeling protein [73]. This interaction could modulate the gene expression responsible for melanoma progression.

5.3. Differentiation

Epithelial-to-mesenchymal transition is a complex biological process by which immotile epithelial cells switch to motile mesenchymal cells. Mesenchymal cells are more invasive, more aggressive, and frequently display resistance to therapies. Melanocytes derive from neural crest epithelium through a first EMT. However, because they reside in the epidermis, melanocytes retain some epithelial cell attributes such as the expression of E-cadherin. Melanoma can also retain a certain degree of the epithelial phenotype, but can further switch to a more mesenchymal phenotype with exacerbated invasive properties and a strong resistance to TTs [74].

Over the last decade, numerous studies have involved ubiquitination in the regulation of EMT. The role of the F-box family was particularly well-studied in various types of cancer [75]. For instance, FBXW7 can suppress cell migration and invasion by negatively regulating the transcription factor SNAIL in human non-small cell lung cancer (NSCLC) [54]. As FBXW7 is frequently downregulated in cancer cell lines, functional studies revealed that a higher level of FBXW7 dramatically inhibited migration and invasiveness of renal cell carcinoma [76]. SKP2, a member of the F-box/LRR-repeat protein (FBXL) subfamily, is known to participate in degradative ubiquitination of the cyclin-dependent kinase inhibitor p27^{kip1}, a negative cell cycle regulator. Therefore, the inhibition of SKP2 in diverse cancers, including cutaneous [77,78] and uveal melanomas [79,80], was reported to inhibit cell proliferation in vitro and suppress tumor development in vivo. In 2014, a study revealed that the levels of SKP2 were elevated by TGF-β1 treatment in human melanoma cells [81]. It is known that TGF-β1 induces EMT [82]. Increased levels of SKP2 were accompanied with AKT and c-Myc activation during EMT [81]. Recently, the RING finger protein 128 (RNF128), an E3 ligase from the RING family, was described to favor melanoma development by inducing EMT [83]. The authors showed that RNF128 was downregulated in melanoma compared to peripheral normal tissue. The downregulation of RNF128 promoted melanoma cell proliferation in vitro and in vivo, through the degradative ubiquitination of CD44 and cortactin (CTTN). These two factors can activate the Wnt pathway, previously described as a critical axis involved in EMT and stemness in melanoma [75,83].

5.4. Antitumor Immunity

An increasing number of studies reveal a closer connection between the microbiota and cancer immunity, particularly the capability of the microbiota to regulate the expression of the cancer immune checkpoints [84]. Recently, Li et al. demonstrated that an alteration of intestinal microbiota in $Rnf5^{-/-}$ mice may have a role in antitumor immunity [85]. RING finger protein 5 (RNF5) is a E3 ubiquitin ligase, localized in the endoplasmic reticulum (ER) membrane and implicated in numerous cell processes, including the ER quality control system, through ubiquitination of misfolded proteins. Li et al. showed that RNF5 regulated the antitumor immunity and controlled melanoma tumor growth. A significant reduction of the unfolded protein response (UPR) components was seen in the response to RNF5 deletion, related with inflammasome increase, recruitment and activation of dendritic cells and T-cells, and the reduced expression of antimicrobial peptides (AMPs) in intestinal epithelial cells. Decreased AMPs might cause imbalance in the gut microbiota composition and promote a pro-inflammatory tumor micro-environment. The importance of the gut microbiota in the control of tumor growth in $Rnf5^{-/-}$ mice was confirmed by an antibiotic cocktail treatment that prevented tumor growth inhibition. Their data demonstrated that RNF5 loss, linked with an altered UPR signaling, coincided with variations in gut microbiota composition, activation of antitumor immunity, and consequently, efficient melanoma growth inhibition [85].

6. Deubiquitination and Melanoma

Protein ubiquitination processes can be reversed by deubiquitinating enzymes, which cleave the isopeptide bond between ubiquitin and its substrate [86]. These enzymes fall into two main categories: the cysteine proteases comprising the ubiquitin C-terminus hydrolases (UCHs), ubiquitin-specific proteases (USPs), ovarian tumor proteases (OTUs), Machado–Josephin domain proteases (MJDs), and the metalloprotease Jab1/MPN/Mov34 (JAMM) domain containing metalloisopeptidase [87]. Dysregulation of the DUB, and the consequent alteration of the ubiquitin system, are involved in the increase of the oncogene effects and/or decrease in the tumor suppressor activity in cancers in general, and in melanoma specifically.

6.1. Tumor Suppressors

BAP1 (BRCA-associated protein 1) is a nuclear deubiquitinase belonging to UCH family. BAP1 acts as tumor suppressor and is involved in many crucial cellular processes [88]. Germline mutations of BAP1 have been associated with hereditary predisposition to multiple cancers, including uveal melanoma (UM) and cutaneous melanoma (CM). Individuals who carry the mutated BAP1 gene develop melanocytic lesions later in life, and some of those benign lesions can transform into cutaneous melanomas [89]. BAP1 has been demonstrated to be involved in DNA damage and deubiquitination of the histone H2A, a histone family related to cell differentiation and organism development, and associated with cancer [90,91]. More recently, Webster et al. showed that BAP1 deletion in melanocytes cooperated with the oncogenic form of BRAF to promote melanoma growth in mice [92].

Interestingly, the loss of BAP1 was associated with apoptosis in a large set of cell types, but not in melanocytes and mesothelial cells, where its inactivation favored tumorigenesis, demonstrating a cell-specific tumor suppressor function of BAP1 [93]. BAP1 was also reported to exert its tumor suppressor function through the Hippo pathway that plays a key role in uveal melanoma [94].

Despite this, a recent meta-analysis based on TCGA dataset described opposite roles of BAP1 in survival of uveal and cutaneous melanoma. This analysis showed that low BAP1 mRNA was associated with a better overall survival (OS) in CM patients, particularly in older patients, in contrast with a poor OS in UM patients [95]. This analysis was in contrast with preceding studies, where the depletion of BAP1 expression indicated a worse outcome in CM patients [92,96].

Another deubiquitinase that is well-known as tumor suppressor is the cylindromatosis (CYLD) tumor suppressor protein, a UCH deubiquitinase that predominantly removes K63- and M1-linked chains from target proteins [97]. CYLD was shown to deubiquitinate different substrates, such as the proto-oncogene BCL-3 (B-cell chronic lymphatic leukemia protein 3), preventing its nuclear translocation and accumulation, which is associated with activation of NF-κB-dependent gene transcription and cell proliferation [98].

CYLD is suppressed in human melanoma cells, by the transcription factor SNAIL1. Loss of CYLD stimulates cellular proliferation, migration, and invasion by triggering BCL-3 nucleus translocation and activation of cyclin D1 and N-cadherin [99].

Recently, the role of CYLD was investigated in a murine model (Grm1) for spontaneous melanoma development [100]. The authors demonstrated that CYLD-knockout mice displayed increased tumor growth compared to wild-type mice. CYLD-deficiency appeared to favor lymphatic angiogenesis [100].

6.2. Tumor Promoters

Another deubiquitinase family critical for cancer progression is the ubiquitin-specific peptidases (USPs) family. USP deubiquitinases are involved in various aspects of the tumorigenesis process, including the regulation of transcription factors, apoptosis-related factors, DNA repair activity, histone modifications, and cell cycle progression [87,101].

The ubiquitin-specific protease USP4 appears as a regulator of different cellular pathways and targets a variety of substrates. It was found that the expression of the USP4 was upregulated in melanoma tissues and cell lines [102]. Impairing the expression of USP4 inhibits the invasive and migratory ability of melanoma cells. This phenotype correlates with a downregulation of N-cadherin and upregulation of E-cadherin, suggesting that EMT could be reversed. These data indicate that USP4 may act as an oncogene [102].

Very recently, Guao et al. showed that Spautin-1, a small-molecule autophagy inhibitor, capable of inhibiting the deubiquitinating activity of USP10 and USP13, induced cell cycle arrest in G2 phase and increased cell apoptosis in melanoma cell lines [102]. These results reveal the potential interest of USP10/USP13 targeting by Spautin-1 as an anti-melanoma strategy [103].

7. Ubiquitination and Resistance

Despite the conspicuous clinical response of BRAF-mutated melanoma to BRAF inhibitors and the dramatic response rate of immune checkpoint therapies, the prognosis of melanoma patients remains unfavorable, mainly due to the development of drug resistance. In this last part of the review, we discuss the involvement of the ubiquitination system toward melanoma drugs and immune checkpoint therapy resistance.

7.1. Drugs Resistance

In the past few years, some actors have been identified as crucial players in melanoma drug resistance, like NEDD4 [103]. NEDD4 belongs to a subfamily of HECT E3 ligases and mediates substrate ubiquitination and proteasomal degradation, as well as receptor-mediated endocytosis. NEDD4 exhibits an oncogenic function. Indeed, the inhibition of

NEDD4 ubiquitination activity promotes the PTEN stabilization, which can induce an antiproliferative response in melanoma [104]. Very recently, Yang et al. demonstrated that the voltage-dependent anion-selective channel (VDAC) 2 and 3, during erastin-induced ferroptosis in melanoma cells, were ubiquitinated by NEDD4 and sent to degradation. The knockdown of NEDD4 increased the VDAC2/3 protein level, with a consequent improvement of erastin sensitivity in melanoma cell lines and in the mice xenograft model [105]. These results uncover the crucial role of NEDD4 in the negative regulation of erastin-induced ferroptosis in melanoma.

In 2015, Kim et al. identified the ubiquitin ligase RNF125 as a crucial component of the innate and adaptive resistance in BRAFi-resistant melanomas [106]. RNF125 is a RING-type E3 ubiquitin ligase that acts as a positive regulator in T-cell activation, but a negative one in the antiviral innate immunity [107,108]. A decreased level of RNF125 transcript in BRAFi-resistant melanoma cells conferred a growth advantage in the presence of BRAFi. The inhibition of Janus kinase 1 (JAK1) activity due to ubiquitination by RNF125 decreased EGFR expression at the transcriptomic and protein levels, overcoming BRAFi resistance in melanoma cells [106]. These data suggest an important role of RNF125 in reducing the growth of BRAFi-resistant melanoma by the dysregulation of JAK and EGFR.

The same team recently reported that RNF4 promotes tumorigenesis and confers resistance to targeted therapies in melanoma [109]. RNF4 is a SUMO-dependent E3 ubiquitin ligase implicated in cancer that regulates the tumorigenesis of melanoma. Mechanistically, RNF4 seems to bind, ubiquitinate, and increase the expression of eIF2α. Moreover, the author showed that the RNF4–eIF2α axis plays an important role in the resistance of melanoma cells toward BRAFi [109].

As part of the RING-type family and HECT family, the F-box E3 ligase family member FBXO42 was also recently described as involved in the resistance of melanoma to targeted therapies [110]. Using the CRISPR–Cas9-mediated genome-wide screen, the authors identified FBXO42 loss as a driver of trametinib (MEK inhibitor) resistance in NRAS-mutated melanoma.

Data in the literature indicate that ubiquitin-specific peptidases (USPs), the main members of the deubiquitinase family, are involved in DNA damage repair activity, suggesting that USPs may be linked to drug resistance during cancer treatment. USPs are investigated as possible targets to develop inhibitors for cancer prevention [101]. Recently, a study described how the depletion of USP28 favored resistance to BRAF inhibitor therapies. USP28 deubiquitinated and stabilized FBXW7, a component of the SCF ubiquitin ligase complex that controls the degradation of BRAF [111]. Therefore, USP28 depletion increased BRAF protein levels and melanoma cell resistance to BRAF inhibitors [57]. These results show that USP28 is a key factor in ERK pathway activation and in resistance to BRAF inhibitors in vitro and in vivo.

Increased activity of USP14, a proteasome-associated DUB, was observed in melanoma cells and in melanoma patients compared to normal skin and nevi b-AP15, a selective USP14 inhibitor; the USP14 reduced proliferation of melanoma cells independent of the mutational cell status. The selective inhibitor b-AP15 also showed anti-melanoma activity in a mouse model of a BRAFi-resistant tumor, suggesting that USP14 is a possible target in melanoma with acquired resistance to targeted therapies [112].

A genetic screen of the whole-genome shRNA library led to the identification of two negative regulators of resistance to Vemurafenib in BRAF^{V600E}-expressing melanoma cells: neurofibromin 1 (NF1) and CUL3 [113]. The authors showed that loss of CUL3, a core component of the SCF E3 ubiquitin ligase complex, activates Rac1 leading to MAPKi resistance. Inhibition of the SRC family could reverse resistance induced by CUL3 depletion via the inactivation of the Rac1 protein [113]. These data highlight the SRC-Rac1 signaling axis as a new mechanism implicated in BRAFi resistance.

7.2. Resistance to ICTs

As for targeted therapies, patients with melanoma also develop resistance to immunotherapies. Antibody inhibitors against PD-1 or its ligand (PD-L1) have become commonly used to treat various types of cancer [114]. Recently, Meng et al. described a regulatory mechanism of PD-1 and demonstrated its critical role in antitumor immunity [115]. FBXO38, a component of a SCF E3 ligase complex, was reported to induce K48-linked polyubiquitination of PD-1 and cause its proteasomal degradation. In vivo experiments in mice showed that FBXO38 knockdown led to faster tumor progression along with a higher PD-1 expression level. This study highlights the clinical potential of FBXO38 as it offers an alternative method to block the PD-1 pathway [115].

In the same way, Otubain 1 (OTUB1) is a deubiquitinase member of the ovarian tumor (OTU) domain family that specifically cleaves K48-linked polyubiquitin chains, regulates many cancer associated signaling pathways, and has a critical role in cancer initiation and progression [116]. In 2019, it was shown that OTUB1 is a crucial controller of the activation and function of CD8 T-cells and Natural Killer (NK) cells in immune responses against cancer [117]. Indeed, the deletion of OTUB1 in T-lymphocytes or NK cells increased their anti-melanoma activity, establishing its key role as a regulator of antitumor immunity and as a potential target to improve immunotherapy [117].

Very recently, Scortegagna et al. identified the role of the E3 ubiquitin ligase SIAH2 (Seven in absentia homolog 2) in the regulation of T-regulatory (Treg) cells [118]. In $Siah2^{-/-}$ nude mice inoculated with melanoma cells, tumor-infiltrating Treg cells were dramatically less proliferative, leading to the inhibition of tumor growth, compared to Treg from wild-type mice. Moreover, the tumor growth was drastically reduced when $Siah2^{-/-}$ mice were challenged with anti-PD-1 treatment [118]. The authors concluded that SIAH2 controls Treg-cell recruitment and its loss in the host sensitizes melanoma to anti-PD-1 treatment. Thus, targeting SIAH2 could be beneficial to impair melanoma growth and development. The Ronai lab is currently developing SIAH1/2 inhibitors, able to affect melanoma cell viability, that could further be used in combination with targeted or immune checkpoint therapies [119].

Furthermore, in the immunotherapy context, Mezzadra et al. recently demonstrated that loss of chemokine-like factor (CKLF)-like MARVEL transmembrane domain containing family member 6 (CMTM6) decreased PD-L1 protein levels in melanoma cells [120]. At molecular level, the authors showed that CMTM6 interacted with PD-L1 and protected it from degradative ubiquitination. In agreement with this observation, CMTM6, by increasing PD-L1-expression, enhances the ability of tumor cells to inhibit the function of T-cells [120]. Thus, targeting CMTM6 to increase PD-L1 ubiquitination and degradation has a potential value as a therapeutic strategy to improve the immune response of melanoma cells (Table 2).

Table 2. Deubiquitinating enzymes and their roles in melanoma progression.

Family	Gene	Substrate	Pathway	Function in melanoma		Refs
UCH	BAP1	Histone H2A	DNA double-strand break repair	Cell differentiation	Tumor suppressor	[83–89]
	CYLD	BCL-3	N-cadherin expression	Proliferation, migration, invasion and lymph angiogenesis	Tumor suppressor	[93]
		-	Angiogenesis			[95]
USP	USP4	-	EMT	Migration and invasion	Tumor promoter	[97]
	USP10/13	p53	p53	Proliferation	Tumor promoter	[98,99]
	USP14	Proteasome substrates	UPS	Proliferation	Resistance promotion	[109]
	USP28	Fbw7	MAPK	BRAF inhibitor resistance	Resistance prevention	[108]

Table 2. *Cont.*

Family	Gene	Substrate	Pathway	Function in melanoma		Refs
OTU	OTUB1	UBE2N	DNA double-strand breaks repair	Initiation and progression	Tumor promoter	[113]
		AKT	CD8 T cells and NK cells activation	Immune cell activation		[114]

UCH: ubiquitin C-terminus hydrolase; BAP1: BRCA-associated Protein 1; CYLD: cylindromatosis tumor suppressor protein; OTU: ovarian tumor protease; USP: ubiquitin-specific protease; EMT: epithelial-to-mesenchymal transition; UPS: ubiquitin-proteasome system.

8. Conclusions and Future Directions

An increasing number of studies have demonstrated the critical role of ubiquitination in cancer development, progression, and resistance to therapies, and this also holds true in melanoma. As a major post-translational modification, ubiquitination controls the expression and function of proteins. This level of regulation should be considered in addition to gene expression levels to clearly understand the processes of melanoma development.

Since ubiquitination is involved in most of the cellular processes that are deregulated in tumor cells, targeting ubiquitination has appeared to be a rational therapeutic strategy in cancers. However, the pleiotropic role of ubiquitination also raises concerns about possible adverse effects, unless an enzyme that is specifically expressed in the considered neoplasm is targeted.

Proteasome inhibitors (Bortezomib, Carfilzomib, Ixazomib) were one of the first drugs, which interfere with ubiquitination processes, that were successfully used in clinical trial for multiple myeloma [121]. With an overall response rate of 23.7% (18.7–29.4), and a median duration of response of 7.8 months (5.6–9.2), Carfilzomib was shown to be a safe and effective treatment option for patients with relapsed multiple myeloma refractory, when compared to Bortezomib, Thalidomide, or Lenalidomide [122]. The first reversible and orally administered proteasome inhibitor, Ixazomib, was approved by the FDA in 2015 [123]. Ixazomib showed an overall response rate of 27% at the maximum tolerated dose. It appears to be less toxic, with an excellent tolerability, when compared to Bortezomib [123]. Of note, no beneficial effects were observed in metastatic malignant melanoma patients treated with Bortezomib [124]. Basically, each step of the ubiquitination process can be pharmacologically targeted. Indeed, several component targeting E1 ubiquitin-activating enzymes have been described. Among them, Pevonedistat is being used in clinical trials for acute myeloid leukemia and melanoma [125]. Because of the absence of a classical druggable site, few inhibitors of E2 ubiquitin-conjugating enzymes have been described so far, and none are in clinical trial [126]. Concerning the E3 ligases, as they are considered as the pivotal enzyme in the ubiquitination process, efforts have allowed the discovery of specific inhibitors. For instance, an inhibitor of MDM2, a key regulator of p53 stability, has been approved in clinic for liver and pancreatic cancer [4]. Among the FDA-approved E3 modulators, Thalidomide and Lenalidomide have shown no significant responses in their respective phase II studies [127,128].

Finally, deubiquitinating enzymes that reverse ubiquitination are also the target of inhibitors. Pimozide, an USP1 inhibitor, is in clinical trial for glioblastoma [129].

However, the successful use of ubiquitination process inhibitors has probably been limited because of the lack of specificity of the drugs used. Recently, approaches hijacking the ubiquitin-proteasome system (UPS) have emerged to overcome specificity and redundancy problems. The first one uses ubiquitin variants (UbVs) that were designed to improve potency and specificity toward UPS enzymes. However, the delivery of these engineered proteins to the cells remains challenging. The second one is an approach gaining increasing interest because it can potentially target 97% of the reputable, undruggable proteins. This approach, called proteolysis-targeting-chimera (PROTAC) uses heterobifunctional compounds that foster the formation of a complex between an E3 ligase and the target protein, promoting ubiquitination and degradation of the latter. Virtually, this approach might be used to target and destroy any protein essential in tumor development.

Today, the few clinical trials using inhibitors of the UPS have shown no clear objective benefits in patients with melanoma. Nevertheless, recent reports indicating that ubiquitination affects responses to targeted and immune therapies might prompt the evaluation of inhibitors of ubiquitination process in combination with current treatments. The PROTAC approach, specifically targeting the epigenetic processes or key oncogenic pathways, also deserves further investigation in the context of melanoma [130,131].

Author Contributions: Conceptualization, F.S., S.G. and N.H.; validation, C.B. and R.B.; writing—original draft preparation, F.S., S.G. and N.H.; writing—review and editing, N.E.-H. and C.P.; supervision, C.B. and R.B.; project administration, R.B. All authors have read and agreed to the published version of the manuscript.

Funding: This research received no external funding.

Institutional Review Board Statement: Not applicable.

Informed Consent Statement: Not applicable.

Data Availability Statement: No new data were created or analyzed in this study. Data sharing is not applicable to this article.

Conflicts of Interest: The authors declare no conflict of interest.

Abbreviations

AKT: A Serine/Threonine Kinase; AMPs: Antimicrobial Peptides; APC/C: Anaphase-Promoting Complex/Cyclosome; ATG: Autophagy-related protein; BAP1: BRCA1-Associated Protein 1; BCL3: B-cell chronic lymphatic leukemia protein 3; BRAF: Rapidly Accelerated Fibrosarcoma B-type; BRCA1: Breast Cancer 1; BRG1: Brahma-Related Gene-1; c-CBL: Casitas B-lineage lymphoma; CD147: Cluster of Differentiation 147; CDK6: Cyclin Dependent Kinase 6; CKLF: Chemokine-Like Factor; CM: Cutaneous Melanoma; CMTM6: Chemokine-like factor (CKLF)-like MARVEL Transmembrane domain containing family member 6; c-Myc: Avian Myelocytomatosis virus oncogene cellular homolog; CRISPR: Clustered Regularly Interspaced Short Palindromic Repeats; CTLA4: Cytotoxic T-Lymphocyte-associated antigen 4; CTTN: Cortactin; CUL: Cullin Protein; CYLD: Cylindromatosis tumor suppressor protein; DUBs: Deubiquitinating enzymes; EGFR: Epidermal Growth Factor Receptor; ELK1: Ets-Like protein 1; EMT: Epithelial-to-Mesenchymal Transition; ER: Endoplasmic Reticulum; ERK: Extracellular signal-Regulated Kinase; FAT10: human leukocyte antigen F locus Adjacent Transcript 10; FBXW7: F-box and WD repeat-containing 7 protein; FBXL: F-box/LRR-repeat protein; FBXO: F-box Only protein; FRA1: Fos-Related Antigen 1; FZR1: Fizzy-Related protein 1; GSK: Glycogen Synthase Kinase; HACE1: ankyrin repeat-containing E3 ubiquitin-protein ligase 1; HECT: Homology to E6-AP C-Terminus; ICTs: Immune Checkpoint Therapies; ITCH: Itchy E3 ubiquitin-protein ligase; ITGAV: Integrin subunit Alpha V; ITGB1: Integrin Beta-1; ISG15: interferon-stimulated gene 15; JAK1: Janus Kinase 1; JAMM: Metalloprotease Jab1/MPN/Mov34; MAPK: Mitogen-Activated Protein Kinase; MDM2: Mouse Double Minute 2; MEK: MAPK/Erk1 Kinase; MITF: Microphthalmia-associated Transcription Factor; MJDs: Machado–Josephin domain proteases; NEDD: Neural precursor cell Expressed Developmentally Down-regulated protein; NF1: Neurofibromin 1; NK: Natural Killer; NRAS: Neuroblastoma; RAS: viral oncogene homolog; PARK2: Parkinson Protein 2; PD1: Programmed cell death protein 1; PHD: Plant Homeodomain; PP2A: Protein serine/threonine Phosphatase 2A; PROTAC: proteolysis-targeting-chimera; PTEN: Phosphatase and Tensin homolog; OTUs: Ovarian Tumor proteases; OTUB1: Otubain 1; OS: overall survival; RBX1: RING box protein 1; RING: Really Interesting New Gene; RNF: RING finger protein; TGF: Transforming Growth Factor; TRAF6: Tumor Necrosis Factor Receptor-associated Factor 6; TRIM63: Tripartite Motif-containing protein 63; TTs: Targeted Therapies; Treg: T-regulatory; SCF: Skp1, Cullins, F-box proteins; SIAH2: Seven In Absentia Homolog 2; SKP: S-phase Kinase-associated Protein; SMAD7: Mothers against decapentaplegic homolog 7; SOX10: SRY-related HMG box-containing factor 10; SUMO: Small Ub-related Modifier; Ub: Ubiquitin; UBC: Ub-conjugating; UBE: Ub-conjugating enzyme E; UBL: Ub-like proteins; UbVs: Ubiquitin Variants; UCHs: Ubiquitin C-terminus Hydrolases; UEV1A: Ubiquitin-conjugating Enzyme Variant 1A; UFM1: Ub-Fold Modifier; UM: Uveal Melanoma; UPR: Unfolded Protein Response; UPS: Ubiquitin-Proteasome System; URM1: Ub-Related Modifier

1; USPs: Ubiquitin-Specific Proteases; VDAC: Voltage-Dependent Anion-selective Channel; Wnt: Wingless-related integration site.

References

1. Swatek, K.N.; Komander, D. Ubiquitin modifications. *Cell Res.* **2016**, *26*, 399–422. [CrossRef]
2. Senturk, E.; Manfredi, J.J. Mdm2 and tumorigenesis: Evolving theories and unsolved mysteries. *Genes Cancer* **2012**, *3*, 192–198. [CrossRef] [PubMed]
3. Ma, J.; Guo, W.; Li, C. Ubiquitination in melanoma pathogenesis and treatment. *Cancer Med.* **2017**, *6*, 1362–1377. [CrossRef]
4. Deng, L.; Meng, T.; Chen, L.; Wei, W.; Wang, P. The role of ubiquitination in tumorigenesis and targeted drug discovery. *Signal Transduct. Target. Ther.* **2020**, *5*, 11. [CrossRef] [PubMed]
5. Popovic, D.; Vucic, D.; Dikic, I. Ubiquitination in disease pathogenesis and treatment. *Nat. Med.* **2014**, *20*, 1242–1253. [CrossRef] [PubMed]
6. Long, G.V.; Stroyakovskiy, D.; Gogas, H.; Levchenko, E.; de Braud, F.; Larkin, J.; Garbe, C.; Jouary, T.; Hauschild, A.; Grob, J.-J.; et al. Dabrafenib and trametinib versus dabrafenib and placebo for Val600 BRAF-mutant melanoma: A multicentre, double-blind, phase 3 randomised controlled trial. *Lancet* **2015**, *386*, 444–451. [CrossRef]
7. Long, G.V.; Stroyakovskiy, D.; Gogas, H.; Levchenko, E.; de Braud, F.; Larkin, J.; Garbe, C.; Jouary, T.; Hauschild, A.; Grob, J.J.; et al. Combined BRAF and MEK inhibition versus BRAF inhibition alone in melanoma. *N. Engl. J. Med.* **2014**, *371*, 1877–1888. [CrossRef]
8. LoRusso, P.M.; Schalper, K.; Sosman, J. Targeted therapy and immunotherapy: Emerging biomarkers in metastatic melanoma. *Pigment Cell Melanoma Res.* **2019**. [CrossRef]
9. Hauschild, A.; Grob, J.-J.; Demidov, L.V.; Jouary, T.; Gutzmer, R.; Millward, M.; Rutkowski, P.; Blank, C.U.; Miller, W.H.; Kaempgen, E.; et al. Dabrafenib in BRAF-mutated metastatic melanoma: A multicentre, open-label, phase 3 randomised controlled trial. *Lancet* **2012**, *380*, 358–365. [CrossRef]
10. McArthur, G.A.; Chapman, P.B.; Robert, C.; Larkin, J.; Haanen, J.B.; Dummer, R.; Ribas, A.; Hogg, D.; Hamid, O.; Ascierto, P.A.; et al. Safety and efficacy of vemurafenib in BRAF(V600E) and BRAF(V600K) mutation-positive melanoma (BRIM-3): Extended follow-up of a phase 3, randomised, open-label study. *Lancet. Oncol.* **2014**, *15*, 323–332. [CrossRef]
11. Hodi, F.S.; O'Day, S.J.; McDermott, D.F.; Weber, R.W.; Sosman, J.A.; Haanen, J.B.; Gonzalez, R.; Robert, C.; Schadendorf, D.; Hassel, J.C.; et al. Improved survival with ipilimumab in patients with metastatic melanoma. *N. Engl. J. Med.* **2010**, *363*, 711–723. [CrossRef]
12. Wolchok, J.D.; Chiarion-Sileni, V.; Gonzalez, R.; Rutkowski, P.; Grob, J.-J.; Cowey, C.L.; Lao, C.D.; Wagstaff, J.; Schadendorf, D.; Ferrucci, P.F.; et al. Overall Survival with Combined Nivolumab and Ipilimumab in Advanced Melanoma. *N. Engl. J. Med.* **2017**, *377*, 1345–1356. [CrossRef]
13. Sharma, P.; Hu-Lieskovan, S.; Wargo, J.A.; Ribas, A. Primary, Adaptive, and Acquired Resistance to Cancer Immunotherapy. *Cell* **2017**, *168*, 707–723. [CrossRef]
14. Kruger, S.; Ilmer, M.; Kobold, S.; Cadilha, B.L.; Endres, S.; Ormanns, S.; Schuebbe, G.; Renz, B.W.; D'Haese, J.G.; Schloesser, H.; et al. Advances in cancer immunotherapy 2019—Latest trends. *J. Exp. Clin. Cancer Res.* **2019**, *38*, 1–11. [CrossRef] [PubMed]
15. Schachter, J.; Ribas, A.; Long, G.V.; Arance, A.; Grob, J.J.; Mortier, L.; Daud, A.; Carlino, M.S.; McNeil, C.; Lotem, M.; et al. Pembrolizumab versus ipilimumab for advanced melanoma: Final overall survival results of a multicentre, randomised, open-label phase 3 study (KEYNOTE-006). *Lancet* **2017**, *390*, 1853–1862. [CrossRef]
16. Pickart, C.M. Mechanisms underlying ubiquitination. *Annu. Rev. Biochem.* **2001**, *70*, 503–533. [CrossRef] [PubMed]
17. Satija, Y.K.; Bhardwaj, A.; Das, S. A portrayal of E3 ubiquitin ligases and deubiquitylases in cancer. *Int. J. cancer* **2013**, *133*, 2759–2768. [CrossRef] [PubMed]
18. Komander, D.; Rape, M. The ubiquitin code. *Annu. Rev. Biochem.* **2012**, *81*, 203–229. [CrossRef]
19. Chau, V.; Tobias, J.W.; Bachmair, A.; Marriott, D.; Ecker, D.J.; Gonda, D.K.; Varshavsky, A. A multiubiquitin chain is confined to specific lysine in a targeted short-lived protein. *Science* **1989**, *243*, 1576–1583. [CrossRef] [PubMed]
20. Pickart, C.M.; Fushman, D. Polyubiquitin chains: Polymeric protein signals. *Curr. Opin. Chem. Biol.* **2004**, *8*, 610–616. [CrossRef]
21. Deng, L.; Wang, C.; Spencer, E.; Yang, L.; Braun, A.; You, J.; Slaughter, C.; Pickart, C.; Chen, Z.J. Activation of the IkappaB kinase complex by TRAF6 requires a dimeric ubiquitin-conjugating enzyme complex and a unique polyubiquitin chain. *Cell* **2000**, *103*, 351–361. [CrossRef]
22. Wang, C.; Deng, L.; Hong, M.; Akkaraju, G.R.; Inoue, J.; Chen, Z.J. TAK1 is a ubiquitin-dependent kinase of MKK and IKK. *Nature* **2001**, *412*, 346–351. [CrossRef]
23. Winston, J.T.; Strack, P.; Beer-Romero, P.; Chu, C.Y.; Elledge, S.J.; Harper, J.W. The SCFbeta-TRCP-ubiquitin ligase complex associates specifically with phosphorylated destruction motifs in IkappaBalpha and beta-catenin and stimulates IkappaBalpha ubiquitination in vitro. *Genes Dev.* **1999**, *13*, 270–283. [CrossRef]
24. Margottin-Goguet, F.; Hsu, J.Y.; Loktev, A.; Hsieh, H.M.; Reimann, J.D.R.; Jackson, P.K. Prophase destruction of Emi1 by the SCF(betaTrCP/Slimb) ubiquitin ligase activates the anaphase promoting complex to allow progression beyond prometaphase. *Dev. Cell* **2003**, *4*, 813–826. [CrossRef]

25. Walsh, M.C.; Lee, J.; Choi, Y. Tumor necrosis factor receptor-associated factor 6 (TRAF6) regulation of development, function, and homeostasis of the immune system. *Immunol. Rev.* **2015**, *266*, 72–92. [CrossRef] [PubMed]
26. Yuan, T.; Yan, F.; Ying, M.; Cao, J.; He, Q.; Zhu, H.; Yang, B. Inhibition of Ubiquitin-Specific Proteases as a Novel Anticancer Therapeutic Strategy. *Front. Pharmacol.* **2018**, *9*, 1–10. [CrossRef]
27. Wilkinson, K.D. DUBs at a glance. *J. Cell Sci.* **2009**, *122*, 2325–2329. [CrossRef]
28. Fuchs, S.Y.; Spiegelman, V.S.; Kumar, K.G.S. The many faces of beta-TrCP E3 ubiquitin ligases: Reflections in the magic mirror of cancer. *Oncogene* **2004**, *23*, 2028–2036. [CrossRef]
29. Liu, J.; Suresh Kumar, K.G.; Yu, D.; Molton, S.A.; McMahon, M.; Herlyn, M.; Thomas-Tikhonenko, A.; Fuchs, S.Y. Oncogenic BRAF regulates beta-Trcp expression and NF-kappaB activity in human melanoma cells. *Oncogene* **2007**, *26*, 1954–1958. [CrossRef]
30. Santra, M.K.; Wajapeyee, N.; Green, M.R. F-box protein FBXO31 mediates cyclin D1 degradation to induce G1 arrest after DNA damage. *Nature* **2009**, *459*, 722–725. [CrossRef]
31. Lee, E.K.; Lian, Z.; D'Andrea, K.; Letrero, R.; Sheng, W.; Liu, S.; Diehl, J.N.; Pytel, D.; Barbash, O.; Schuchter, L.; et al. The FBXO4 tumor suppressor functions as a barrier to BRAFV600E-dependent metastatic melanoma. *Mol. Cell. Biol.* **2013**, *33*, 4422–4433. [CrossRef]
32. Valimberti, I.; Tiberti, M.; Lambrughi, M.; Sarcevic, B.; Papaleo, E. E2 superfamily of ubiquitin-conjugating enzymes: Constitutively active or activated through phosphorylation in the catalytic cleft. *Sci. Rep.* **2015**, *5*, 14849. [CrossRef]
33. Hormaechea-Agulla, D.; Kim, Y.; Song, M.S.; Song, S.J. New Insights into the Role of E2s in the Pathogenesis of Diseases: Lessons Learned from UBE2O. *Mol. Cells* **2018**, *41*, 168–178. [CrossRef] [PubMed]
34. Hosseini, S.M.; Okoye, I.; Chaleshtari, M.G.; Hazhirkarzar, B.; Mohamadnejad, J.; Azizi, G.; Hojjat-Farsangi, M.; Mohammadi, H.; Shotorbani, S.S.; Jadidi-Niaragh, F. E2 ubiquitin-conjugating enzymes in cancer: Implications for immunotherapeutic interventions. *Clin. Chim. Acta* **2019**, *498*, 126–134. [CrossRef] [PubMed]
35. Gorlov, I.; Orlow, I.; Ringelberg, C.; Hernando, E.; Ernstoff, M.S.; Cheng, C.; Her, S.; Parker, J.S.; Thompson, C.L.; Gerstenblith, M.R.; et al. Identification of gene expression levels in primary melanoma associated with clinically meaningful characteristics. *Melanoma Res.* **2018**, *28*, 380–389. [CrossRef] [PubMed]
36. Ueki, T.; Park, J.-H.; Nishidate, T.; Kijima, K.; Hirata, K.; Nakamura, Y.; Katagiri, T. Ubiquitination and downregulation of BRCA1 by ubiquitin-conjugating enzyme E2T overexpression in human breast cancer cells. *Cancer Res.* **2009**, *69*, 8752–8760. [CrossRef]
37. Hu, W.; Xiao, L.; Cao, C.; Hua, S.; Wu, D. UBE2T promotes nasopharyngeal carcinoma cell proliferation, invasion, and metastasis by activating the AKT/GSK3β/β-catenin pathway. *Oncotarget* **2016**, *7*, 15161–15172. [CrossRef]
38. Zhang, W.; Zhang, Y.; Yang, Z.; Liu, X.; Yang, P.; Wang, J.; Hu, K.; He, X.; Zhang, X.; Jing, H. High expression of UBE2T predicts poor prognosis and survival in multiple myeloma. *Cancer Gene Ther.* **2019**, *26*, 347–355. [CrossRef]
39. Dikshit, A.; Jin, Y.J.; Degan, S.; Hwang, J.; Foster, M.W.; Li, C.-Y.; Zhang, J.Y. UBE2N Promotes Melanoma Growth via MEK/FRA1/SOX10 Signaling. *Cancer Res.* **2018**, *78*, 6462–6472. [CrossRef]
40. Kraft, S.; Moore, J.B.; Muzikansky, A.; Scott, K.L.; Duncan, L.M. Differential UBE2C and HOXA1 expression in melanocytic nevi and melanoma. *J. Cutan. Pathol.* **2017**, *44*, 843–850. [CrossRef]
41. Liu, L.; Zhao, J.; Pan, B.; Ma, G.; Liu, L. UBE2C overexpression in melanoma and its essential role in G2/M transition. *J. Cancer* **2019**, *10*, 2176–2184. [CrossRef]
42. Cappadocia, L.; Lima, C.D. Ubiquitin-like Protein Conjugation: Structures, Chemistry, and Mechanism. *Chem. Rev.* **2018**, *118*, 889–918. [CrossRef]
43. Mo, Y.Y.; Moschos, S.J. Targeting Ubc9 for cancer therapy. *Expert Opin. Ther. Targets* **2005**, *9*, 1203–1216. [CrossRef]
44. Moschos, S.J.; Mo, Y.-Y. Role of SUMO/Ubc9 in DNA damage repair and tumorigenesis. *J. Mol. Histol.* **2006**, *37*, 309–319. [CrossRef]
45. Moschos, S.J.; Smith, A.P.; Mandic, M.; Athanassiou, C.; Watson-Hurst, K.; Jukic, D.M.; Edington, H.D.; Kirkwood, J.M.; Becker, D. SAGE and antibody array analysis of melanoma-infiltrated lymph nodes: Identification of Ubc9 as an important molecule in advanced-stage melanomas. *Oncogene* **2007**, *26*, 4216–4225. [CrossRef] [PubMed]
46. Xu, W.; Gong, L.; Haddad, M.M.; Bischof, O.; Campisi, J.; Yeh, E.T.H.; Medrano, E.E. Regulation of microphthalmia-associated transcription factor MITF protein levels by association with the ubiquitin-conjugating enzyme hUBC9. *Exp. Cell Res.* **2000**, *255*, 135–143. [CrossRef]
47. Cheli, Y.; Giuliano, S.; Guiliano, S.; Botton, T.; Rocchi, S.; Hofman, V.; Hofman, P.; Bahadoran, P.; Bertolotto, C.; Ballotti, R. Mitf is the key molecular switch between mouse or human melanoma initiating cells and their differentiated progeny. *Oncogene* **2011**, *30*, 2307–2318. [CrossRef] [PubMed]
48. Bertolotto, C.; Lesueur, F.; Giuliano, S.; Strub, T.; De Lichy, M.; Bille, K.; Dessen, P.; D'Hayer, B.; Mohamdi, H.; Remenieras, A.; et al. A SUMOylation-defective MITF germline mutation predisposes to melanoma and renal carcinoma. *Nature* **2011**, *480*, 94–98. [CrossRef] [PubMed]
49. Wang, P.; Li, Y.; Ma, Y.; Zhang, X.; Li, Z.; Yu, W.; Zhu, M.; Wang, J.; Xu, Y.; Xu, A. Comprehensive Investigation into the Role of Ubiquitin-Conjugating Enzyme E2S in Melanoma Development. *J. Invest. Dermatol.* **2021**, *141*, 374–384. [CrossRef]
50. Gajan, A.; Martin, C.E.; Kim, S.; Joshi, M.; Michelhaugh, S.K.; Sloma, I.; Mittal, S.; Firestine, S.; Shekhar, M.P.V. Alternative Splicing of RAD6B and Not RAD6A is Selectively Increased in Melanoma: Identification and Functional Characterization. *Cells* **2019**, *8*, 1375. [CrossRef]

51. Sarma, A.; Gajan, A.; Kim, S.; Gurdziel, K.; Mao, G.; Nangia-Makker, P.; Shekhar, M.P.V. RAD6B loss disrupts expression of melanoma phenotype in part by inhibiting WNT/beta-catenin signaling. *Am. J. Pathol.* **2020**, 112490. [CrossRef] [PubMed]
52. Berndsen, C.E.; Wolberger, C. New insights into ubiquitin E3 ligase mechanism. *Nat. Struct. Mol. Biol.* **2014**, *21*, 301–307. [CrossRef] [PubMed]
53. Lin, J.; Ji, A.; Qiu, G.; Feng, H.; Li, J.; Li, S.; Zou, Y.; Cui, Y.; Song, C.; He, H.; et al. FBW7 is associated with prognosis, inhibits malignancies and enhances temozolomide sensitivity in glioblastoma cells. *Cancer Sci.* **2018**, *109*, 1001–1011. [CrossRef] [PubMed]
54. Zhang, Y.; Zhang, X.; Ye, M.; Jing, P.; Xiong, J.; Han, Z.; Kong, J.; Li, M.; Lai, X.; Chang, N.; et al. FBW7 loss promotes epithelial-to-mesenchymal transition in non-small cell lung cancer through the stabilization of Snail protein. *Cancer Lett.* **2018**, *419*, 75–83. [CrossRef] [PubMed]
55. Shimizu, K.; Nihira, N.T.; Inuzuka, H.; Wei, W. Physiological functions of FBW7 in cancer and metabolism. *Cell. Signal.* **2018**, *46*, 15–22. [CrossRef]
56. Aydin, I.T.; Melamed, R.D.; Adams, S.J.; Castillo-Martin, M.; Demir, A.; Bryk, D.; Brunner, G.; Cordon-Cardo, C.; Osman, I.; Rabadan, R.; et al. FBXW7 mutations in melanoma and a new therapeutic paradigm. *J. Natl. Cancer Inst.* **2014**, *106*, dju107. [CrossRef]
57. Saei, A.; Palafox, M.; Benoukraf, T.; Kumari, N.; Jaynes, P.W.; Iyengar, P.V.; Muñoz-Couselo, E.; Nuciforo, P.; Cortés, J.; Nötzel, C.; et al. Loss of USP28-mediated BRAF degradation drives resistance to RAF cancer therapies. *J. Exp. Med.* **2018**, *215*, 1913–1928. [CrossRef]
58. Wan, L.; Chen, M.; Cao, J.; Dai, X.; Yin, Q.; Zhang, J.; Song, S.-J.; Lu, Y.; Liu, J.; Inuzuka, H.; et al. The APC/C E3 Ligase Complex Activator FZR1 Restricts BRAF Oncogenic Function. *Cancer Discov.* **2017**, *7*, 424–441. [CrossRef]
59. Yin, Q.; Wyatt, C.J.; Han, T.; Smalley, K.S.M.; Wan, L. ITCH as a potential therapeutic target in human cancers. *Semin. Cancer Biol.* **2020**, 1–14. [CrossRef]
60. Yin, Q.; Han, T.; Fang, B.; Zhang, G.; Zhang, C.; Roberts, E.R.; Izumi, V.; Zheng, M.; Jiang, S.; Yin, X.; et al. K27-linked ubiquitination of BRAF by ITCH engages cytokine response to maintain MEK-ERK signaling. *Nat. Commun.* **2019**, *10*, 1870. [CrossRef]
61. Montagnani, V.; Maresca, L.; Apollo, A.; Pepe, S.; Carr, R.M.; Fernandez-Zapico, M.E.; Stecca, B. E3 ubiquitin ligase PARK2, an inhibitor of melanoma cell growth, is repressed by the oncogenic ERK1/2-ELK1 transcriptional axis. *J. Biol. Chem.* **2020**, *295*, 16058–16071. [CrossRef] [PubMed]
62. Wang, S.; Wu, Y.; Xu, Y.; Tang, X. miR-10b promoted melanoma progression through Wnt/β-catenin pathway by repressing ITCH expression. *Gene* **2019**, *710*, 39–47. [CrossRef]
63. Cheng, Y.; Chen, G.; Martinka, M.; Ho, V.; Li, G. Prognostic significance of Fbw7 in human melanoma and its role in cell migration. *J. Investig. Dermatol.* **2013**, *133*, 1794–1802. [CrossRef]
64. Rambow, F.; Job, B.; Petit, V.; Gesbert, F.; Delmas, V.; Seberg, H.; Meurice, G.; Van Otterloo, E.; Dessen, P.; Robert, C.; et al. New Functional Signatures for Understanding Melanoma Biology from Tumor Cell Lineage-Specific Analysis. *Cell Rep.* **2015**, *13*, 840–853. [CrossRef] [PubMed]
65. Nihal, M.; Wood, G.S. c-CBL regulates melanoma proliferation, migration, invasion and the FAK-SRC-GRB2 nexus. *Oncotarget* **2016**, *7*, 53869–53880. [CrossRef] [PubMed]
66. Torrino, S.; Visvikis, O.; Doye, A.; Boyer, L.; Stefani, C.; Munro, P.; Bertoglio, J.; Gacon, G.; Mettouchi, A.; Lemichez, E. The E3 ubiquitin-ligase HACE1 catalyzes the ubiquitylation of active Rac1. *Dev. Cell* **2011**, *21*, 959–965. [CrossRef]
67. Goka, E.T.; Lippman, M.E. Loss of the E3 ubiquitin ligase HACE1 results in enhanced Rac1 signaling contributing to breast cancer progression. *Oncogene* **2015**, *34*, 5395–5405. [CrossRef] [PubMed]
68. Gao, Z.F.; Wu, Y.N.; Bai, Z.T.; Zhang, L.; Zhou, Q.; Li, X. Tumor-suppressive role of HACE1 in hepatocellular carcinoma and its clinical significance. *Oncol. Rep.* **2016**, *36*, 3427–3435. [CrossRef]
69. Zhou, Z.; Zhang, H.-S.; Zhang, Z.-G.; Sun, H.-L.; Liu, H.-Y.; Gou, X.-M.; Yu, X.-Y.; Huang, Y.-H. Loss of HACE1 promotes colorectal cancer cell migration via upregulation of YAP1. *J. Cell. Physiol.* **2019**, *234*, 9663–9672. [CrossRef]
70. El-Hachem, N.; Habel, N.; Naiken, T.; Bziouech, H.; Cheli, Y.; Beranger, G.E.; Jaune, E.; Rouaud, F.; Nottet, N.; Reinier, F.; et al. Uncovering and deciphering the pro-invasive role of HACE1 in melanoma cells. *Cell Death Differ.* **2018**, *25*, 2010–2022. [CrossRef]
71. Zheng, Y.; Chen, H.; Zhao, Y.; Zhang, X.; Liu, J.; Pan, Y.; Bai, J.; Zhang, H. Knockdown of FBXO22 inhibits melanoma cell migration, invasion and angiogenesis via the HIF-1α/VEGF pathway. *Investig. New Drugs* **2020**, *38*, 20–28. [CrossRef] [PubMed]
72. Wu, B.; Liu, Z.-Y.; Cui, J.; Yang, X.-M.; Jing, L.; Zhou, Y.; Chen, Z.-N.; Jiang, J.-L. F-Box Protein FBXO22 Mediates Polyubiquitination and Degradation of CD147 to Reverse Cisplatin Resistance of Tumor Cells. *Int. J. Mol. Sci.* **2017**, *18*, 212. [CrossRef]
73. Habel, N.; El-Hachem, N.; Soysouvanh, F.; Hadhiri-Bzioueche, H.; Giuliano, S.; Nguyen, S.; Horák, P.; Gay, A.-S.; Debayle, D.; Nottet, N.; et al. FBXO32 links ubiquitination to epigenetic reprograming of melanoma cells. *Cell Death Differ.* **2021**. [CrossRef]
74. Li, F.Z.; Dhillon, A.S.; Anderson, R.L.; McArthur, G.; Ferrao, P.T. Phenotype Switching in Melanoma: Implications for Progression and Therapy. *Front. Oncol.* **2015**, *5*, 31. [CrossRef]
75. Song, Y.; Lin, M.; Liu, Y.; Wang, Z.W.; Zhu, X. Emerging role of F-box proteins in the regulation of epithelial-mesenchymal transition and stem cells in human cancers. *Stem Cell Res. Ther.* **2019**, *10*, 1–11. [CrossRef] [PubMed]
76. He, H.; Dai, J.; Xu, Z.; He, W.; Wang, X.; Zhu, Y.; Wang, H. Fbxw7 regulates renal cell carcinoma migration and invasion via suppression of the epithelial-mesenchymal transition. *Oncol. Lett.* **2018**, *15*, 3694–3702. [CrossRef]

77. Li, Q.; Murphy, M.; Ross, J.; Sheehan, C.; Carlson, J.A. Skp2 and p27kip1 expression in melanocytic nevi and melanoma: An inverse relationship. *J. Cutan. Pathol.* **2004**, *31*, 633–642. [CrossRef] [PubMed]
78. Liu, S.; Yamauchi, H. p27-Associated G1 arrest induced by hinokitiol in human malignant melanoma cells is mediated via down-regulation of pRb, Skp2 ubiquitin ligase, and impairment of Cdk2 function. *Cancer Lett.* **2009**, *286*, 240–249. [CrossRef]
79. Katagiri, Y.; Hozumi, Y.; Kondo, S. Knockdown of Skp2 by siRNA inhibits melanoma cell growth in vitro and in vivo. *J. Dermatol. Sci.* **2006**, *42*, 215–224. [CrossRef] [PubMed]
80. Zhao, H.; Pan, H.; Wang, H.; Chai, P.; Ge, S.; Jia, R.; Fan, X. SKP2 targeted inhibition suppresses human uveal melanoma progression by blocking ubiquitylation of p27. *Oncol. Targets. Ther.* **2019**, *12*, 4297–4308. [CrossRef] [PubMed]
81. Qu, X.; Shen, L.; Zheng, Y.; Cui, Y.; Feng, Z.; Liu, F.; Liu, J. A signal transduction pathway from TGF-β1 to SKP2 via Akt1 and c-Myc and its correlation with progression in human melanoma. *J. Investig. Dermatol.* **2014**, *134*, 159–167. [CrossRef] [PubMed]
82. Larue, L.; Bellacosa, A. Epithelial-mesenchymal transition in development and cancer: Role of phosphatidylinositol 3' kinase/AKT pathways. *Oncogene* **2005**, *24*, 7443–7454. [CrossRef] [PubMed]
83. Wei, C.-Y.; Zhu, M.-X.; Yang, Y.-W.; Zhang, P.-F.; Yang, X.; Peng, R.; Gao, C.; Lu, J.-C.; Wang, L.; Deng, X.-Y.; et al. Downregulation of RNF128 activates Wnt/β-catenin signaling to induce cellular EMT and stemness via CD44 and CTTN ubiquitination in melanoma. *J. Hematol. Oncol.* **2019**, *12*, 21. [CrossRef] [PubMed]
84. Dai, Z.; Zhang, J.; Wu, Q.; Fang, H.; Shi, C.; Li, Z.; Lin, C.; Tang, D.; Wang, D. Intestinal microbiota: A new force in cancer immunotherapy. *Cell Commun. Signal.* **2020**, *18*, 1–16. [CrossRef] [PubMed]
85. Li, Y.; Tinoco, R.; Elmén, L.; Segota, I.; Xian, Y.; Fujita, Y.; Sahu, A.; Zarecki, R.; Marie, K.; Feng, Y.; et al. Gut microbiota dependent anti-tumor immunity restricts melanoma growth in Rnf5 −/− mice. *Nat. Commun.* **2019**, *10*. [CrossRef]
86. Nicholson, B.; Leach, C.A.; Goldenberg, S.J.; Francis, D.M.; Kodrasov, M.P.; Tian, X.; Shanks, J.; Sterner, D.E.; Bernal, A.; Mattern, M.R.; et al. Characterization of ubiquitin and ubiquitin-like-protein isopeptidase activities. *Protein Sci.* **2008**, *17*, 1035–1043. [CrossRef] [PubMed]
87. McClurg, U.L.; Robson, C.N. Deubiquitinating enzymes as oncotargets. *Oncotarget* **2015**, *6*, 9657–9668. [CrossRef]
88. Ventii, K.H.; Devi, N.S.; Friedrich, K.L.; Chernova, T.A.; Tighiouart, M.; Van Meir, E.G.; Wilkinson, K.D. BRCA1-associated protein-1 is a tumor suppressor that requires deubiquitinating activity and nuclear localization. *Cancer Res.* **2008**, *68*, 6953–6962. [CrossRef] [PubMed]
89. Wiesner, T.; Obenauf, A.C.; Murali, R.; Fried, I.; Griewank, K.G.; Ulz, P.; Windpassinger, C.; Wackernagel, W.; Loy, S.; Wolf, I.; et al. Germline mutations in BAP1 predispose to melanocytic tumors. *Nat. Genet.* **2011**, *43*, 1018–1021. [CrossRef]
90. Scheuermann, J.C.; de Ayala Alonso, A.G.; Oktaba, K.; Ly-Hartig, N.; McGinty, R.K.; Fraterman, S.; Wilm, M.; Muir, T.W.; Müller, J. Histone H2A deubiquitinase activity of the Polycomb repressive complex PR-DUB. *Nature* **2010**, *465*, 243–247. [CrossRef] [PubMed]
91. Yu, H.; Pak, H.; Hammond-Martel, I.; Ghram, M.; Rodrigue, A.; Daou, S.; Barbour, H.; Corbeil, L.; Hébert, J.; Drobetsky, E.; et al. Tumor suppressor and deubiquitinase BAP1 promotes DNA double-strand break repair. *Proc. Natl. Acad. Sci. USA* **2014**, *111*, 285–290. [CrossRef]
92. Webster, J.D.; Pham, T.H.; Wu, X.; Hughes, N.W.; Li, Z.; Totpal, K.; Lee, H.-J.; Calses, P.C.; Chaurushiya, M.S.; Stawiski, E.W.; et al. The tumor suppressor BAP1 cooperates with BRAFV600E to promote tumor formation in cutaneous melanoma. *Pigment Cell Melanoma Res.* **2019**, *32*, 269–279. [CrossRef]
93. He, M.; Chaurushiya, M.S.; Webster, J.D.; Kummerfeld, S.; Reja, R.; Chaudhuri, S.; Chen, Y.-J.; Modrusan, Z.; Haley, B.; Dugger, D.L.; et al. Intrinsic apoptosis shapes the tumor spectrum linked to inactivation of the deubiquitinase BAP1. *Science* **2019**, *364*, 283–285. [CrossRef]
94. Lee, H.-J.; Pham, T.; Chang, M.T.; Barnes, D.; Cai, A.G.; Noubade, R.; Totpal, K.; Chen, X.; Tran, C.; Hagenbeek, T.; et al. The tumor suppressor BAP1 regulates the Hippo pathway in pancreatic ductal adenocarcinoma. *Cancer Res.* **2020**, *80*, 1656–1668. [CrossRef]
95. Liu-Smith, F.; Lu, Y. Opposite Roles of BAP1 in Overall Survival of Uveal Melanoma and Cutaneous Melanoma. *J. Clin. Med.* **2020**, *9*, 411. [CrossRef]
96. Kumar, R.; Taylor, M.; Miao, B.; Ji, Z.; Njauw, J.C.-N.; Jönsson, G.; Frederick, D.T.; Tsao, H. BAP1 has a survival role in cutaneous melanoma. *J. Invest. Dermatol.* **2015**, *135*, 1089–1097. [CrossRef]
97. Sato, Y.; Goto, E.; Shibata, Y.; Kubota, Y.; Yamagata, A.; Goto-Ito, S.; Kubota, K.; Inoue, J.; Takekawa, M.; Tokunaga, F.; et al. Structures of CYLD USP with Met1- or Lys63-linked diubiquitin reveal mechanisms for dual specificity. *Nat. Struct. Mol. Biol.* **2015**, *22*, 222–229. [CrossRef]
98. Massoumi, R.; Podda, M.; Fässler, R.; Paus, R. Cylindroma as tumor of hair follicle origin. *J. Investig. Dermatol.* **2006**, *126*, 1182–1184. [CrossRef] [PubMed]
99. Massoumi, R.; Kuphal, S.; Hellerbrand, C.; Haas, B.; Wild, P.; Spruss, T.; Pfeifer, A.; Fässler, R.; Bosserhoff, A.K. Down-regulation of CYLD expression by Snail promotes tumor progression in malignant melanoma. *J. Exp. Med.* **2009**, *206*, 221–232. [CrossRef] [PubMed]
100. De Jel, M.M.; Schott, M.; Lamm, S.; Neuhuber, W.; Kuphal, S.; Bosserhoff, A.-K. Loss of CYLD accelerates melanoma development and progression in the Tg(Grm1) melanoma mouse model. *Oncogenesis* **2019**, *8*, 56. [CrossRef] [PubMed]
101. Young, M.-J.; Hsu, K.-C.; Lin, T.E.; Chang, W.-C.; Hung, J.-J. The role of ubiquitin-specific peptidases in cancer progression. *J. Biomed. Sci.* **2019**, *26*, 42. [CrossRef] [PubMed]

102. Guo, W.; Ma, J.; Pei, T.; Zhao, T.; Guo, S.; Yi, X.; Liu, Y.; Wang, S.; Zhu, G.; Jian, Z.; et al. Up-regulated deubiquitinase USP4 plays an oncogenic role in melanoma. *J. Cell. Mol. Med.* **2018**, *22*, 2944–2954. [CrossRef] [PubMed]
103. Zou, X.; Levy-Cohen, G.; Blank, M. Molecular functions of NEDD4 E3 ubiquitin ligases in cancer. *Biochim. Biophys. Acta—Rev. Cancer* **2015**, *1856*, 91–106. [CrossRef]
104. Aronchik, I.; Kundu, A.; Quirit, J.G.; Firestone, G.L. The antiproliferative response of indole-3-carbinol in human melanoma cells is triggered by an interaction with NEDD4-1 and disruption of wild-type PTEN degradation. *Mol. Cancer Res.* **2014**, *12*, 1621–1634. [CrossRef]
105. Yang, Y.; Luo, M.; Zhang, K.; Zhang, J.; Gao, T.; Connell, D.O.; Yao, F.; Mu, C.; Cai, B.; Shang, Y.; et al. Nedd4 ubiquitylates VDAC2/3 to suppress erastin-induced ferroptosis in melanoma. *Nat. Commun.* **2020**, *11*, 433. [CrossRef] [PubMed]
106. Kim, H.; Frederick, D.T.; Levesque, M.P.; Cooper, Z.A.; Feng, Y.; Krepler, C.; Brill, L.; Samuels, Y.; Hayward, N.K.; Perlina, A.; et al. Downregulation of the Ubiquitin Ligase RNF125 Underlies Resistance of Melanoma Cells to BRAF Inhibitors via JAK1 Deregulation. *Cell Rep.* **2015**, *11*, 1458–1473. [CrossRef]
107. Zhao, H.; Li, C.C.; Pardo, J.; Chu, P.C.; Liao, C.X.; Huang, J.; Dong, J.G.; Zhou, X.; Huang, Q.; Huang, B.; et al. A novel E3 ubiquitin ligase TRAC-1 positively regulates T cell activation. *J. Immunol.* **2005**, *174*, 5288–5297. [CrossRef] [PubMed]
108. Arimoto, K.; Takahashi, H.; Hishiki, T.; Konishi, H.; Fujita, T.; Shimotohno, K. Negative regulation of the RIG-I signaling by the ubiquitin ligase RNF125. *Proc. Natl. Acad. Sci. USA* **2007**, *104*, 7500–7505. [CrossRef] [PubMed]
109. Avitan-Hersh, E.; Feng, Y.; Oknin Vaisman, A.; Abu Ahmad, Y.; Zohar, Y.; Zhang, T.; Lee, J.S.; Lazar, I.; Sheikh Khalil, S.; Feiler, Y.; et al. Regulation of eIF2α by RNF4 Promotes Melanoma Tumorigenesis and Therapy Resistance. *J. Invest. Dermatol.* **2020**, *140*, 2466–2477. [CrossRef]
110. Nagler, A.; Vredevoogd, D.W.; Alon, M.; Cheng, P.F.; Trabish, S.; Kalaora, S.; Arafeh, R.; Goldin, V.; Levesque, M.P.; Peeper, D.S.; et al. A genome-wide CRISPR screen identifies FBXO42 involvement in resistance toward MEK inhibition in NRAS-mutant melanoma. *Pigment Cell Melanoma Res.* **2020**, *33*, 334–344. [CrossRef]
111. Schülein-Völk, C.; Wolf, E.; Zhu, J.; Xu, W.; Taranets, L.; Hellmann, A.; Jänicke, L.A.; Diefenbacher, M.E.; Behrens, A.; Eilers, M.; et al. Dual regulation of Fbw7 function and oncogenic transformation by Usp28. *Cell Rep.* **2014**, *9*, 1099–1109. [CrossRef] [PubMed]
112. Didier, R.; Mallavialle, A.; Ben Jouira, R.; Domdom, M.A.; Tichet, M.; Auberger, P.; Luciano, F.; Ohanna, M.; Tartare-Deckert, S.; Deckert, M. Targeting the Proteasome-Associated Deubiquitinating Enzyme USP14 Impairs Melanoma Cell Survival and Overcomes Resistance to MAPK-Targeting Therapies. *Mol. Cancer Ther.* **2018**, *17*, 1416–1429. [CrossRef]
113. Vanneste, M.; Feddersen, C.R.; Varzavand, A.; Zhu, E.Y.; Foley, T.; Zhao, L.; Holt, K.H.; Milhem, M.; Piper, R.; Stipp, C.S.; et al. Functional Genomic Screening Independently Identifies CUL3 as a Mediator of Vemurafenib Resistance via Src-Rac1 Signaling Axis. *Front. Oncol.* **2020**, *10*, 442. [CrossRef] [PubMed]
114. Han, Y.; Liu, D.; Li, L. PD-1/PD-L1 pathway: Current researches in cancer. *Am. J. Cancer Res.* **2020**, *10*, 727–742.
115. Meng, X.; Liu, X.; Guo, X.; Jiang, S.; Chen, T.; Hu, Z.; Liu, H.; Bai, Y.; Xue, M.; Hu, R.; et al. FBXO38 mediates PD-1 ubiquitination and regulates anti-tumour immunity of T cells. *Nature* **2018**, *564*, 130–135. [CrossRef]
116. Saldana, M.; VanderVorst, K.; Berg, A.L.; Lee, H.; Carraway, K.L. Otubain 1: A non-canonical deubiquitinase with an emerging role in cancer. *Endocr. Relat. Cancer* **2019**, *26*, R1–R14. [CrossRef]
117. Zhou, X.; Yu, J.; Cheng, X.; Zhao, B.; Manyam, G.C.; Zhang, L.; Schluns, K.; Li, P.; Wang, J.; Sun, S.-C. The deubiquitinase Otub1 controls the activation of CD8+ T cells and NK cells by regulating IL-15-mediated priming. *Nat. Immunol.* **2019**, *20*, 879–889. [CrossRef] [PubMed]
118. Scortegagna, M.; Hockemeyer, K.; Dolgalev, I.; Poźniak, J.; Rambow, F.; Li, Y.; Feng, Y.; Tinoco, R.; Otero, D.C.; Zhang, T.; et al. Siah2 control of T-regulatory cells limits anti-tumor immunity. *Nat. Commun.* **2020**, *11*, 99. [CrossRef] [PubMed]
119. Feng, Y.; Sessions, E.H.; Zhang, F.; Ban, F.; Placencio-Hickok, V.; Ma, C.T.; Zeng, F.Y.; Pass, I.; Terry, D.B.; Cadwell, G.; et al. Identification and characterization of small molecule inhibitors of the ubiquitin ligases Siah1/2 in melanoma and prostate cancer cells. *Cancer Lett.* **2019**, *449*, 145–162. [CrossRef] [PubMed]
120. Mezzadra, R.; Sun, C.; Jae, L.T.; Gomez-Eerland, R.; De Vries, E.; Wu, W.; Logtenberg, M.E.W.; Slagter, M.; Rozeman, E.A.; Hofland, I.; et al. Identification of CMTM6 and CMTM4 as PD-L1 protein regulators. *Nature* **2017**, *549*, 106–110. [CrossRef]
121. Merin, N.; Kelly, K. Clinical Use of Proteasome Inhibitors in the Treatment of Multiple Myeloma. *Pharmaceuticals* **2014**, *8*, 1–20. [CrossRef] [PubMed]
122. Thompson, J.L. Carfilzomib: A second-generation proteasome inhibitor for the treatment of relapsed and refractory multiple myeloma. *Ann. Pharmacother.* **2013**, *47*, 56–62. [CrossRef]
123. Richardson, P.G.; Zweegman, S.; O'Donnell, E.K.; Laubach, J.P.; Raje, N.; Voorhees, P.; Ferrari, R.H.; Skacel, T.; Kumar, S.K.; Lonial, S. Ixazomib for the treatment of multiple myeloma. *Expert Opin. Pharmacother.* **2018**, *19*, 1949–1968. [CrossRef] [PubMed]
124. Markovic, S.N.; Geyer, S.M.; Dawkins, F.; Sharfman, W.; Albertini, M.; Maples, W.; Fracasso, P.M.; Fitch, T.; Lorusso, P.; Adjei, A.A.; et al. A phase II study of bortezomib in the treatment of metastatic malignant melanoma. *Cancer* **2005**, *103*, 2584–2589. [CrossRef] [PubMed]
125. Bhatia, S.; Pavlick, A.C.; Boasberg, P.; Thompson, J.A.; Mulligan, G.; Pickard, M.D.; Faessel, H.; Dezube, B.J.; Hamid, O. A phase I study of the investigational NEDD8-activating enzyme inhibitor pevonedistat (TAK-924/MLN4924) in patients with metastatic melanoma. *Investig. New Drugs* **2016**, *34*, 439–449. [CrossRef]
126. Wertz, I.E.; Wang, X. From Discovery to Bedside: Targeting the Ubiquitin System. *Cell Chem. Biol.* **2019**, *26*, 156–177. [CrossRef]

127. Pawlak, W.Z.; Legha, S.S. Phase II study of thalidomide in patients with metastatic melanoma. *Melanoma Res.* **2004**, *14*, 57–62. [CrossRef]
128. Glaspy, J.; Atkins, M.B.; Richards, J.M.; Agarwala, S.S.; O'Day, S.; Knight, R.D.; Jungnelius, J.U.; Bedikian, A.Y. Results of a multicenter, randomized, double-blind, dose-evaluating phase 2/3 study of lenalidomide in the treatment of metastatic malignant melanoma. *Cancer* **2009**, *115*, 5228–5236. [CrossRef]
129. Altun, M.; Kramer, H.B.; Willems, L.I.; McDermott, J.L.; Leach, C.A.; Goldenberg, S.J.; Kumar, K.G.S.; Konietzny, R.; Fischer, R.; Kogan, E.; et al. Activity-Based Chemical Proteomics Accelerates Inhibitor Development for Deubiquitylating Enzymes. *Chem. Biol.* **2011**, *18*, 1401–1412. [CrossRef]
130. Sun, X.; Gao, H.; Yang, Y.; He, M.; Wu, Y.; Song, Y.; Tong, Y.; Rao, Y. PROTACs: Great opportunities for academia and industry. *Signal Transduct. Target. Ther.* **2019**, *4*, 64. [CrossRef]
131. Vogelmann, A.; Robaa, D.; Sippl, W.; Jung, M. Proteolysis targeting chimeras (PROTACs) for epigenetics research. *Curr. Opin. Chem. Biol.* **2020**, *57*, 8–16. [CrossRef] [PubMed]

Review

Melanoma Single-Cell Biology in Experimental and Clinical Settings

Hans Binder [1], Maria Schmidt [1], Henry Loeffler-Wirth [1], Lena Suenke Mortensen [1] and Manfred Kunz [2,*]

[1] Interdisciplinary Center for Bioinformatics, University of Leipzig, 04107 Leipzig, Germany; binder@izbi.uni-leipzig.de (H.B.); schmidt@izbi.uni-leipzig.de (M.S.); wirth@izbi.uni-leipzig.de (H.L.-W.); mortensen@izbi.uni-leipzig.de (L.S.M.)
[2] Department of Dermatology, Venereology and Allergology, University of Leipzig Medical Center, Philipp-Rosenthal-Str. 23-25, 04103 Leipzig, Germany
* Correspondence: Manfred.Kunz@medizin.uni-leipzig.de; Tel.: +49-341-97-18610; Fax: +49-341-97-18609

Abstract: Cellular heterogeneity is regarded as a major factor for treatment response and resistance in a variety of malignant tumors, including malignant melanoma. More recent developments of single-cell sequencing technology provided deeper insights into this phenomenon. Single-cell data were used to identify prognostic subtypes of melanoma tumors, with a special emphasis on immune cells and fibroblasts in the tumor microenvironment. Moreover, treatment resistance to checkpoint inhibitor therapy has been shown to be associated with a set of differentially expressed immune cell signatures unraveling new targetable intracellular signaling pathways. Characterization of T cell states under checkpoint inhibitor treatment showed that exhausted $CD8^+$ T cell types in melanoma lesions still have a high proliferative index. Other studies identified treatment resistance mechanisms to targeted treatment against the mutated BRAF serine/threonine protein kinase including repression of the melanoma differentiation gene microphthalmia-associated transcription factor (MITF) and induction of AXL receptor tyrosine kinase. Interestingly, treatment resistance mechanisms not only included selection processes of pre-existing subclones but also transition between different states of gene expression. Taken together, single-cell technology has provided deeper insights into melanoma biology and has put forward our understanding of the role of tumor heterogeneity and transcriptional plasticity, which may impact on innovative clinical trial designs and experimental approaches.

Keywords: melanoma; single-cell transcriptome sequencing; treatment response; pseudotime analysis

1. Melanoma Biology, Clinics and Treatment

Melanoma is a highly aggressive cutaneous neoplasia, which has been intensively analyzed by molecular techniques in the past few years [1,2]. Indeed, a number of mutational analyses have been performed and identified key driver mutations among which mutant *BRAF*V600 is the most prevalent, affecting almost 50% of all melanoma patients [3–5]. Mutant *BRAF*V600 leads to an activation of the classical mitogen-activated protein kinase (MAPK) pathway with downstream targets being mitogen-activated extracellular signal-regulated kinases (MEK) 1/2 and extracellular-signal regulated kinases (ERK) 1/2. Promising treatment responses were obtained by targeting this pathway on the level of BRAF kinase and MEK1/2, which has been a mainstay of melanoma therapy in recent years [1,2,6]. BRAF-targeted treatment includes small molecule inhibitors vemurafenib, dabrafenib, and encorafenib, directed against activated (mutated) BRAF kinase, which has significantly improved the survival rate of affected patients. Overall treatment success is hampered by the fact that a significant number of patients show primary resistance (~20%) and also secondary resistance, which occurs in the vast majority of patients. The currently used treatment options mainly consist of combination treatments of BRAF inhibition combined with MEK1/2 inhibition, which is not only more effective but also reduces side effects such as the development of epidermal neoplasias and exanthemas [7]. Cobimetinib, trametinib, and binimetinib are currently used as MEK1/2 inhibitors in combination therapy. The 5-year overall survival rate of combination therapy has reached 50%, which may be regarded as a major breakthrough for this highly aggressive tumor [8]. Still, the majority of patients develop a secondary resistance [9]. More recently, adjuvant treatment after complete tumor eradication in stage III (lymph node metastasis) has been approved using this combination of treatment, and neo-adjuvant (pre-operation) treatment studies are under way [10,11].

The mechanisms underlying primary and secondary resistance to targeted treatment have been an area of intensive investigations in recent years [12–23]. Among the most prominent cellular mechanisms are switches to *NRAS* mutations [15,17,23], aberrant *BRAF* splicing [14,15], *BRAF* amplifications [12,13,15–17], *MAP2K1* (*MEK1*) mutations [13,17], *PTEN* and *PIK3CA* mutations [17], and *COT* overexpression [21].

Principally, mechanisms of treatment resistance are heterogeneous but show many overlapping patterns in different studies. An earlier study found NRAS and PDGFR overexpression in a number of melanoma cell lines after development of treatment resistance to BRAF inhibitor PLX4032 in vitro [23]. In one of the most comprehensive subsequent studies, 45 patients were analyzed by whole-exome sequencing before BRAF inhibitor (vemurafenib or dabrafenib) treatment, after early (less than 12 weeks) and late development of resistance [17]. Top resistance variants were *NRAS* mutations, *BRAF* amplifications, *MEK1* and *MEK2* mutations, and *PTEN* mutations/amplifications. *MEK1* and *PTEN* mutations were partly already present before treatment.

A similar study analyzed 59 metastatic melanoma lesions from patients treated with dabrafenib or vemurafenib [15]. Authors performed a targeted genetic screen of *NRAS*, *BRAF*, *MEK1*, *MEK2*, and *AKT1* genetic variants. Resistance mechanisms were found in 58% of progressing tumors, with *BRAF* splice variants, *BRAF* amplifications, and *NRAS* and *MEK1/2* mutations being present in 8–32% of cases. In another study, *BRAF* amplifications were found in 4 out of 20 melanoma patients, and *NRAS* mutations in 5 out of 20 melanoma patients, under treatment with vemurafenib, as determined by whole-exome sequencing and quantitative polymerase chain reaction (PCR) [16]. *BRAF* genetic amplifications were also a major mechanism of secondary treatment resistance in a study on 28 melanoma samples resistant to combined BRAF and MEK inhibition, as determined by targeted sequencing of *BRAF*, *NRAS*, *KRAS*, *MEK1*, and *MEK2* [12]. Overall, 8 out of 28 samples showed very high numbers of *BRAF* amplifications (ultra-amplifications). Subsequent in vitro studies showed that *BRAF* ultra-amplified melanoma cell lines may become addicted to BRAF/MEK1 inhibition, as cells died after drug-removal [12]. This might be of relevance for clinical settings and might speak for drug holidays to enhance later treatment response.

In an analysis of 10 patients under combined treatment with dabrafenib and trametinib, genetic resistance mechanisms were found in 9 out of 11 progressing tumors analyzed by a focused PCR panel for *BRAF*, *NRAS*, *MEK1/2*, and *AKT1* [13]. *BRAF* amplifications were found in 4, and *MEK1/2* mutations in 3 samples. In a smaller study analyzing 5 patients that developed acquired resistance to combined BRAF and MEK1/2 inhibition (dabrafenib, trametinib), a new mutation in *MEK2* was observed in one patient, and *BRAF* amplification and alternative *BRAF* splicing were found in two other patients [14]. The pathogenic role of the new *MEK2* mutation was verified via in vitro experiments. *BRAF*-mutant melanomas may also acquire resistance through activation of the EGFR pathway, as shown in a study on melanoma patients treated with vemurafenib or dabrafenib, a finding that has been observed earlier in colon cancer [19]. *EGFR* expression was shown to be related to *SOX10* downregulation, and in vitro *SOX10*-low cells were enriched in the presence of BRAF inhibition in vitro. This phenomenon was reversed after drug removal, which also suggests drug-holidays being useful in re-sensitizing cells to BRAF inhibition. Taken together, the mentioned studies underline that resistance mechanisms in melanoma to targeted treatment use different mechanisms but center around re-activated MAPK or PTEN-AKT1 pathways.

Studies on transcriptional mechanisms of primary resistance to targeted treatment revealed a MITF-low/NF-κB-high transcriptional phenotype which could be linked to specific gene expression profiles in cell lines and patient biopsies, and a MITF-low/AXL-high phenotype [20,22]. In vitro, combined treatment of cell lines with BRAF inhibition and an AXL inhibitor significantly reduced melanoma cell viability of MITF-low/AXL-high cells, supporting the functional relevance of these findings [20]. In a large-scale study using RNA-sequencing of metastatic melanoma samples, transcriptomic patterns of 48 single-drug or double-drug disease progressors were compared with patient-matched baseline melanoma tissues [18]. Transcriptomic patterns of treatment resistance involved differential gene expression of tumor and stromal genes. Among up-regulated genes in resistant lesions were *c-MET*, *IL-8*, *c-FOS*, macrophage marker *CD163*, chemokine *CCL8*, and *NFKBIA*.

However, these transcriptional mechanisms are incompletely understood as the underlying data mostly originates from bulk sequencing studies; thus, they do not reflect clonal structures and are only partly recapitulating selection processes. Overall, primary and secondary resistance mechanisms to targeted therapy may be either due to genetic changes (mutations, amplifications) or changes in gene expression of specific pathways [24].

Major progress was made in the field of immunotherapies in melanoma. Immunotherapies, in particular immunecheckpoint inhibition (ICI), targeting the cytotoxic T lymphocyte antigen 4 (CTLA-4), programmed cell death protein 1 (PD-1), and programmed cell death protein ligand 1 (PD-L1) have been approved in recent years in a number of different cancers including malignant melanoma [25]. However, a larger number of patients did not respond to these treatments (60% in case of PD-1 inhibition, 80% for CTLA-4 inhibition) as a primary resistance. Treatment response rates could slightly be enhanced by a combination of anti-PD1 and anti-CTLA4 treatment [26].

The underlying mechanisms for primary and secondary treatment resistance to immunotherapies have been studied in recent years and include a number of different mechanisms [27]. In one of the earliest studies addressing this issue, immune markers of anti-CTLA4 treatment response of melanoma patients were analyzed [28]. Pre-treatment tumors of overall 110 patients were analyzed by whole-exome sequencing. Transcriptome data were generated for 40 patients. Mutational load, neoantigen load, and transcriptomes of cytolytic activity were associated with treatment response. Enhanced expression of granzyme A (*GRZMA*) and perforin 1 (*PRF1*) were associated with responses, as were *CTLA-4* and *PD-L2* expression. In a parallel study of another group, melanoma exomes from 64 patients treated with CTLA-4-blocking antibodies were analyzed by whole-exome sequencing [29]. Mutational load alone was not sufficient to predict treatment benefit. Neoepitope analysis identified neoantigen landscapes with a strong treatment response. Further, the predicted neoantigens were able to activate T cells from patients treated with anti-CTLA4 antibodies in in vitro experiments.

Hugo and co-workers performed a large-scale study on 28 metastatic melanoma lesions, 27 of which were pre-treatment lesions, and analyzed gene expression patterns of responding versus non-responding lesions [30]. Overall, the mutational load of tumors correlated with patient survival (but not with tumor response). Among the genes that were upregulated in non-responding lesions were mesenchymal transition genes such as *AXL*, *WNT5A*, and *TWIST*, as well as immunosuppressive genes such as *IL10*, *VEGFA*, and *VEGFC*. Resistant lesions showed a gene expression signature called IPRES (innate anti-PD1 resistance), which is comprised of 26 transcriptomic signatures including mesenchymal transition, wound healing, and angiogenesis.

In a first study on secondary treatment resistance, samples from paired baseline and relapsing lesions in four patients were analyzed [31]. By use of whole-exome sequencing it was shown that resistant lesions in two patients carried mutations in interferon-receptor-associated Janus kinase 1 (*JAK1*) or Janus kinase 2 (*JAK2*) genes, associated with the deletion of the wild-type allele. A third patient showed a truncating mutation in the beta-2-microglobulin (*B2M*) gene, which is part of the MHC-I complex.

In a later large-scale analysis of treatment resistance, 54 samples with CTLA4- blockade followed by anti-PD1 treatment were analyzed by a 12-marker immunohistochemistry panel and NanoString® technology (of 795 immune-related genes) (nanoString, Seattle, WA, USA) [32]. This study showed that individual protein markers and gene expression patterns in early on-treatment biopsies were predictive of responses for the checkpoint blockage. Among markers for treatment response to anti-PD1 treatment were CD8, CD4, CD3, PD-1, PD-L1, and LAG3 protein expression in responders versus non-responders in early on-treatment samples. In the NanoString® analyses of response to anti-PD1 treatment, up-regulation of HLA-molecules, IFN-γ pathway effectors, and different chemokines were observed.

In a subsequent study, 68 patients with advanced melanoma were investigated before and after anti-PD-1 treatment by whole-exome and transcriptome analysis [33]. Responders under treatment experienced a so-called mutation contraction, which means that the number of clonal and subclonal variants decreased on therapy in these patients. Transcriptomic analyses showed an increase in gene expressions patterns of $CD8^+$ T cells, NK cells, and M1 macrophages in responders as compared to non-responders.

Recently, pre-treatment tumors taken from 144 metastatic melanoma patient were analyzed by whole-exome and whole-transcriptome sequencing, and mutational and transcriptomic features were assessed for correlation with response to anti-PD1 treatment [34]. Interestingly, there was no significant association of specific gene mutations to response or resistance to treatment. Regarding gene expression, 4 of the 13 MHC-II associated HLA genes were significantly upregulated in responders. Significantly enriched pathways in responders were IFN-γ response, allograft rejection, complement, inflammatory response, and interleukin (IL6)-JAK-STAT3 signaling. Signatures for T cells, B cells, macrophages, $CD8^+$ cytotoxic, and exhausted $CD4^+$ T cells were also enriched. Interestingly, there were differences between patients with previous exposure to anti-CTLA4 treatment and those who were naïve to this treatment with a higher expression of immune-related pathways in in responders of the anti-CTLA4 pre-treated group. Among prominent immune genes were *CXCL9*, *CXCL10*, and *CXCR3*, among prominent immune markers were CD20, CD163, CD4, FOXP3, and CTLA-4.

In a more recent study, authors built an immune predictive score called IMPRES, based on a gene pattern analysis of spontaneously regressing neuroblastomas, to predict immune checkpoint inhibitor response in melanoma [35]. Overall, 18 immune checkpoint genes were chosen and high expression of *HVEM* (a member of the tumor necrosis factor receptor superfamily), *CD27* and *CD40* were associated with better response rates, while immune inhibitory molecules such as *CD276*, *TIM-3*, and *VISTA* were associated with worse response. This signature was tested in an own melanoma data set of 41 patients of the authors under immune checkpoint blockage and on other data sets [30,32]. In particular, *PD-1/OX40L* expression was predictive for anti-PD1 treatment response. However, the predictive capacity of the IMPRES score is controversially discussed [36].

Taken together, a significant number of genetic and genomic studies on mechanisms of treatment response and resistance under immune checkpoint inhibition support the notion of immune cell patterns, HLA molecules and chemokines as major drivers of response.

Recurrences and treatment failures of melanoma may not only derive from global changes in gene patterns but also from intra-tumor heterogeneity and the outgrowth of pre-existing treatment-resistant clones. Moreover, evidence has also been provided that tumor cell plasticity mediated by an activated tissue microenvironment secreting TNF-α and other immune modulators may cause resistance [37,38]. Transcriptional and epigenetic states may change during treatment and impact on recurrences and treatment resistance [37,39].

Multiple subclonal mutations, gene expression patterns, or epigenetic mechanisms may be present in tumor lesions and create a genetically heterogeneous population of tumor cells. In addition, the tumor microenvironment can impact on melanoma biology, in particular on predisposed subclones or subclones that may be re-programmed transcriptionally. Here, we summarize current knowledge on the analysis of melanoma heterogeneity through single-cell RNA-seq (scRNA-seq) technology, with an emphasis on treatment response and resistance.

2. Clonal Heterogeneity in Melanoma

Clonal heterogeneity is currently regarded as one of the most relevant factors for treatment resistance and recurrence of malignant tumors [40]. The model of a clonal evolution of tumors with many molecularly heterogeneous subclones had been suggested in earlier reports, at a time when the molecular basis of tumor heterogeneity could not be analyzed in more detail [41]. Based on current knowledge, many of the recurrences and treatment failures of metastatic tumors derive at least in part from this clonal heterogeneity in tumor lesions consisting of different molecular subclones [42,43].

In melanoma, intra-tumor heterogeneity has been described for the presence or absence of *BRAF* mutations, but more detailed analyses on mutational patterns were still lacking at that time [44].

The molecular heterogeneity in melanoma lesions has been analyzed recently in more detail by use of whole-genome sequencing of distinct macrodissected tumor areas of primary melanomas and metastases [45]. In this study, 8 melanoma samples of primary melanomas and lymph node metastases were analyzed with multiregion sequencing of 41 regions. On average, 489 non-synonymous mutations were observed of which 13% were heterogeneously distributed. MAPK pathway genes (*BRAF*, *NRAS*, and *NF1*) were frequently mutated throughout all tumor regions (truncal mutations). Mutational tumor heterogeneity was associated with patient survival, with higher heterogeneity leading to shorter overall survival in this limited cohort of patients. Phylogenetic trees showed that 88% of driver mutations as derived from the catalogue of somatic mutations in cancer (Cosmic) database were truncal mutations, supporting their role in melanoma biology. Further analyses with larger sample sets and consecutive biopsies may help to understand the biological and clinical impact of this intra-tumor heterogeneity. Heterogeneously distributed mutations were found in subclones for *PIK3CA*, *PIK3R1*, *PTEN*, *MSN*, *JAK2*, *JAK3*, *NOTCH2*, and *IDH1*, with little overlap between the different samples.

In a subsequent study, authors compared mutational patterns of melanomas with signs of chronic sun damage (CSD melanomas) with high and low sun damage [46]. Ultra-deep sequencing was performed for 72 in situ and invasive melanomas for 40 cancer-associated genes. One sample set of an individual patient was analyzed in more detail regarding 5 regions in the primary tumor and 7 in in-transit metastases. There were no significant differences regarding the transcriptomes as determined by RNA-seq. Whole-exome sequencing showed that the vast majority of all mutation (96%) were found in all lesions and were regarded as truncal mutations, which comprised *KIT* and *CTNN1* mutations. In total, 60 genes were carrying non-truncal mutations, only four (*COL3A1*, *CTNNB1*, *FOXO3*, and *SRC1*) belonged to the Cancer Gene Census (https://cancer.sanger.ac.uk/census), and the majority was thus regarded as passenger mutations. Interestingly, phylogenetic trees showed that mutations in primary lesions did not appear earlier than in in-transit metastases.

In a recent paper on melanoma, tumor heterogeneity has been simulated in vivo by an admixture of 0.05% of A375 BRAF inhibitor-resistant melanoma cells to 99.95% of A375 BRAF inhibitor-sensitive melanoma cells [47]. This mixture was subcutaneously injected into mice. After treatment with the BRAF inhibitor vemurafenib, the number of resistant cells significantly increased in the overall regressing tumors, basically laying the foundations for relapse and secondary resistance of these tumors [47]. This phenomenon is in agreement with clinical findings for metastatic melanomas. However, based on current knowledge, selection of subclonal populations during treatment response are not the only mechanisms that support treatment resistance. Resistance may also derive from drug-induced re-programming [48].

The prognostic relevance of intra-tumor heterogeneity has recently been emphasized, as higher heterogeneity was associated with worse outcomes [49]. Authors used a clonal heterogeneity analysis tool (CHAT) to estimate intra-tumor heterogeneity, and CIBER-SORT to analyze the immune cell composition from a cohort of 402 melanoma patients of TCGA [49,50]. More heterogeneous tumors were associated with gene patterns indicating less CD8[+] T cells, T follicular cells, and M1 macrophages, while gene patterns of tumor-promoting M2 macrophages were enhanced. Highly heterogeneous tumors also had lower *PD1* and *PD-L1* expression and a lower expression of genes of cytotoxic pathways. These data were confirmed by others, showing that indeed intra-tumor heterogeneity plays an important role in patient survival, a finding that was further validated in a murine melanoma model with B16 melanoma cells [51].

Taken together, the mentioned studies have provided strong evidence for a prognostically relevant genetic heterogeneity in melanoma, either in primary lesions or in metastases. A deeper understanding of this heterogeneity may be achieved by recently developed single-cell technologies.

3. Single-Cell Technology

3.1. Principles of Single-Cell Individualization

Single-cell technology is based on the individualization of cells using different technologies. For a further in depth understanding, the reader is referred to a number of excellent recent reviews [52,53]. One of the first technologies addressing single-cell transcriptomics was introduced by the company Fluidigm® (Fluidigm, South San Francisco, CA, USA). This technology is based on a complex microfluidics system. Single cells are captured on an integrated fluidic circuit RNA-seq chip within the Fluidigm® C1 system. Cell capture, cell lysis, mRNA reverse transcription, and cDNA amplification are performed within the system. Subsequent next-generation sequencing may be performed by Illumina® (Illumina, San Diego, CA, USA) sequencing technology [54,55]. This technology allowed the analysis of 96, and later 384, cells at a time. One major advantage of this technology lies in the fact that whole transcriptomes could be analyzed with complete mRNAs (in the 96-cell format). Other microfluidic systems were introduced, e.g., by 10xGenomics® (10x Genomics, Pleasanton, CA, USA), based on a direct integration of single cells in an emulsion that harbors an individual cell, gel beads covered with molecular identifiers, and capture oligonucleotides. In principle, this technology allows an unlimited number of cells to be analyzed (5000–10,000 cells are recommended). Sequencing is limited to 3′-primed ends of the respective mRNAs and sequencing depth is generally lower compared to the Fluidigm® system. Apart from these widely used techniques, a number of individually established technologies are in use in different laboratories. Recent technologies also include sampling of cells into multi-well plates with subsequent lysis and library preparation in a multi-well format using the SmartSeq 2® (Illumina, San Diego, CA, USA) protocol to overcome 3′-end bias.

3.2. Single-Cell Data Processing and Analysis

Bioinformatics analysis is crucial for extracting knowledge from scRNA-seq data in order to discover the heterogeneity of cell populations in space and time and to understand the underlying molecular mechanisms on tissue, cell and gene levels (Figure 1). A variety of tools have been designed to conduct bulk RNA-seq data analyses, but many of them cannot be directly applied to scRNA-seq [56,57]. Except short-read mapping, almost all data analyses such as differential expression, cell clustering, and gene regulatory network inference have certain disparities between scRNA-seq and bulk RNA-seq techniques. Because of the low amount of starting material, scRNA-seq has limitations regarding data quality due to comparatively low capture efficiency and high dropouts. It produces noisier and sparser data compared to bulk RNA-seq raising substantial challenges for computational analysis. Downstream analysis can be split into two orthogonal views, namely focusing either onto the cells as the functional unit or onto genes or gene programs. Whereas cell-based analysis commonly performs clustering and describes pseudo-temporal behavior of the data, gene-based analysis typically extracts differentially expressed genes, gene sets, and gene regulatory networks. In both situations, scRNA-seq also raises new conceptual challenges, namely to merge 'traditional' differential gene expression analysis of bulk samples with cell-type differentiation, diversity analysis, and counting, as performed traditionally using methods such as FACS (fluorescence-activated cell sorting) or using whole-genome gene expression as a marker instead of single fluorescent labels to identify a cell type. Such joint analyses of cell- and gene-level information provide novel insights regarding genomic regulation of cell-type specific programs and regarding cell-types, particularly in terms of continuously varying states during development of tissues in health and/or disease. Such views enable extracting (pseudo-)temporal information from cross sectional data, estimating interactions between different cell types on gene and molecular levels, and, in consequence, specifying tissue architecture, e.g., in terms of tumor microenvironment and physiological state of the bystander cells.

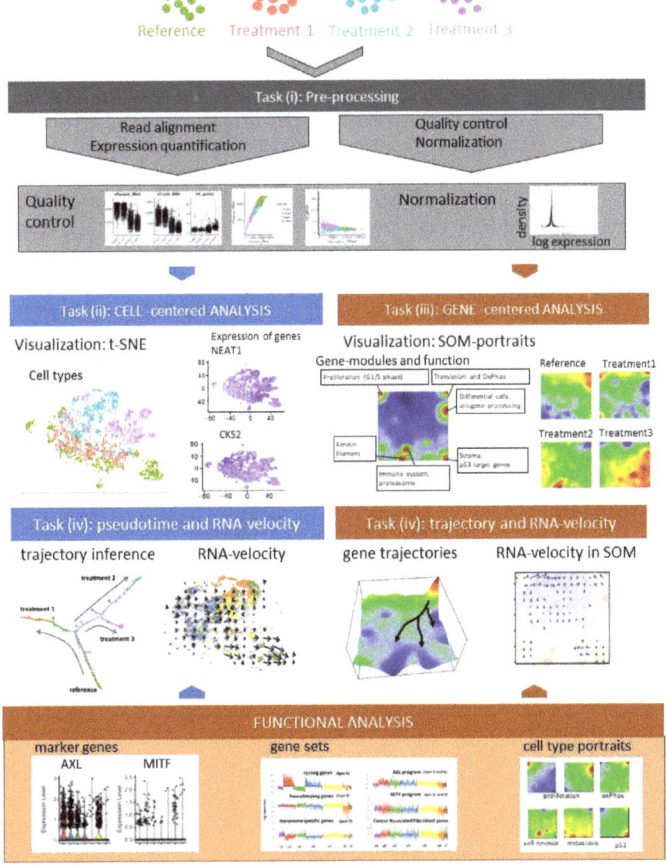

Figure 1. Principles of single-cell analyses based on melanoma cells analyses: A schematic representation of single-cell analyses is shown. Analysis starts with classical read alignment and quality control and normalization measures as in bulk RNA-seq. Subsequent analysis of transcriptomic cell clusters is performed by t-distributed stochastic neighbor embedding (t-SNE) as described in the text. Individual genes (*NEAT1*, *CKS2*) may be mapped onto clonal structures. Alternatively, self-organizing maps may be chosen, which represents a gene-based clustering method of cellular subclones. Pseudotime dynamics shows different trajectories of treatment resistance under three different treatment conditions which may also be demonstrated by RNA-velocity analysis. Marker genes for treatment resistance are found in different subclones and are part of larger gene sets or cell type portraits.

Bioinformatics analysis workflow of scRNA-seq data may be divided into five major tasks (i–v), which still raise a series of methodical and conceptual challenges and therefore is under permanent development [58].

i. Preprocessing aims at removing the effect of all factors without relevance for the expected biological effects. It includes read alignment, expression quantification, quality control, technical bias correction, and normalization. Mapping tools originally developed for bulk RNA-seq are mostly applicable also to scRNA-seq data. Further steps include quality control and filtering of unwanted genes and cells (e.g., cells expressing only a few genes); imputing missing values, batch correction (reducing systematic measurement biases between different runs and/or treatment groups), and normalizing gene expression (reducing unwanted variance between cells due to capture efficiency, sequencing depth, dropouts, and other technical effects). Technical noise of scRNA-seq is a common problem due to the low starting material and challenging experimental protocols. Detailed descriptions and recommendations of suited program-tools have recently been published.

ii. Cell typing and diversity analysis aims at disentangling cell identities and their functional impact in the respective tissues. It includes clustering of cellular transcriptomes and their assignment to cell types (also called populations) in a supervised or unsupervised way. The former classification approach uses cell-type gene signatures taken from previous studies to assign the new data to these 'known' cell types. The latter class-discovery approach splits new data into de-novo groups of cells. In a second step, these new groups are related to known cell types by applying previous cell type signatures and statistical enrichment techniques, thus linking unsupervised with supervised approaches. Classifying cells into types or physiological states is essential for many secondary analyses to characterize the tumor microenvironment by composition of immune cells and/or to extract varying fractions of tumor cells from different developmental stages. For this task and scRNA-seq in general, reliable reference systems with a resolution down to cell states are required. Depending on the research question, even intermediate transition states might be of interest. Reference cell atlases of cell types of different healthy and cancer tissues, of immune cells and of melanoma-related cell types extracted from previous melanoma studies, have been published in a number of reports [50,59,60] and have put an emphasis on immune cells in these settings [61–63].

iii. Gene module and marker extraction, functional analysis, and network inference aim at understanding gene regulation of cells on the gene level including aberrant effects due to genetic defects, external stimuli leading to treatment resistance and intrinsic evolutionary adaptations on tissue level. This task analyses co-expression of groups of genes, characterizes their functional context, and infers gene networks. Gene networks affect interactions between different cell types and/or signaling pathways. Beyond simple changes in average gene expression between cell types (or across bulk-collected libraries), scRNA-seq enables a high granularity of changes in expression. Particularly, cell type-specific alterations in cell state across samples are of special interest. These analyses deliver individual marker genes and sets of signature genes characterizing the different cell types and states, and, in addition, genes reflecting interactions between the cell types in the complex microenvironments of the respective tissue type. Appropriate methods to modularize transcriptional programs are non-negative matrix normalization (NMF) [64] or self-organizing-maps (SOM) [65].

iv. Analysis of developmental trajectories in terms of pseudotime and RNA velocity aim at deducing time-dependent aspects of tissue development and cancer progression from cross-sectional scRNA-seq data. scRNA-seq experiments provide snapshot data, which resolves the molecular heterogeneity of cell cultures and tissues with single cell resolution under static conditions (see task (ii)). Given, that each cell is measured only once, one needs computational methods to deduce developmental trajectories on cellular level from time-independent data. The pseudotime model assumes that single-cell transcriptomes can be understood as a series of microscopic states of cellular development that exist in parallel at the same (real) time in the cell culture or tissue under study. Moreover, the model assumes that the temporal development smoothly and continuously changes transcriptional states in small and densely distributed steps so that the similarity of transcriptional characteristics can serve as a proxy of time, called pseudotime. It scales development in units of values between zero and unities for the start and end points, respectively. The pseudotime algorithm typically aligns the cells along a trajectory in reduced multi-dimensional space where a large variety of projection algorithms can be applied, differing regarding criteria such as cellular ordering, topology, scalability and usability [66]. Each method has its own characteristics in terms of the underlying algorithm, produced outputs and regarding the topology of the pseudotime trajectory (e.g., predefined linear, multibranched, cyclic, or 'inferred from the data'). 'RNA-velocity' provides another independent approach to infer developmental trajectories from static scRNA-seq data [67,68]. It directly 'forecasts' the transcriptional state of a cell based on the relation between spliced and unspliced mRNA in terms of a directional change of cell state in cell-diversity space (task (v)). RNA-velocity provides a vector-field reflecting transcriptional changes of each cell, which can be transferred into developmental trajectories joining sources and sinks of mRNA abundance in cell-state and gene-state space.

v. Dimension reduction, visualization of cell- and gene-state space, and data portrayals aim at enabling the intuitive perception of complex data in order to extract 'hidden' information and to support hypothesis development and testing. scRNA-seq data are high-dimensional data (ten-thousands of transcripts multiplied with ten-to-hundred thousand of cells multiplied with a multitude of biological conditions), which is difficult to visualize in its original form. Dimension reduction and appropriate visualization are therefore important challenges in all four tasks listed above. Conceptually, two perpendicular types of information have to be considered, namely cell- and gene-centered views on the scRNA transcriptomes as addressed in tasks II and III, respectively [61,69]. For the view on cell diversity, different methods projecting multi-dimensional cell-transcriptomes data into two dimensions are in use, such as Principal Component Analysis (PCA), t-distributed stochastic neighbor embedding (t-SNE) and Uniform Manifold Approximation and Projection (UMAP) [70,71]. These methods produce point clouds in cell similarity space visualizing mutual similarities between the single-cell transcriptomes in terms of colored clusters of cells (task II) and/or of colored expression levels of selected gene markers and signatures in the individual cell transcriptomes (task III). For visualization of transcriptomic landscapes in gene state space, we developed the expression portrayal method based on self-organizing map (SOM) machine learning. Such landscapes support identification of modules of co-expressed genes, of their mutual network topology and of their functional context [72,73].

3.3. Single-Cell Exome-Seq

Single-cell technology has also been applied to exomes. An earlier exome sequencing study on renal cell carcinoma identified 260 mutations in 25 single cells, but could not reveal a clonal structure in this tumor [74]. This may be due to the relatively small number of cells analyzed. Interestingly, many of the newly identified mutated genes had not been described before in renal cell carcinoma. In a whole-genome single-cell sequencing study on lymphoblastic leukemia, targeted sequencing was performed of a panel of single nucleotide variants (SNVs), deletions, and IgH sequences in 1,479 single tumor cells from six acute lymphoblastic leukemia (ALL) patients [75]. A clonal structure of the individual samples could be identified, consisting of 1 to 5 different clones.

A sequencing study for combined genomic DNA and mRNA analysis of the same cell was performed for a mouse embryonic stem cell line [76]. The discrimination between the DNA and mRNA libraries was relying on the use of two different amplification protocols and different molecular adaptors. Authors compared copy numbers with gene expression data and found that copy number variations appeared to influence variability in gene expression among cells. This study showed for the first time that parallel DNA and RNA analyses may in principle be possible for one individual cell, but it is still far from routine use. Overall, single-cell whole-genome or exome sequencing (exome-seq) is principally more challenging than scRNA-seq analysis due to the high number of amplification-derived artifacts. Some recent publications have described the key issues of this technology [77]. By use of single-cell exome-seq technology, a phylogenetic tree of metastasis development has been built for colon carcinoma [78]. Authors showed that metastasis development appeared to be a late event in primary tumors after accumulation of a larger set of mutations. Interestingly, there was no obvious overlap regarding the accumulation of mutations before metastasis in different samples, and the first metastasis-specific mutations also did not overlap between samples. Authors used a FACS-based technology to separate their cells. A more recent study used exome-sequencing technology for the analysis of a limited number of genes using the Tapestri® platform (Mission Bio, South San Francisco, CA, USA) to unravel the clonal diversity of T-cell acute lymphoblastic leukemia (T-ALL) [79]. The panel contained 110 genes and tested more than 100,000 cells of 25 samples. Longitudinal samples showed clones with a minor presence at diagnosis that, at later stages, developed into relevant major clones. This technology may be of particular relevance for hematological malignancies but may also be used in solid tumors.

4. Single-Cell Analyses in Melanoma

4.1. Primary Melanomas, Lymph Node Metastases and Cell Lines

scRNA-seq has been applied in a significant number of studies on malignant melanoma (Table 1; Figure 2). The first major scRNA-seq study analyzing melanoma tissues investigated 19 samples of primary melanomas and metastatic lesions [80]. A significant intertumor heterogeneity was observed for melanoma cells in these tissues, while the immune cells in these analyses showed a relative homogeneous gene expression pattern [80]. Major subgroups of transcriptional heterogeneity were associated with cell cycle, spatial context of cells, and a drug-resistance program (MITF-low/AXL-high signature). Authors used single-cell signatures of T cell, B cells, fibroblasts, macrophages, and endothelial cells derived from this study and mapped them onto gene patterns of bulk sequences of 471 melanoma samples present in the Cancer Genome Atlas (TCGA). They then searched for genes expressed by cells of one type that may influence or reflect the proportion of cells of a different cell type in the tumor. By this means they showed that the abundance of cancer-associated fibroblasts (CAF) is predictive of the phenotype, and that fibroblast signatures influence the presence of specific immune cell signatures. Moreover, they identified single cells with an AXL-high/MITF-low signature in an AXL-low/MITF-high population, which would have been missed in bulk sequencing and may give rise to treatment resistance. The AXL/MITF dichotomy has been supported by a later study re-analyzing these data by a new software called Cyclum to identify latent periodic developmental processes [81].

Table 1. Summary of single-cell melanoma transcriptomics and proteomics studies and main outcome.

No	Melanoma Samples	Experimental or Clinical Set-Up	Characteristics of Clonal Structure	Main Findings	References
1.	Primary melanomas and metastases ($n = 19$)	Untreated	Clonal signatures of cell cycle, spatial context, drug-resistance programs	Presence of AXL-high/MITF-low population in a AXL-low/MITF-high cluster; single-cell signatures with prognostic relevance	[80]
2.	Melanoma cell lines representing different stages of differentiation ($n = 8$)	Untreated	Cell clones with SOX9 and SOX10 high expression and transitional cells, knockdown of SOX10 affects clonal structure	Transition between gene networks instead of selection of individual clones (transcriptional plasticity)	[82]
3.	Melanoma short-term cultures (BRAF and/or NRAS mutant) ($n = 3$)	Untreated	Clonal structure of cell cycle, stromal, OxPhos, pigmentation genes	Four different clonal structures with additional subclonal structures and stem cell-like subclones	[65]
4.	Samples from 32 metastatic melanoma patients ($n = 48$)	Anti-PD1 inhibitor treatment of patients, either alone or in combination with anti-CTLA4 treatment	CD8$^+$ T cells clones consisted of memory/survival (TCF7$^+$) and exhaustion (CD38$^+$) clones, respectively	TCF7$^+$/CD8$^+$ T cells are crucial for treatment response	[83]
5.	Human melanoma samples ($n = 33$)	Clinical samples under anti-CTLA4 treatment	Clonal immune exclusion program: CDK4/CDK6 expression, JAK-STAT3 signaling, TNF pathway, senescence-associated programs, Myc targets	CDK4/CDK6 inhibitor treatment of resistant clones improved survival of mice in a murine melanoma model	[84]
6.	Human melanoma samples ($n = 25$)	Anti-PD-1 inhibitor treatment of patients, either alone or in combination with anti-CTLA4 treatment	CD4$^+$/CD8$^+$ T cells with clusters of resting, transitional and exhausted T cells	Dysfunctional (exhausted) CD8+ T cells are still proliferative and showed tumor reactivity ex vivo	[85]
7.	Tumor tissue of melanoma cell line mouse xenografts (minimal residual disease) ($n = 3$)	Murine xenograft model, BRAFi treatment	Minimal residual disease with 4 different transcriptional subpopulations (pigmented, SMC, NCSC, invasive cells)	Enrichment of neuronal stem cells population after BRAFi treatment; successful treatment with retinoid receptor inhibitor	[86]
8.	A375 and 451Lu melanoma cell lines ($n = 2$)	BRAFi treatment	Patterns of resistance are present in parental cells and vice versa	Identification of a pre-resistant state at the tip of the parental population	[64]
9.	Melanoma cell line A375 ($n = 1$)	BRAFi treatment after CRISPR/Cas interference with MAPK pathway	Clonal selection of treatment resistant clones	Resistance-mediating positions in MAPK genes were mostly located around *MEK1*E203K or *KRAS*Q61	[87]
10.	BRAF-mutant melanoma cell lines ($n = 3$)	BRAFi treatment; testing of 13 different proteomic markers with single-cell barcode chip technology	Increased clonal heterogeneity under treatment	Activation of MEK/ERK and NF-κB p65 signaling in resitant clones; NF-κB inhibitor increased sensitivity of cells	[88]
11.	BRAF-mutant melanoma cell line ($n = 1$)	BRAFi treatment; testing of 19 different proteomic markers with single-cell barcode chip technology	Drug-induced clonal cell states changes with NGFR/AXL or MITF, MART1 patterns	Two different trajectories of treatment resistance of MITF-high and MITF- low cells	[89]

Abbreviations: BRAFi, BRAF inhibitor; SMC, starved-like melanoma cells, NCSC, neural crest stem cells; MAPK, mitogen-activated protein kinases; NGFR, nerve growth factor receptor; MITF, microphthalmia-associated transcription factor.

Melanoma

Tumors
Heterogeneity:
donors, stages, location, treatment

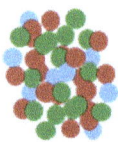

Tumor cells and microenvironment (TME):
Melanocytes, immune cell infiltration (T-, B-, Tregs, NKs, macrophages), fibroblasts, endothelial cells

Changing TME
- Immune editing/evasion
- Immune cell composition
- Immune checkpoint activation/deactivation
- T-cell exhaustion

Diversity: Cell types

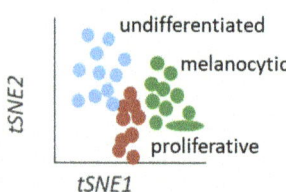

Cell lines
heterogeneous regarding:
genetics, culture conditions, treatment

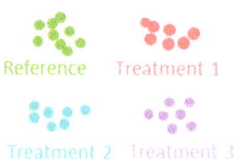

Tumor cells
Melanocytes of different types (MITF/AXL-programs, proliferation, stemness)

Changing tumour cell programs
- melanocyte-vs-mesenchymal
- AXL-vs-MITF
- Proliferation/stemness
- Stages of differentiation (neural crest, melanocytic, transitory)

Pseudo-Dynamic: Development

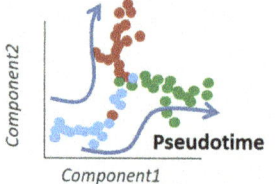

Figure 2. Schematic representation of single-cell analyses in melanoma samples. Either melanoma tumors or cell lines underwent single-cell sequencing analyses, which unraveled different types of cells and levels of heterogeneity in melanoma lesions and mechanisms of treatment resistance, e.g., mediated by T cell exclusion or T cell exhaustion programs under immune checkpoint therapy. Changes in cellular programs in tumor cells were also identified in cell culture studies supporting a role of the dichotomy of the AXL and MITF programs for treatment response and resistance.

Our group has analyzed the transcriptomes of 92 single cells cultured from a patient biopsy of a *BRAF* wild type/*NRAS* wild type melanoma metastasis by scRNA-seq [65]. We used self-organizing maps (SOM) to identify sub-clones and found gene patterns of proliferation, oxidative phosphorylation, pigmentation, and cellular stroma [65]. These categories could be further refined, especially regarding cell cycle genes referring to different stages of cell cycle such as G1, S, and G2/M phase. In principle, every cell showed an individual gene pattern. Interestingly, gene expression patterns overlapped with those of clinical gene expression studies with associated patient survival data, further emphasizing the clinical relevance of these single-cell analyses [82]. Cellular heterogeneity was less pronounced in *BRAF* mutant/*NRAS* wild type and *BRAF* wild type/*NRAS* mutant cultures. In order to identify new treatment options based on gene expression patterns, kinome expression patterns across sub-populations were analyzed. Cell cycle kinases

CDK4 and CDK2 were consistently highly expressed in a majority of cells, suggesting that both might be interesting targets. Indeed, treatment of melanoma cell cultures cells with CDK4 inhibitor palbociclib reduced cell proliferation to a similar extent as MAPK inhibitors. Finally, a low abundant subclone with high expression of an ABC transporter module, surface markers CD271 and CD133, and multiple aldehyde dehydrogenases (ALDHs), was identified. These findings support a role of cancer stem cells in melanoma biology, which has been described for other tumor entities [90,91]. Thus, single-cell gene expression patterns may provide new treatment targets above BRAF/MAPK inhibitor treatment.

In another report, authors addressed the question whether melanoma cells may shift between different states of differentiation from a melanocytic on one end and a mesenchymal-like state at the other end of differentiation [82]. Authors studied 10 melanoma cultures using scRNA-seq and found shared gene regulatory networks that underlie the extreme melanocytic and mesenchymal states which are both present in an intermediate state. Among both states SOX9 (de-differentiated stage) and SOX10 (differentiated stages) play an important role. The intermediate state shared some transcriptional regulons such as SOX10, TFAP2, and MITF with the melanocytic state, but also with the mesenchymal state such as FOSL1, IRF3, and STAT1. The transcriptional state had functional consequences, as it determined the migratory capacity of cells. After *SOX10* knockdown, cells monitored in time-series and analyzed by pseudotime analysis, showed a sequential transition between both extreme states (with SOX10 and SOX9 expression). Thus, this intermediate state indeed exists and is characterized by a distinct gene regulator network rather than by heterogeneous mixture of cells, further supporting the notion of a transcriptional plasticity between different melanoma cell states.

4.2. Treatment Resistance Under Immune Checkpoint Inhibition

Analysis of treatment resistance and response has been a focus area of a number of single-cell studies [83–85,88]. In one of the earlier studies, scRNA-seq analyses were performed for 33 human melanoma tumors, and a T cell signature was identified that allowed to classify hundreds of bulk-sequenced tumors as tumors harboring a seed (T-cell)-exclusion program [84]. This exclusion program was then mapped onto ipilimumab and anti-PD1 treated samples analyzed by scRNA-seq to identify co-expressed genes in individual cells. The T cell exclusion program included transcriptional patterns of apoptosis, JAK-STAT3 signaling, TNF pathway, senescence-association, Myc targets, and p53 binding. Indeed, melanoma lesions expressed features of this program as determined by multicolor immunofluorescence. Among the genes tested were *TP53* (up), *JUN* (down), *MYC* (up), and *HLA-A* (down). The presence of the treatment resistance program also correlated with checkpoint inhibitor response in melanoma patients in an independent sample set. Finally, blockage of CDK4/CDK6 kinases, which were part of the resistance program, inhibited melanoma cells growth in vitro and in vivo in a melanoma mouse model. Taken together, single-cell analyses allowed the identification of a malignant cell program that is associated with T cell exclusion and is predictive for checkpoint inhibitor resistance that maybe targeted by CDK4/CDK6 inhibition.

In another study, single-cell transcriptomes were generated via 48 tumor samples from 32 metastatic melanoma patients using a Smart-seq2 protocol [83]. Biopsies were taken at baseline and under anti-PD1 inhibitor treatment, either alone or in combination with anti-CTLA4 treatment, including two patients with anti-CTLA4 treatment alone. CD45$^+$ cells were used to define an 11-cluster transcriptomic pattern. Two clusters were more prominent in responder lesions and in non-responder lesions. Treatment resistant clusters were enriched for genes linked T cell exhaustion (*LAG3*, *PDCD1*, *HAVCR2*, *TIGIT*, *CD38*) and cell cycle genes (*CDK1*, *CCNB1*, *MKI67*, and *CDK4*). Individual markers of responders were *LTB*, *TCF7*, and *CCR7*, and of non-responders were *CCL3*, *CD38*, and *HAVCR2*. Authors then focused their analyses on CD8$^+$ T cells, which consisted of two clonal states, memory/survival state, and exhaustion state, called CD8_G and CD8_B cells, respectively. Prominent populations of response were TCF7$^+$/CD8$^+$ T cells (TCF7 is part of Wnt signaling and crucial for differentiation and self-renewal). Further analysis via cell-sorting showed that CD39/TIM3 discriminated exhausted from memory/effector cells, which was verified in a B16-F10 murine melanoma model. T cell receptor (TCR) analysis showed that enriched TCRs were more common in exhausted clusters. Together, this study may help to select patients for anti-PD1 therapy based on subclonal T cell states, which may be of relevance for clinical trials.

A more recent study focused on dysfunctional T cells in melanoma lesions under immune checkpoint therapy [85]. In this study, 25 melanoma samples were analyzed by scRNA-seq with a focus on CD4$^+$ and CD8 T$^+$ cells in patients with prior treatment against CTLA-4 or PD-1, or a combination of both. Immune cell subtypes were widely shared across patients, but their relative abundance differed considerably between patients, even when disease stage and treatment background were matched. In particular, CD8$^+$ T cells partly transitioned into a dysfunctional T cell pool characterized by the expression of *PDCD1*, *LAG3*, and molecules shared with CD4$^+$ Treg (e.g., *CSF1*, *ZBED2*). Interestingly, however, single-cell TCR sequencing and expression of cell cycle genes showed that these so-called dysfunctional T cells had the highest levels of clonal expansion. Ex vivo cultured tumor-infiltrating lymphocytes (TIL) from melanoma patients showed that tumor reactivity correlated with a CD8$^+$ T cell dysfunctional state. Collectively, these data suggests that the dysfunctional CD8$^+$ T cells are dynamically differentiating and are an active cell compartment with tumor reactivity in patients. Models of regulation of this T cell compartment should help to create innovative treatment approaches.

These data were partly re-analyzed (8 non-treated melanoma patients) in a subsequent study [92]. Here, authors addressed the question of a spatiotemporal activity of IFN-γ as a major mediator of tumor immunity. First, a Myc-driven B cell lymphoma and a B16F10 murine tumor model were used. When injecting OVA antigen-positive and negative B16F10 melanoma cells into mice, mosaic tumors were generated. By co-injection of CD8$^+$ OVA-specific T cells, a homogenous expression of MHC class I, and PD-L1 upregulation on tumor cells was induced, irrespective of a close proximity of T cells and melanoma cells, supporting the notion of a distant activity of immune cells. As mentioned, by reanalysis of the abovementioned clinical single-cell data, it was shown that CD8$^+$ T cells are indeed the major source of IFN-γ, and interferon-signatures were found in different cell populations such as macrophages and neutrophils (melanoma cells were sparse in these samples). These findings suggest that tumor cells in human melanomas might also be targeted by distant immune cells in the microenvironment.

4.3. Treatment Resistance under Targeted Treatment

To identify markers of resistance against BRAF inhibitor (BRAFi) treatment, a new analysis software was developed that outperformed existing platforms regarding large complex substructures and large numbers of sampled cells [64]. The software was termed SAKE, which stands for scRNA-seq analysis and klustering evaluation. To further test this software, melanoma cell lines 451Lu and A375 were analyzed either as parental or BRAF inhibitor (vemurafenib)-resistant cells. t-SNE analysis showed that four populations may be separated, but individual cell clones with gene patterns of parental cells existed in resistant cells and vice versa (without obvious enrichment). By use of differential gene expression analysis the major differentially expressed gene with upregulation in resistant cells was shown to be *DCT* (dopachrome tautomerase). Sorting of cells from parental cells revealed that DCT-enriched cells were more resistant to BRAF inhibition than the whole culture. In a final set of experiments, authors observed a transitional population characterized by *ENT5A*, *AXL*, *GFR*, *PDGFRB*, and *JUN* expression, which was localized at the tip of the parental population proximal to the resistant population, indicating a pre-resistant state as described earlier by others [48]. Without prior knowledge, SAKE identified this intermediate population, characterized by *AXL*, *JUN*, *NGFR*, *WNT5A*, *FGFR1*, and *NRG1* expression. By testing of copy number variations in single cells as a surrogate marker for genetic heterogeneity, it was found that this transitional (pre-resistant) population was derived from several unrelated clonal lineages and most likely reflects a transient stage rather than a particular clone. Taken together, *DCT* was identified as a marker for individual resistant clones in untreated populations and together with mechanisms of transient gene regulation towards resistance may be an interesting therapeutic target.

In another report, CRISPR RNA-guided deaminase technology was combined with CROP-seq (CRISPR droplet sequencing) technology to introduce mutations in 3 genes of the MAPK pathway in A375 melanoma cells, namely *NRAS*, *KRAS* and *MAP2K1* (*MEK1*) [87]. Overall, 420 sgRNAs were introduced into the melanoma cells. Subsequent drug response was tested against BRAF inhibitor vemurafenib. Enrichment of individual sgRNAs under treatment indicated treatment resistance. Most positive findings referred to sgRNAs targeting *MEK1* in the E203 codon region, which is a well-known resistance region. Apart from this, the most significant results were observed for mutations induced in the vicinity of Q61 in the *KRAS* gene, which has already been shown in other studies. Further transcriptomic analysis of resistant clones showed enhanced expression for *CD74*, *HLA-DRA*, *SLC26A2*, *HLA-DRB1*, *FOS*, and *HLA-DPA1* for *MEK1*E203K-related clones and *CXCL1*, *IL-8*, *CXCL2*, *SOD2*, and *CCL2* for *KRAS*Q61-related clones. Taken together, this study established a new platform that may be extended to other target genes and tumor entities to uncover mechanisms of resistance to targeted treatment.

In a recent report, an experimental setting is described recapitulating minimal residual disease after targeted treatment. In this study, subcutaneously injected mice with *BRAF*V600E mutant melanoma cells were treated with BRAF inhibitor dabrafenib [86]. Single-cell analyses were performed for minimal residual disease after transplanted tumors regressed under treatment. In the subclonal structure of minimal residual disease, for 4 different cell states were enriched such as NCSC (neural crest stem cells), invasive cells, SMC (starved-like melanoma cells), and pigmented cells, among which SMC showed the most significant enrichment under treatment. Single cell trajectories as derived from pseudotime analyses showed that an early proliferative state developed via two different developmental trajectories into NCSC and SMC cells. By use of multiplexed immunohistochemistry (IHC) of melanoma lesions, it was demonstrated that murine melanoma xenografts showed a specific spatial pattern for the different cell states marked by different discriminative markers. In further in vitro experiments, the transition into the NCSC state was cell-autonomous and reversible, tested by drug exposure and subsequent drug removal. Finally, computational analysis of gene regulatory networks showed that another component of the gene regulatory network of minimal residual disease is the retinoid X receptor-γ. Consequently, inhibition of this receptor by the small molecule inhibitor HX531 led to significantly longer survival of mice under dabrafenib treatment, with a significant percentage (20%) of mice being tumor-free even after 4 months of treatment. Together, treatment resistance appears to develop along different developmental trajectories identified by single-cell transcriptomics, a finding which may be exploited for new treatment approaches.

In a study on BRAFi treatment of different melanoma cell lines, RNA-seq data of 18 melanoma cell lines were included [88]. Nine cell lines were used to define different levels of BRAFi sensitivity. Drug resistant cells showed a low melanocytic cell signature, and elevated levels of neural crest and mesenchymal genes as well as genes of activated JNK and NF-κB pathways. Based on the analysis of different *NGFR* and *MRT-1* expression, a cluster of highly plastic cell lines under BRAFi treatment of brief (3d) or prolonged (71–90 d) inhibition was defined. These cells developed signatures of NCSC and epithelial-to-mesenchymal transition genes and genes of elevated invasiveness and migration. Using a Markov model for prediction, authors showed that the clusters underwent both cell state interconversion and drug selection. In a subsequent single-cell analysis, single-cell barcode chip technology (SNBC) was used to analyze 13 different proteomic markers (including NGFR, TNFR, MART-1, JNK, pERK, and pNF-κB p65). It was demonstrated for one of these cell lines that BRAFi treatment increased cellular heterogeneity at day 3 and 6 of treatment, which was reminiscent of cell state transitions in other systems [93]. There was a negative correlation between NGFR and MITF/MART-1 expression at day 3. At day 6, an activation of MEK/ERK and NF-κB p65 signaling was observed, suggestive for a role of both pathways for an adaptive cell state transition. Indeed, by use of specific inhibitors (trametinib, MEK inhibitor; and JSH23, NF-κB p65 translocation inhibitor), an additional growth arrest was found in these cells under BRAFi treatment. However, a combination of vemurafenib and trametinib did not halt the neural crest transition, and resistance emerged after prolonged treatment. Only the triple combination of vemurafenib, trametinib, and the JSH23 inhibitor kept the cells in a drug-sensitive state, which argues for the strong role of NF-κB p65 in treatment resistance.

These experiments were further extended in a more recent study of the same group, analyzing a larger number of parameters in single cells by use of the same microchamber technology [89]. Among these parameters were MITF, pERK1, p-NF-κB, KI67, NGFR, HIF1α, LDH, and glucose. A BRAF-mutant melanoma cell line was treated with BRAFi, and analyses were made at different time points (days/D0, D1, D3, and D5). Trajectories of BRAFi resistance were measured. Two different trajectories (upper and lower) were observed, characterized by either Ki67 and NGFR/AXL expression or MITF, MART-1 expression. Authors then isolated MITF-high and MITF-low cells from this cell culture and treated cells with BRAFi. Both cell types again used different trajectories for treatment resistance. Together, these results suggest that, upon drug treatment, MITF-high and low cells use distinct trajectories of treatment resistance. Finally, critical point analysis was performed. Here, "critical point" stands for a point of irreversible development. Two different cell clusters were identified that characterized the regions near such tipping points of both trajectories. One cluster showed high network connectivity in a pathway that included MITF, PFK, p-LKB, PKM-2, and LDH-2, while in the other cluster, TNFR, N-cadherin, and p-NF-κB were dominant. Consequently, inhibition of PKM2 and NF-κB with specific inhibitors showed different sensitivities in both cell types, and a combination of both inhibitors with BRAFi was more effective than double combinations. Taken together, the different heterogeneous drug-response trajectories improved our understanding of resistance development, which may have an impact on effective therapy combinations in future.

5. Spatial Sequencing in Melanoma

In order to disentangle the spatiotemporal organization of single-cell analyses, recent experimental approaches tried to analyze near-single-cell transcriptomes in situ. By use of so-called spatial transcriptomics, gene expression patterns were generated from tissue biopsies and analyzed by classical next-generation sequencing [94,95]. Indeed, spatial resolution does not allow single-cell cell resolution, but is at present limited to an area of 100×100 micrometers per spot. Further technological advances will surely go into the direction of single-cell resolution. For melanoma, a study about four lymph node metastases, based on an individual array system, has been published [94]. Overall, 286 tissue domains were analyzed per section (as duplicates), and a total of 2200 domains were investigated that measured 3000 transcripts per domain. Two different gene panels (factors) were observed in the four samples. Melanoma-A consisted of *CD63*, *PMEL*, and *S1000A1*, while Melanoma-B consisted of *S100B*, *FTH1*, and *AEBP1* expression. The factors were heterogeneously distributed among the 4 samples. Melanoma A was present only in samples 1, 2, and 4. Mapping of the gene expression patterns of 284 spots revealed 4 functional clusters, which overlapped with areas annotated by histopathology. Functional clusters included stromal tissue, tumor tissue, lymphoid tissue, and lymphoid tissue at the tumor border. Four genes were used to generate spatial heatmaps mapping to the 4 tissue clusters. This work showed that spatial sequencing in melanoma appears to be possible and provides reasonable results. Further refinement is needed to improve spatial resolution and sequencing depth.

In a more recent work, a more advanced spatial transcriptomic technology was applied to skin squamous cells carcinoma [96]. Transcriptomes of more than 8000 spots across 12 sections were analyzed, and 967 genes per spots were obtained. Spot expression patterns were consistent with the gross histologic architecture of lesions including tumor keratinocytes, tumor stroma, uninvolved stoma and adnexal areas, cancer-associated fibroblasts, and endothelial cells. The 10x Genomics® Visium Spatial Gene Expression Kit® was used for two additional patients with higher resolution. The leading edge of these tumors was composed of two different populations of tumor-specific keratinocytes and basal tumor cells. An immune landscape could further be defined, and it was shown that PD-L1 and PD-L2 were exclusively expressed by migrating dendritic cells (DC) in the tumor vicinity. These analyses identified multiple cell types involved in immunosuppressive mechanisms in DC, exhausted T cells, and Tregs, allowing for a refinement of the local tumor structures. In an extension of these analyses using the NicheNet software (https://github.com/saeyslab/nichenetr; GitHub, Inc., San Francisco, CA, USA)), molecules for specific cell-cell interactions were predicted [97]. Thus far, no such study has been published for primary melanoma lesions.

6. Single-Cell Sequencing of Copy Number Variations

Single-cell exome-sequencing has been performed in melanoma cell line COLO829 across 1475 cells [98]. Analysis was done using the chromium single-cell CNV solution (10× Genomics®) to sequence gDNA. Individual cells exhibited extensive copy number differences showing that this cell line was at least composed of 4 major clusters. Overall, 114 copy number variations were identified with ploidies of 2, 3, and 4, respectively. Chromosomal aberrations were observed for different chromosomes, e.g., for chromosome 18, present in group A and D, and a loss in groups B and C. Subclones emerged from chromosomal losses and gains. Taken together, in line with bulk sequencing reports, major chromosomal aberrations form in melanoma cells in a time-dependent manner, giving rise to heterogeneous cell populations.

7. Perspectives

The published data and further improvements of the mentioned technologies hold great promise for the analysis of melanoma and other tumors in the future. Moreover, the limited availability of fresh tumor tissue for many tumors will profit from the single-cell-analysis of frozen archival material with technologies that are currently under development [99]. Spatial sequencing will not only provide information about tumor heterogeneity but also unravel the spatial composition of different cell populations, which may be of particular relevance for immune checkpoint inhibitor treatment. Finally, emerging techniques of single-cell exome-sequencing, with the advent of customized technologies will further improve our knowledge about the emergence of resistant clones with specific genetic features, as has already been shown in hematological malignancies.

Author Contributions: H.B. and M.K. were involved in conceptualization, writing and draft preparation of the manuscript, M.S., L.S.M., and H.L.-W. were involved in writing and draft preparation. All authors have read and agreed to the published version of the manuscript.

Funding: We acknowledge support from Leipzig University for Open Access Publishing.

Institutional Review Board Statement: Not applicable.

Informed Consent Statement: Not applicable.

Data Availability Statement: Data available in publicly accessible repositories. For details, see cited references.

Conflicts of Interest: M. Kunz has received honoraria from the Speakers Bureau of Roche Pharma and travel support from Novartis Pharma GmbH and Bristol-Myers Squibb GmbH. All other authors declare no conflict of interest.

References

1. Bai, X.; Flaherty, K.T. Targeted and immunotherapies in BRAF mutant melanoma: Where we stand and what to expect. *Br. J. Dermatol.* **2020**. [CrossRef] [PubMed]
2. Schadendorf, D.; Van Akkooi, A.C.J.; Berking, C.; Griewank, K.G.; Gutzmer, R.; Hauschild, A.; Stang, A.; Roesch, A.; Ugurel, S. Melanoma. *Lancet* **2018**, *392*, 971–984. [CrossRef]
3. Cancer Genome Atlas Network. Genomic Classification of Cutaneous Melanoma. *Cell* **2015**, *161*, 1681–1696. [CrossRef] [PubMed]
4. Hodis, E.; Watson, I.R.; Kryukov, G.V.; Arold, S.T.; Imielinski, M.; Theurillat, J.-P.; Nickerson, E.; Auclair, D.; Li, L.; Place, C.; et al. A landscape of driver mutations in melanoma. *Cell* **2012**, *150*, 251–263. [CrossRef]
5. Krauthammer, M.; Kong, Y.; Bacchiocchi, A.; Evans, P.; Pornputtapong, N.; Wu, C.; McCusker, J.P.; Ma, S.; Cheng, E.; Straub, R.; et al. Exome sequencing identifies recurrent mutations in NF1 and RASopathy genes in sun-exposed melanomas. *Nat. Genet.* **2015**, *47*, 996–1002. [CrossRef]
6. Davies, M.A.; Flaherty, K.T. Melanoma in 2017: Moving treatments earlier to move further forwards. *Nat. Rev. Clin. Oncol.* **2018**, *15*, 75–76. [CrossRef]
7. Grimaldi, A.M.; Simeone, E.; Ascierto, P.A. The role of MEK inhibitors in the treatment of metastatic melanoma. *Curr. Opin. Oncol.* **2014**, *26*, 196–203. [CrossRef]
8. Robert, C.; Grob, J.J.; Stroyakovskiy, D.; Karaszewska, B.; Hauschild, A.; Levchenko, E.; Chiarion Sileni, V.; Schachter, J.; Garbe, C.; Bondarenko, I.; et al. Five-Year Outcomes with Dabrafenib plus Trametinib in Metastatic Melanoma. *N. Engl. J. Med.* **2019**, *381*, 626–636. [CrossRef]
9. Menzies, A.M.; Long, G.V. Systemic treatment for BRAF-mutant melanoma: Where do we go next? *Lancet Oncol.* **2014**, *15*, e371–e381. [CrossRef]
10. Dummer, R.; Brase, J.C.; Garrett, J.; Campbell, C.D.; Gasal, E.; Squires, M.; Gusenleitner, D.; Santinami, M.; Atkinson, V.; Mandalà, M.; et al. Adjuvant dabrafenib plus trametinib versus placebo in patients with resected, BRAFV600-mutant, stage III melanoma (COMBI-AD): Exploratory biomarker analyses from a randomised, phase 3 trial. *Lancet Oncol.* **2020**, *21*, 358–372. [CrossRef]
11. Amaria, R.N.; Menzies, A.M.; Burton, E.M.; Scolyer, R.A.; Tetzlaff, M.T.; Antdbacka, R.; Ariyan, C.; Bassett, R.; Carter, B.; Daud, A.; et al. Neoadjuvant systemic therapy in melanoma: Recommendations of the International Neoadjuvant Melanoma Consortium. *Lancet Oncol.* **2019**, *20*, e378–e389. [CrossRef]
12. Moriceau, G.; Hugo, W.; Hong, A.; Shi, H.; Kong, X.; Yu, C.C.; Koya, R.C.; Samatar, A.A.; Khanlou, N.; Braun, J.; et al. Tunable-combinatorial Mechanisms of Acquired Resistance Limit the Efficacy of BRAF/MEK Co-targeting but Result in Melanoma Drug Addiction. *Cancer Cell* **2015**, *27*, 240–256. [CrossRef] [PubMed]
13. Long, G.V.; Fung, C.; Menzies, A.M.; Pupo, G.M.; Carlino, M.S.; Hyman, J.; Shahheydari, H.; Tembe, V.; Thompson, J.F.; Saw, R.P.; et al. Increased MAPK reactivation in early resistance to dabrafenib/trametinib combination therapy of BRAF-mutant metastatic melanoma. *Nat. Commun.* **2014**, *5*, 5694. [CrossRef] [PubMed]
14. Wagle, N.; Van Allen, E.M.; Treacy, D.J.; Frederick, D.T.; Cooper, Z.A.; Taylor-Weiner, A.; Rosenberg, M.; Goetz, E.M.; Sullivan, R.J.; Farlow, D.N.; et al. MAP kinase pathway alterations in BRAF-mutant melanoma patients with acquired resistance to combined RAF/MEK inhibition. *Cancer Discov.* **2014**, *4*, 61–68. [CrossRef]
15. Rizos, H.; Menzies, A.M.; Pupo, G.M.; Carlino, M.S.; Fung, C.; Hyman, J.; Haydu, L.E.; Mijatov, B.; Becker, T.M.; Boyd, S.C.; et al. BRAF inhibitor resistance mechanisms in metastatic melanoma: Spectrum and clinical impact. *Clin. Cancer Res.* **2014**, *20*, 1965–1977. [CrossRef] [PubMed]
16. Shi, H.; Hugo, W.; Kong, X.; Hong, A.; Koya, R.C.; Moriceau, G.; Chodon, T.; Guo, R.; Johnson, D.B.; Dahlman, K.B.; et al. Acquired resistance and clonal evolution in melanoma during BRAF inhibitor therapy. *Cancer Discov.* **2014**, *4*, 80–93. [CrossRef]
17. Van Allen, E.M.; Wagle, N.; Sucker, A.; Treacy, D.J.; Johannessen, C.M.; Goetz, E.M.; Place, C.S.; Taylor-Weiner, A.; Whittaker, S.; Kryukov, G.V.; et al. The genetic landscape of clinical resistance to RAF inhibition in metastatic melanoma. *Cancer Discov.* **2014**, *4*, 94–109. [CrossRef]
18. Hugo, W.; Shi, H.; Sun, L.; Piva, M.; Song, C.; Kong, X.; Moriceau, G.; Hong, A.; Dahlman, K.B.; Johnson, D.B.; et al. Non-genomic and Immune Evolution of Melanoma Acquiring MAPKi Resistance. *Cell* **2015**, *162*, 1271–1285. [CrossRef]
19. Sun, C.; Wang, L.; Huang, S.; Heynen, G.J.J.E.; Prahallad, A.; Robert, C.; Haanen, J.; Blank, C.; Wesseling, J.; Willems, S.M.; et al. Reversible and adaptive resistance to BRAF(V600E) inhibition in melanoma. *Nature* **2014**, *508*, 118–122. [CrossRef]
20. Müller, J.; Krijgsman, O.; Tsoi, J.; Robert, L.; Hugo, W.; Song, C.; Kong, X.; Possik, P.A.; Cornelissen-Steijger, P.D.M.; Geukes Foppen, M.H.; et al. Low MITF/AXL ratio predicts early resistance to multiple targeted drugs in melanoma. *Nat. Commun.* **2014**, *5*, 5712. [CrossRef]
21. Johannessen, C.M.; Boehm, J.S.; Kim, S.Y.; Thomas, S.R.; Wardwell, L.; Johnson, L.A.; Emery, C.M.; Stransky, N.; Cogdill, A.P.; Barretina, J.; et al. COT drives resistance to RAF inhibition through MAP kinase pathway reactivation. *Nature* **2010**, *468*, 968–972. [CrossRef] [PubMed]
22. Konieczkowski, D.J.; Johannessen, C.M.; Abudayyeh, O.; Kim, J.W.; Cooper, Z.A.; Piris, A.; Frederick, D.T.; Barzily-Rokni, M.; Straussman, R.; Haq, R.; et al. A melanoma cell state distinction influences sensitivity to MAPK pathway inhibitors. *Cancer Discov.* **2014**, *4*, 816–827. [CrossRef] [PubMed]
23. Nazarian, R.; Shi, H.; Wang, Q.; Kong, X.; Koya, R.C.; Lee, H.; Chen, Z.; Lee, M.-K.; Attar, N.; Sazegar, H.; et al. Melanomas acquire resistance to B-RAF(V600E) inhibition by RTK or N-RAS upregulation. *Nature* **2010**, *468*, 973–977. [CrossRef] [PubMed]

24. Kunz, M.; Hölzel, M. The impact of melanoma genetics on treatment response and resistance in clinical and experimental studies. *Cancer Metastasis Rev.* **2017**, *36*, 53–75. [CrossRef]
25. Hirsch, L.; Zitvogel, L.; Eggermont, A.; Marabelle, A. PD-Loma: A cancer entity with a shared sensitivity to the PD-1/PD-L1 pathway blockade. *Br. J. Cancer* **2019**, *120*, 3–5. [CrossRef]
26. Larkin, J.; Chiarion-Sileni, V.; Gonzalez, R.; Grob, J.-J.; Rutkowski, P.; Lao, C.D.; Cowey, C.L.; Schadendorf, D.; Wagstaff, J.; Dummer, R.; et al. Five-Year Survival with Combined Nivolumab and Ipilimumab in Advanced Melanoma. *N. Engl. J. Med.* **2019**, *381*, 1535–1546. [CrossRef]
27. Bagchi, S.; Yuan, R.; Engleman, E.G. Immune Checkpoint Inhibitors for the Treatment of Cancer: Clinical Impact and Mechanisms of Response and Resistance. *Annu. Rev. Pathol.* **2020**. [CrossRef]
28. Van Allen, E.M.; Miao, D.; Schilling, B.; Shukla, S.A.; Blank, C.; Zimmer, L.; Sucker, A.; Hillen, U.; Foppen, M.H.G.; Goldinger, S.M.; et al. Genomic correlates of response to CTLA-4 blockade in metastatic melanoma. *Science* **2015**, *350*, 207–211. [CrossRef]
29. Snyder, A.; Wolchok, J.D.; Chan, T.A. Genetic basis for clinical response to CTLA-4 blockade. *N. Engl. J. Med.* **2015**, *372*, 783. [CrossRef]
30. Hugo, W.; Zaretsky, J.M.; Sun, L.; Song, C.; Moreno, B.H.; Hu-Lieskovan, S.; Berent-Maoz, B.; Pang, J.; Chmielowski, B.; Cherry, G.; et al. Genomic and Transcriptomic Features of Response to Anti-PD-1 Therapy in Metastatic Melanoma. *Cell* **2016**, *165*, 35–44. [CrossRef]
31. Zaretsky, J.M.; Garcia-Diaz, A.; Shin, D.S.; Escuin-Ordinas, H.; Hugo, W.; Hu-Lieskovan, S.; Torrejon, D.Y.; Abril-Rodriguez, G.; Sandoval, S.; Barthly, L.; et al. Mutations Associated with Acquired Resistance to PD-1 Blockade in Melanoma. *N. Engl. J. Med.* **2016**, *375*, 819–829. [CrossRef] [PubMed]
32. Chen, P.-L.; Roh, W.; Reuben, A.; Cooper, Z.A.; Spencer, C.N.; Prieto, P.A.; Miller, J.P.; Bassett, R.L.; Gopalakrishnan, V.; Wani, K.; et al. Analysis of Immune Signatures in Longitudinal Tumor Samples Yields Insight into Biomarkers of Response and Mechanisms of Resistance to Immune Checkpoint Blockade. *Cancer Discov.* **2016**, *6*, 827–837. [CrossRef] [PubMed]
33. Riaz, N.; Havel, J.J.; Makarov, V.; Desrichard, A.; Urba, W.J.; Sims, J.S.; Hodi, F.S.; Martín-Algarra, S.; Mandal, R.; Sharfman, W.H.; et al. Tumor and Microenvironment Evolution during Immunotherapy with Nivolumab. *Cell* **2017**, *171*, 934–949.e16. [CrossRef] [PubMed]
34. Liu, D.; Schilling, B.; Liu, D.; Sucker, A.; Livingstone, E.; Jerby-Arnon, L.; Zimmer, L.; Gutzmer, R.; Satzger, I.; Loquai, C.; et al. Integrative molecular and clinical modeling of clinical outcomes to PD1 blockade in patients with metastatic melanoma. *Nat. Med.* **2019**, *25*, 1916–1927. [CrossRef]
35. Auslander, N.; Zhang, G.; Lee, J.S.; Frederick, D.T.; Miao, B.; Moll, T.; Tian, T.; Wei, Z.; Madan, S.; Sullivan, R.J.; et al. Robust prediction of response to immune checkpoint blockade therapy in metastatic melanoma. *Nat. Med.* **2018**, *24*, 1545–1549. [CrossRef]
36. Carter, J.A.; Gilbo, P.; Atwal, G.S. IMPRES does not reproducibly predict response to immune checkpoint blockade therapy in metastatic melanoma. *Nat. Med.* **2019**, *25*, 1833–1835. [CrossRef]
37. Effern, M.; Glodde, N.; Braun, M.; Liebing, J.; Boll, H.N.; Yong, M.; Bawden, E.; Hinze, D.; Van den Boorn-Konijnenberg, D.; Daoud, M.; et al. Adoptive T Cell Therapy Targeting Different Gene Products Reveals Diverse and Context-Dependent Immune Evasion in Melanoma. *Immunity* **2020**, *53*, 564–580.e9. [CrossRef]
38. Landsberg, J.; Kohlmeyer, J.; Renn, M.; Bald, T.; Rogava, M.; Cron, M.; Fatho, M.; Lennerz, V.; Wölfel, T.; Hölzel, M.; et al. Melanomas resist T-cell therapy through inflammation-induced reversible dedifferentiation. *Nature* **2012**, *490*, 412–416. [CrossRef]
39. Yeon, M.; Kim, Y.; Jung, H.S.; Jeoung, D. Histone Deacetylase Inhibitors to Overcome Resistance to Targeted and Immuno Therapy in Metastatic Melanoma. *Front. Cell Dev. Biol.* **2020**, *8*, 486. [CrossRef]
40. Dagogo-Jack, I.; Shaw, A.T. Tumour heterogeneity and resistance to cancer therapies. *Nat. Rev. Clin. Oncol.* **2018**, *15*, 81–94. [CrossRef]
41. Nowell, P.C. The clonal evolution of tumor cell populations. *Science* **1976**, *194*, 23–28. [CrossRef] [PubMed]
42. Barrett, M.T.; Lenkiewicz, E.; Evers, L.; Holley, T.; Ruiz, C.; Bubendorf, L.; Sekulic, A.; Ramanathan, R.K.; Von Hoff, D.D. Clonal evolution and therapeutic resistance in solid tumors. *Front. Pharmacol.* **2013**, *4*, 2. [CrossRef] [PubMed]
43. Aparicio, S.; Caldas, C. The implications of clonal genome evolution for cancer medicine. *N. Engl. J. Med.* **2013**, *368*, 842–851. [CrossRef] [PubMed]
44. Yancovitz, M.; Litterman, A.; Yoon, J.; Ng, E.; Shapiro, R.L.; Berman, R.S.; Pavlick, A.C.; Darvishian, F.; Christos, P.; Mazumdar, M.; et al. Intra- and inter-tumor heterogeneity of BRAF(V600E))mutations in primary and metastatic melanoma. *PLoS ONE* **2012**, *7*, e29336. [CrossRef] [PubMed]
45. Harbst, K.; Lauss, M.; Cirenajwis, H.; Isaksson, K.; Rosengren, F.; Törngren, T.; Kvist, A.; Johansson, M.C.; Vallon-Christersson, J.; Baldetorp, B.; et al. Multiregion Whole-Exome Sequencing Uncovers the Genetic Evolution and Mutational Heterogeneity of Early-Stage Metastatic Melanoma. *Cancer Res.* **2016**, *76*, 4765–4774. [CrossRef]
46. Sanna, A.; Harbst, K.; Johansson, I.; Christensen, G.; Lauss, M.; Mitra, S.; Rosengren, F.; Häkkinen, J.; Vallon-Christersson, J.; Olsson, H.; et al. Tumor genetic heterogeneity analysis of chronic sun-damaged melanoma. *Pigment Cell Melanoma Res.* **2020**, *33*, 480–489. [CrossRef]
47. Obenauf, A.C.; Zou, Y.; Ji, A.L.; Vanharanta, S.; Shu, W.; Shi, H.; Kong, X.; Bosenberg, M.C.; Wiesner, T.; Rosen, N.; et al. Therapy-induced tumour secretomes promote resistance and tumour progression. *Nature* **2015**, *520*, 368–372. [CrossRef]

48. Shaffer, S.M.; Emert, B.L.; Reyes Hueros, R.A.; Cote, C.; Harmange, G.; Schaff, D.L.; Sizemore, A.E.; Gupte, R.; Torre, E.; Singh, A.; et al. Memory Sequencing Reveals Heritable Single-Cell Gene Expression Programs Associated with Distinct Cellular Behaviors. *Cell* **2020**, *182*, 947–959.e17. [CrossRef]
49. Lin, Z.; Meng, X.; Wen, J.; Corral, J.M.; Andreev, D.; Kachler, K.; Schett, G.; Chen, X.; Bozec, A. Intratumor Heterogeneity Correlates With Reduced Immune Activity and Worse Survival in Melanoma Patients. *Front. Oncol.* **2020**, *10*. [CrossRef]
50. Newman, A.M.; Liu, C.L.; Green, M.R.; Gentles, A.J.; Feng, W.; Xu, Y.; Hoang, C.D.; Diehn, M.; Alizadeh, A.A. Robust enumeration of cell subsets from tissue expression profiles. *Nat. Methods* **2015**, *12*, 453–457. [CrossRef]
51. Wolf, Y.; Bartok, O.; Patkar, S.; Eli, G.B.; Cohen, S.; Litchfield, K.; Levy, R.; Jiménez-Sánchez, A.; Trabish, S.; Lee, J.S.; et al. UVB-Induced Tumor Heterogeneity Diminishes Immune Response in Melanoma. *Cell* **2019**, *179*, 219–235.e21. [CrossRef] [PubMed]
52. Lim, B.; Lin, Y.; Navin, N. Advancing Cancer Research and Medicine with Single-Cell Genomics. *Cancer Cell* **2020**, *37*, 456–470. [CrossRef] [PubMed]
53. Aldridge, S.; Teichmann, S.A. Single cell transcriptomics comes of age. *Nat. Commun.* **2020**, *11*, 4307. [CrossRef] [PubMed]
54. Renaud, G.; Stenzel, U.; Maricic, T.; Wiebe, V.; Kelso, J. deML: Robust demultiplexing of Illumina sequences using a likelihood-based approach. *Bioinformatics* **2015**, *31*, 770–772. [CrossRef] [PubMed]
55. Renaud, G.; Kircher, M.; Stenzel, U.; Kelso, J. freeIbis: An efficient basecaller with calibrated quality scores for Illumina sequencers. *Bioinformatics* **2013**, *29*, 1208–1209. [CrossRef]
56. Chen, G.; Ning, B.; Shi, T. Single-Cell RNA-Seq Technologies and Related Computational Data Analysis. *Front. Genet.* **2019**, *10*, 317. [CrossRef]
57. Ji, F.; Sadreyev, R.I. Single-Cell RNA-seq: Introduction to Bioinformatics Analysis. *Curr. Protoc. Mol. Biol.* **2019**, *127*, e92. [CrossRef]
58. Lähnemann, D.; Köster, J.; Szczurek, E.; McCarthy, D.J.; Hicks, S.C.; Robinson, M.D.; Vallejos, C.A.; Campbell, K.R.; Beerenwinkel, N.; Mahfouz, A.; et al. Eleven grand challenges in single-cell data science. *Genome Biol.* **2020**, *21*, 31. [CrossRef]
59. Gentles, A.J.; Newman, A.M.; Liu, C.L.; Bratman, S.V.; Feng, W.; Kim, D.; Nair, V.S.; Xu, Y.; Khuong, A.; Hoang, C.D.; et al. The prognostic landscape of genes and infiltrating immune cells across human cancers. *Nat. Med.* **2015**, *21*, 938–945. [CrossRef]
60. Uhlén, M.; Hallström, B.M.; Lindskog, C.; Mardinoglu, A.; Pontén, F.; Nielsen, J. Transcriptomics resources of human tissues and organs. *Mol. Syst. Biol.* **2016**, *12*, 862. [CrossRef]
61. Hackl, H.; Charoentong, P.; Finotello, F.; Trajanoski, Z. Computational genomics tools for dissecting tumour-immune cell interactions. *Nat. Rev. Genet.* **2016**, *17*, 441–458. [CrossRef] [PubMed]
62. Nieto, P.; Elosua-Bayes, M.; Trincado, J.L.; Marchese, D.; Massoni-Badosa, R.; Salvany, M.; Henriques, A.; Mereu, E.; Moutinho, C.; Ruiz, S.; et al. A Single-Cell Tumor Immune Atlas for Precision Oncology. *bioRxiv* **2020**. [CrossRef]
63. Xie, X.; Liu, M.; Zhang, Y.; Wang, B.; Zhu, C.; Wang, C.; Li, Q.; Huo, Y.; Guo, J.; Xu, C.; et al. Single-cell transcriptomic landscape of human blood cells. *Natl. Sci. Rev.* **2020**. [CrossRef]
64. Ho, Y.-J.; Anaparthy, N.; Molik, D.; Mathew, G.; Aicher, T.; Patel, A.; Hicks, J.; Hammell, M.G. Single-cell RNA-seq analysis identifies markers of resistance to targeted BRAF inhibitors in melanoma cell populations. *Genome Res.* **2018**, *28*, 1353–1363. [CrossRef] [PubMed]
65. Gerber, T.; Willscher, E.; Loeffler-Wirth, H.; Hopp, L.; Schadendorf, D.; Schartl, M.; Anderegg, U.; Camp, G.; Treutlein, B.; Binder, H.; et al. Mapping heterogeneity in patient-derived melanoma cultures by single-cell RNA-seq. *Oncotarget* **2017**, *8*, 846–862. [CrossRef] [PubMed]
66. Saelens, W.; Cannoodt, R.; Todorov, H.; Saeys, Y. A comparison of single-cell trajectory inference methods. *Nat. Biotechnol.* **2019**, *37*, 547–554. [CrossRef]
67. Bergen, V.; Lange, M.; Peidli, S.; Wolf, F.A.; Theis, F.J. Generalizing RNA velocity to transient cell states through dynamical modeling. *Nat. Biotechnol.* **2020**, *38*, 1408–1414. [CrossRef]
68. La Manno, G.; Soldatov, R.; Zeisel, A.; Braun, E.; Hochgerner, H.; Petukhov, V.; Lidschreiber, K.; Kastriti, M.E.; Lönnerberg, P.; Furlan, A.; et al. RNA velocity of single cells. *Nature* **2018**, *560*, 494–498. [CrossRef]
69. Schmidt, M.; Loeffler-Wirth, H.; Binder, H. Developmental scRNAseq Trajectories in Gene- and Cell-State Space-The Flatworm Example. *Genes (Basel)* **2020**, *11*, 1214. [CrossRef]
70. McInnes, L.; Healy, J.; Melville, J. UMAP: Uniform Manifold Approximation and Projection for Dimension Reduction. *arXiv* **2018**, arXiv:1802.03426. Available online: http://arxiv.org/pdf/1802.03426v3 (accessed on 18 September 2020).
71. Kobak, D.; Berens, P. The art of using t-SNE for single-cell transcriptomics. *Nat. Commun.* **2019**, *10*, 5416. [CrossRef] [PubMed]
72. Wirth, H.; Von Bergen, M.; Binder, H. Mining SOM expression portraits: Feature selection and integrating concepts of molecular function. *BioData Min.* **2012**, *5*, 18. [CrossRef] [PubMed]
73. Hopp, L.; Wirth, H.; Fasold, M.; Binder, H. Portraying the expression landscapes of cancer subtypes. *Syst. Biomed.* **2013**, *1*, 99–121. [CrossRef]
74. Xu, X.; Hou, Y.; Yin, X.; Bao, L.; Tang, A.; Song, L.; Li, F.; Tsang, S.; Wu, K.; Wu, H.; et al. Single-cell exome sequencing reveals single-nucleotide mutation characteristics of a kidney tumor. *Cell* **2012**, *148*, 886–895. [CrossRef]
75. Gawad, C.; Koh, W.; Quake, S.R. Dissecting the clonal origins of childhood acute lymphoblastic leukemia by single-cell genomics. *Proc. Natl. Acad. Sci. USA* **2014**, *111*, 17947–17952. [CrossRef]

76. Dey, S.S.; Kester, L.; Spanjaard, B.; Bienko, M.; Van Oudenaarden, A. Integrated genome and transcriptome sequencing of the same cell. *Nat. Biotechnol.* **2015**, *33*, 285–289. [CrossRef]
77. Leung, M.L.; Wang, Y.; Waters, J.; Navin, N.E. SNES: Single nucleus exome sequencing. *Genome Biol.* **2015**, *16*, 55. [CrossRef]
78. Leung, M.L.; Davis, A.; Gao, R.; Casasent, A.; Wang, Y.; Sei, E.; Vilar, E.; Maru, D.; Kopetz, S.; Navin, N.E. Single-cell DNA sequencing reveals a late-dissemination model in metastatic colorectal cancer. *Genome Res.* **2017**, *27*, 1287–1299. [CrossRef]
79. Albertí-Servera, L.; Demeyer, S.; Govaerts, I.; Swings, T.; De Bie, J.; Gielen, O.; Brociner, M.; Michaux, L.M.; Maertens, J.; Uyttebroeck, A.; et al. Single-cell DNA amplicon sequencing reveals clonal heterogeneity and evolution in T-cell acute lymphoblastic leukemia. *Blood* **2020**. [CrossRef]
80. Tirosh, I.; Izar, B.; Prakadan, S.M.; Wadsworth, M.H.; Treacy, D.; Trombetta, J.J.; Rotem, A.; Rodman, C.; Lian, C.; Murphy, G.; et al. Dissecting the multicellular ecosystem of metastatic melanoma by single-cell RNA-seq. *Science* **2016**, *352*, 189–196. [CrossRef]
81. Liang, S.; Wang, F.; Han, J.; Chen, K. Latent periodic process inference from single-cell RNA-seq data. *Nat. Commun.* **2020**, *11*, 1441. [CrossRef] [PubMed]
82. Wouters, J.; Kalender-Atak, Z.; Minnoye, L.; Spanier, K.I.; De Waegeneer, M.; Bravo González-Blas, C.; Mauduit, D.; Davie, K.; Hulselmans, G.; Najem, A.; et al. Robust gene expression programs underlie recurrent cell states and phenotype switching in melanoma. *Nat. Cell Biol.* **2020**, *22*, 986–998. [CrossRef] [PubMed]
83. Sade-Feldman, M.; Yizhak, K.; Bjorgaard, S.L.; Ray, J.P.; De Boer, C.G.; Jenkins, R.W.; Lieb, D.J.; Chen, J.H.; Frederick, D.T.; Barzily-Rokni, M.; et al. Defining T Cell States Associated with Response to Checkpoint Immunotherapy in Melanoma. *Cell* **2018**, *175*, 998–1013.e20. [CrossRef] [PubMed]
84. Jerby-Arnon, L.; Shah, P.; Cuoco, M.S.; Rodman, C.; Su, M.-J.; Melms, J.C.; Leeson, R.; Kanodia, A.; Mei, S.; Lin, J.-R.; et al. A Cancer Cell Program Promotes T Cell Exclusion and Resistance to Checkpoint Blockade. *Cell* **2018**, *175*, 984–997.e24. [CrossRef] [PubMed]
85. Li, H.; Van der Leun, A.M.; Yofe, I.; Lubling, Y.; Gelbard-Solodkin, D.; Van Akkooi, A.C.J.; Van den Braber, M.; Rozeman, E.A.; Haanen, J.B.A.G.; Blank, C.U.; et al. Dysfunctional CD8 T Cells Form a Proliferative, Dynamically Regulated Compartment within Human Melanoma. *Cell* **2019**, *176*, 775–789.e18. [CrossRef] [PubMed]
86. Rambow, F.; Rogiers, A.; Marin-Bejar, O.; Aibar, S.; Femel, J.; Dewaele, M.; Karras, P.; Brown, D.; Chang, Y.H.; Debiec-Rychter, M.; et al. Toward Minimal Residual Disease-Directed Therapy in Melanoma. *Cell* **2018**, *174*, 843–855.e19. [CrossRef] [PubMed]
87. Jun, S.; Lim, H.; Chun, H.; Lee, J.H.; Bang, D. Single-cell analysis of a mutant library generated using CRISPR-guided deaminase in human melanoma cells. *Commun. Biol.* **2020**, *3*, 154. [CrossRef]
88. Su, Y.; Wei, W.; Robert, L.; Xue, M.; Tsoi, J.; Garcia-Diaz, A.; Homet Moreno, B.; Kim, J.; Ng, R.H.; Lee, J.W.; et al. Single-cell analysis resolves the cell state transition and signaling dynamics associated with melanoma drug-induced resistance. *Proc. Natl. Acad. Sci. USA* **2017**, *114*, 13679–13684. [CrossRef]
89. Su, Y.; Ko, M.E.; Cheng, H.; Zhu, R.; Xue, M.; Wang, J.; Lee, J.W.; Frankiw, L.; Xu, A.; Wong, S.; et al. Multi-omic single-cell snapshots reveal multiple independent trajectories to drug tolerance in a melanoma cell line. *Nat. Commun.* **2020**, *11*, 2345. [CrossRef]
90. Cojoc, M.; Mäbert, K.; Muders, M.H.; Dubrovska, A. A role for cancer stem cells in therapy resistance: Cellular and molecular mechanisms. *Semin. Cancer Biol.* **2015**, *31*, 16–27. [CrossRef]
91. Lawson, D.A.; Bhakta, N.R.; Kessenbrock, K.; Prummel, K.D.; Yu, Y.; Takai, K.; Zhou, A.; Eyob, H.; Balakrishnan, S.; Wang, C.-Y.; et al. Single-cell analysis reveals a stem-cell program in human metastatic breast cancer cells. *Nature* **2015**, *526*, 131–135. [CrossRef] [PubMed]
92. Thibaut, R.; Bost, P.; Milo, I.; Cazaux, M.; Lemaître, F.; Garcia, Z.; Amit, I.; Breart, B.; Cornuot, C.; Schwikowski, B.; et al. Bystander IFN-γ activity promotes widespread and sustained cytokine signaling altering the tumor microenvironment. *Nat. Cancer* **2020**, *1*, 302–314. [CrossRef] [PubMed]
93. Mojtahedi, M.; Skupin, A.; Zhou, J.; Castaño, I.G.; Leong-Quong, R.Y.Y.; Chang, H.; Trachana, K.; Giuliani, A.; Huang, S. Cell Fate Decision as High-Dimensional Critical State Transition. *PLoS Biol.* **2016**, *14*, e2000640. [CrossRef] [PubMed]
94. Thrane, K.; Eriksson, H.; Maaskola, J.; Hansson, J.; Lundeberg, J. Spatially Resolved Transcriptomics Enables Dissection of Genetic Heterogeneity in Stage III Cutaneous Malignant Melanoma. *Cancer Res.* **2018**, *78*, 5970–5979. [CrossRef] [PubMed]
95. Crosetto, N.; Bienko, M.; Van Oudenaarden, A. Spatially resolved transcriptomics and beyond. *Nat. Rev. Genet.* **2015**, *16*, 57–66. [CrossRef] [PubMed]
96. Ji, A.L.; Rubin, A.J.; Thrane, K.; Jiang, S.; Reynolds, D.L.; Meyers, R.M.; Guo, M.G.; George, B.M.; Mollbrink, A.; Bergenstråhle, J.; et al. Multimodal Analysis of Composition and Spatial Architecture in Human Squamous Cell Carcinoma. *Cell* **2020**, *182*, 497–514.e22. [CrossRef]
97. Browaeys, R.; Saelens, W.; Saeys, Y. NicheNet: Modeling intercellular communication by linking ligands to target genes. *Nat. Methods* **2020**, *17*, 159–162. [CrossRef]
98. Velazquez-Villarreal, E.I.; Maheshwari, S.; Sorenson, J.; Fiddes, I.T.; Kumar, V.; Yin, Y.; Webb, M.G.; Catalanotti, C.; Grigorova, M.; Edwards, P.A.; et al. Single-cell sequencing of genomic DNA resolves sub-clonal heterogeneity in a melanoma cell line. *Commun. Biol.* **2020**, *3*, 318. [CrossRef]
99. Slyper, M.; Porter, C.B.M.; Ashenberg, O.; Waldman, J.; Drokhlyansky, E.; Wakiro, I.; Smillie, C.; Smith-Rosario, G.; Wu, J.; Dionne, D.; et al. Author Correction: A single-cell and single-nucleus RNA-Seq toolbox for fresh and frozen human tumors. *Nat. Med.* **2020**, *26*, 1307. [CrossRef]

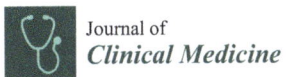

Brief Report

NF1-Dependent Transcriptome Regulation in the Melanocyte Lineage and in Melanoma

Lionel Larribère [1,2,*] and Jochen Utikal [1,2]

1. Skin Cancer Unit, German Cancer Research Center (DKFZ), 69120 Heidelberg, Germany; j.utikal@dkfz.de
2. Department of Dermatology, Venereology and Allergology, University Medical Center Mannheim, Ruprecht-Karl University of Heidelberg, 68167 Mannheim, Germany
* Correspondence: l.larribere@dkfz.de

Abstract: The precise role played by the tumor suppressor gene *NF1* in melanocyte biology and during the transformation into melanoma is not completely understood. In particular, understanding the interaction during melanocyte development between *NF1* and key signaling pathways, which are known to be reactivated in advanced melanoma, is still under investigation. Here, we used RNAseq datasets from either situation to better understand the transcriptomic regulation mediated by an *NF1* partial loss of function. We found that *NF1* mutations had a differential impact on pluripotency and on melanoblast differentiation. In addition, major signaling pathways such as VEGF, senescence/secretome, endothelin, and cAMP/PKA are likely to be upregulated upon *NF1* loss of function in both melanoblasts and metastatic melanoma. In sum, these data bring new light on the transcriptome regulation of the *NF1*-mutated melanoma subgroup and will help improve the possibilities for specific treatment.

Keywords: melanoblast; melanoma; NF1; transcriptome; RNAseq

1. Introduction

The implication of the *NF1*-encoded protein neurofibromin (NF1) in melanocyte biology has been investigated for more than 20 years. Despite its ubiquitous expression, NF1 has been described as regulating lineage-specific mechanisms by interacting with melanocyte-associated genes such as MITF or cKIT [1]. Indeed, *NF1* germline mutations induce neurofibromatosis type 1 syndrome, manifestations of which include defects in neural crest-derived cells such as melanocytes [2]. The embryological origin of these defects was previously described in *Nf1* mouse models. In fact, $Nf1^{+/-}$ or $Nf1^{-/-}$ mice in which mutations were specifically induced in the melanocyte lineage showed hyperpigmentation [3,4]. Moreover, a partial rescue of the belly spot phenotype in $Mitf^{Mi-wh/+}$ or $cKit^{W/+}$ mice was observed when the latter were crossed with $Nf1^{+/-}$ mice [5,6]. These "café-au-lait" macules, which are benign melanocytic lesions, can be observed in almost all patients [7,8], and the cells located in the macules usually carry a second somatic mutation on the wildtype *NF1* allele suggesting a selective advantage to the cell subpopulation [9].

The main described function of NF1 is a GTPase activity which inactivates RAS [10], and RAS deregulation in the melanocyte lineage is known to lead to pigmentation defects [11]. This phenotype can be explained at least in part by the fact that pigmentation's main regulator, MITF, can be phosphorylated by an active RAS-ERK pathway [12]. NF1 can also be phosphorylated by the protein kinase A (PKA), whose pathway is activated by cAMP and plays an important role during melanogenesis [13]. Another NF1 function is to interact with the cytoskeleton structures in order to control lamellopodia formation and actin polymerization. These processes are mainly regulated by RAC1 signaling, and it was recently observed that variable *NF1* expression levels changed the cell migration rate of melanoblasts in an RAC1-dependent manner [14]. Moreover, microtubule network fluctuation as well as FAK activity may also be influenced by NF1 [15–17]. Furthermore, NF1's interaction with cKIT signaling leads to a dysregulation of the melanoblast migration [6].

Interestingly, the migration and invasive phenotype of melanoblasts during development closely resemble the aggressive behavior of melanoma metastases [18–20]. The cell plasticity of lineage-committed melanoblasts is also observed in certain clones of melanoma tumors which have undergone dedifferentiation and which are usually refractory to treatments [21,22]. Recently, miRNAs identified in a human model of melanoblasts were described as potential drivers of melanoma development [23]. Malignant melanoma has been classified in four subgroups according to its main genetic drivers by The Cancer Genome Atlas: mutant *BRAF*, mutant *NRAS*, mutant *NF1*, or triple wild-type tumors [24]. In general, mutant *NF1* melanoma contain WT *BRAF* and WT *NRAS*, and rather carry comutations in the so-called RASopathy genes (*PTPN11* or *RASA2*). These tumors typically appear on chronically sun-exposed skin or in older individuals [25,26]. However, *NF1* mutations can sometime appear concurrently with *BRAF* or *NRAS* mutations. Indeed, a classification in three subgroups has also been suggested: mutant *BRAF*, mutant *NRAS*, non-*BRAF*mut/non-*NRAS*mut [27]. These co-occurring mutations lead to a higher RAS GTPase activity and resistance to BRAF inhibitors [28]. For example, the treatment of melanoma cells with the combination of BRAF inhibitor and MEK inhibitor showed either a loss of *NF1* expression or an acquired mutation [29]. Mutations cooperation between *NF1* and *BRAF* was also described in melanocytic nevi to explain the bypass of oncogene-induced senescence (OIS) and the progression to transformed melanoma [30]. Nevertheless, although 15% of sporadic melanoma bear *NF1* somatic mutations, no targeted treatment has been developed for this patient's subgroup, mainly due to the complexity of the protein.

In this report we intended to analyze the NF1-controlled transcriptome and identify regulated signaling pathways in two independent models: $NF1^{+/-}$ induced pluripotent stem cell-derived melanoblasts and their late stage transformed counterpart, $NF1^{+/-}$ metastatic melanoma.

2. Materials and Methods

2.1. Cell Lines

Three human induced pluripotent stem cell (hiPSC) lines were generated from fibroblasts obtained from skin biopsies of two patients with Neurofibromatosis Type 1 carrying *NF1* mutations (University of Ulm, Ulm, Germany) (one clone from the first patient and two clones from the second patient), and three hiPSC lines were generated from three healthy donors (University Medical Center Mannheim, Mannheim, Germany) (one clone from each patient) according to the ethical regulation. Patients with *NF1* mutations did not present melanoma tumors. The reprogramming protocol was already described by Larribere et al. [31]. Melanoblasts were derived from either *NF1*-mutated or *NF1*-wildtype hiPSC lines following a previously published protocol [1].

2.2. RNA Sequencing and Analysis

Briefly, total RNA was isolated with an RNeasy kit (Qiagen, Hilden, Germany), and DNase I digestion was performed to remove genomic DNA. Illumina sequencing libraries were prepared using the TruSeq Stranded mRNA Library Prep Kit (Illumina, Eindhoven, Netherland) according to the manufacturer's protocol. Briefly, poly(A)+ RNA was purified from 500 ng of total RNA using oligo(dT) beads, fragmented to a median insert length of 155 bp, and converted to cDNA. The ds cDNA fragments were then end-repaired, adenylated on the 3' end, adapter-ligated, and amplified with 15 cycles of PCR. The libraries were quantified using a Qubit ds DNA HS Assay kit (Life Technologies-Invitrogen, Darmstadt, Germany) and validated on an Agilent 4200 TapeStation System (Agilent technologies, Waldbronn, Germany). Based on the Qubit quantification and sizing analysis, multiplexed sequencing libraries were normalized, pooled (4plex), and sequenced on HiSeq 4000 single-read 50 bp with a final concentration of 250 pM (spiked with 1% PhiX control). The tool bcl2fastq (version 2.20.0.422, Illumina, Eindhoven, Netherland) was used for generating the fastq files and demultiplexing.

Gene set enrichment analyses were performed with Ingenuity Pathway Analysis (IPA) (Ingenuity® Systems, Redwood City, CA, USA, www.ingenuity.com) using a Log2-threshold = 2, p-value < 0.05.

2.3. Data from cBioportal Database

The melanoma sample's genomic dataset originated from the Skin Cutaneous Melanoma study (TCGA, Firehose Legacy) in the cBioportal database (Memorial Sloan Kettering Cancer Center, New York, NY, USA). Selected metastatic melanoma samples included patients with distant metastases or metastases in regional lymph nodes, as established by the American Joint Committee on Cancer (AJCC). These samples were divided in two groups according to a high (*NF1*-high, n = 25) or low (*NF1*-low, n = 26) expression level of *NF1* with a z-score threshold of 1. Accordingly, these filtered samples bore either loss-of-function SNPs or heterozygous deletions (*NF1*-low) or no *NF1* mutations (*NF1*-high).

The genomic dataset from the Cancer Cell Line Encyclopedia (Broad, 2019) contained a large range of tumor entities including melanoma cell lines (about 6%). As before, these samples were divided in two groups according to a high (*NF1*-high, n = 64) or low (*NF1*-low, n = 61) *NF1* mRNA expression (z-score relative to diploid samples, threshold = 1).

3. Results and Discussion

3.1. NF1 Mutations Have Differential Impact on Pluripotency and on Differentiation

The transcriptome of NF1-mutated human induced pluripotent stem cells (hiPSCs) was analyzed by RNA sequencing and compared to wildtype control hiPSCs, in order to specifically study the impact of NF1 mutations during reprogramming. The top 20 regulated genes are represented in Figure 1A. Among these genes, one can find regulators of DNA replication (histones), transcription and gene regulation (transcription factors), genes involved in cellular (cytoskeleton) and extracellular matrix structures (cadherin). Genes were also involved in intracellular signal transduction (G protein-coupled receptor (GPCR) and GTPases) or in ion or glucose transport. Genes involved in the WNT, Retinoic Acid, or Fatty Acid Biosynthesis pathways were also reported. We observed genes involved in biological functions such as apoptosis, inflammation, or immune response. Finally, many genes were involved in blood vessels or cardiac function, which is in line with the observed main defects leading to the short survival of Nf1$^{-/-}$ mice [32].

A pathway analysis of the most regulated genes with the IPA software resulted in the following signalings (Figure 1B). Genes involved in pluripotency such as SMAD6, TGFB, WNT2B, WNT3, WNT5A were retrieved, although no phenotypic differences have been observed between NF1-mutated hiPSCs and NF1-WT hiPSCs [31]. These data may argue for a role of WNT and SMAD pathways during NF1-mutated stem cell reprogramming that is less important than other pathways such as FGFR2. Indeed, FGFR signaling controls cell survival, proliferation, embryonic development, and organogenesis by activating MAPK, PI3K/AKT, PLCγ, and STAT pathways [33]. These pathways are also described as interacting with WNT and TGFβ and could in this situation play redundant functions. ILK and more generally the integrin pathway promote several cellular functions such as adhesion, growth, and migration. The involvement of NF1 in migration has for example been established [14,17]. Rho GTPases belong to a subfamily of the Ras superfamily and are therefore expected to interact with NF1 [34]. This study from Upadhyaya et al., already discussed the role of the Rho GTPase pathway in NF1 tumorigenesis. Epithelial-to-mesenchymal transition (EMT) is a biological process that occurs during embryogenesis but also in cancer metastases. During reprogramming, cells will also undergo sequential EMT and mesenchymal-to-epithelial transition (MET), the latter being required for pluripotency acquisition [35]. Pathways activated by RAS (and likely by NF1 loss) have been described as playing a crucial role during EMT and MET. For instance, Arima et al., described the loss of NF1-activated EMT-related signalings and, additionally, that an excessive mesenchymal phenotype may play a role in the development of NF1-associated neurofibromas [36].

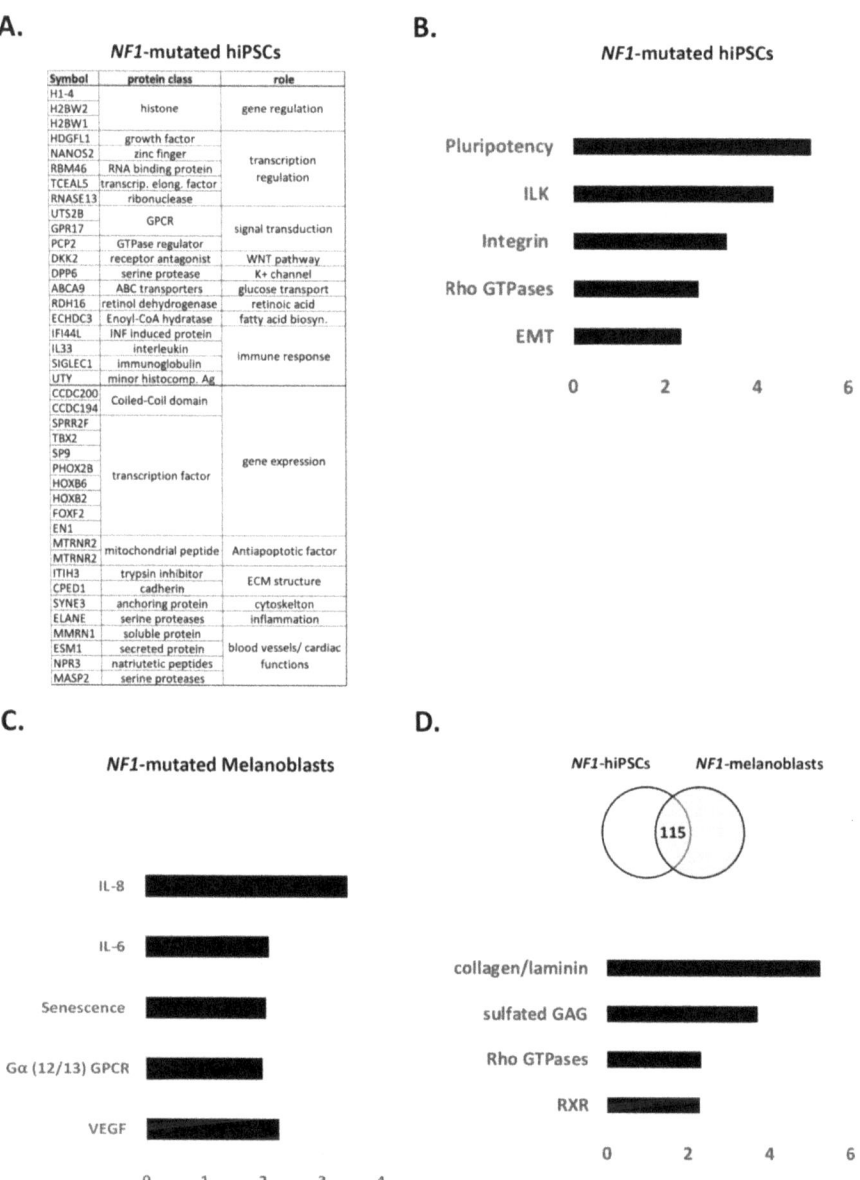

Figure 1. *NF1* mutations have a differential impact on pluripotency and on differentiation. (**A**) Top 20 regulated genes in *NF1*-mutated hiPSCs compared to *NF1*-WT hiPSCs. (**B**) Main regulated signaling pathways in *NF1*-mutated hiPSCs compared to *NF1*-WT hiPSCs. (**C**) Main regulated signaling pathways in *NF1*-mutated melanoblasts compared to *NF1*-WT melanoblasts. (**D**) Common regulated signaling pathways in *NF1*-mutated hiPSCs and in *NF1*-mutated melanoblasts.

Next, we analyzed the transcriptome of melanoblasts differentiated from NF1-mutated hiPSCs and compared it to that of wildtype control melanoblasts [1]. A similar IPA pathway analysis presented the following results (Figure 1C). In contrast to NF1-mutated hiPSCs, regulated genes in NF1-mutated melanoblasts were mainly involved in the senescence, IL-6/8, VEGF, and GPCR pathways. Interestingly, oncogene-induced senescence (OIS) generated by the loss of NF1 expression was described in melanoma cells before [30] and was also observed specifically in melanocytes located in the NF1-associated "café-au-lait" macules [31]. OIS leads to the secretion of a panel of cytokines in the extracellular environment, which includes IL-6/8 acting as a paracrine activation loop, as previously described [37,38]. These data bring additional confirmation of NF1's role in the senescence of melanocytes precursors and in the regulation of the secretome. The involvement of NF1 during melanocyte differentiation was reproduced in a study using NF1$^{+/-}$ embryonic pluripotent stem cells [39]. This NF1 model allowed one to link NF1 mutations to the hyperpigmentation of melanocytes and to replicate the loss of heterozygosity specifically in CALMs.

Although the VEGF pathway does not play a major role in melanoblast differentiation, an essential role of NF1 in controlling endothelial cell proliferation was described [40]. Indeed, the authors of this study showed a reduction of NF1 expression upon VEGF stimulation and the consequent activation of MAPK and PI3K-AKT pathways. Finally, the activation of the GPCR superfamily was observed. In particular, the coupled $G_{\alpha 12/13}$ protein subunit regulates cellular proliferation, movement, and morphology and is also involved in cancer [41]. For example, after the binding of endothelin to its receptor EDNRA, coupled $G_{\alpha q}/G_{\alpha 11}$ and $G_{\alpha 12}/G_{\alpha 13}$ proteins are activated [42]. However, the function of neural crest cells and their derived melanoblasts is dependent on EDNRB activation and on the involvement of coupled $G_{\alpha i}/G_{\alpha 0}$, $G_{\alpha q}/G_{\alpha 11}$, or $G_{\alpha 13}$ subunits. The endothelin signaling leads to the activation of phospholipase Cβ, inhibition of adenyl cyclase, activation of plasma membrane Ca^{2+} channels, and activation of nonreceptor tyrosine kinases [43,44]. Of note, genes encoding for some members of associated G proteins (GNAS, GNAQ, and GNA11) have been described as being mutated in tumors and as being oncogenic drivers of uveal melanoma [45]. It is interesting to retrieve the endothelin receptor coupled G protein since the complex relationship between endothelin signaling and NF1 has already been discussed based on pigmentation transgenic mice models [4]. Indeed, NF1 is likely to play different roles in skin and fur pigmentation [46].

We also analyzed common NF1-induced pathway regulation in hiPSCs and in melanoblasts (Figure 1D). Overlapping regulated genes belong to signalings involved in general cellular functions such as cell differentiation, migration, and adhesion, confirming the pleiotropic role of NF1. For example, collagen, laminin, or sulfated glycosaminoglycans families, which are expressed at the cell membrane and in the extracellular matrix, or the actin network were commonly regulated. The Rho GTPase family, which was described above as being potentially associated to pluripotency function, is also likely to be involved in more general cellular functions concerning Nf1-mutated melanoblasts [34]. Last, the RXR family of nuclear receptors could be regulated by NF1 signaling. For instance, similar ventricular myocyte defects were observed in $Rxr\alpha^{-/-}$ mouse embryos and in embryos with homozygous mutations on *Nf1* [47].

3.2. Role of NF1 in the Gene's Regulation of Melanoblasts and Melanoma

Next, we used the RNAseq dataset of the TCGA Firehose melanoma cohort from the publicly available cBioportal database [48,49]. 161 metastatic melanoma samples were divided in two groups according to a high or low expression level of NF1 mRNA (z-score threshold of 1). Surprisingly, the number of regulated genes between the two groups was not very high (*n* = 229, log2-FC threshold: 2). Consequently, a discrete number of pathways appeared to be overrepresented in NF1-low expressing metastatic melanoma samples: Paxillin, cAMP, and PKA (Figure 2A). The influence of the cAMP/PKA pathway in melanoma development has been described. The MC1R/cAMP pathway controls UV-mediated melanin synthesis, and certain mutations in the MC1R gene lead to pigment defects in people with red hair and fair skin, therefore increasing the risk of melanoma [50]. More recently, structural biology studies on the MC1R/cAMP signaling pathway have focused on its mechanisms for enhancing genomic stability, suggesting pharmacologic opportunities to reduce melanoma risk [51]. The role of the cAMP pathway in melanoma treatment resistance has also been described before. Systematic gain-of-function resistance studies have revealed a cAMP-dependent melanocytic signaling network associated with drug resistance, including GPCR, adenyl cyclase, PKA, and cAMP response element binding protein (CREB) [52]. More recently, an alternative activation of the cAMP pathway in melanocytes has been shown downstream of the G protein-coupled estrogen receptor. This activation led to melanoma cell vulnerability to immunotherapy [53]. However, the specific role of NF1 in melanoma treatment resistance is still unclear. Earlier sensitivity assays of MEK inhibitors in BRAF-WT, NRAS-WT, and NF1-mutated melanoma did not show a high correlation [25,54]. More experimental studies focusing on the exact role of NF1 and cAMP in the context of treatment resistance are needed. Paxillin is involved in cellular adhesion to the extracellular matrix (via binding to focal adhesion kinases, FAK) and therefore contributes to migration. A defect in the paxillin expression can provoke cancer progression [55,56]. Along this line, NF1 is described as interacting with FAK, and its deregulation influences cellular migration [17]. Recently, the loss of NF1 in melanoma cells led to increased migration and metastases formation in vivo [14].

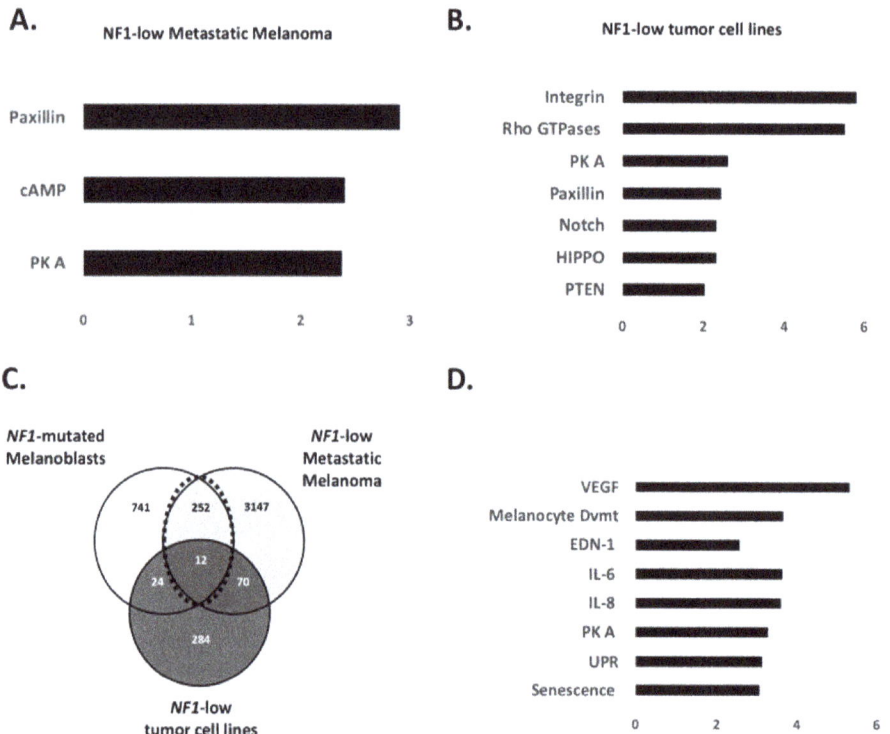

Figure 2. Role of NF1 in the gene's regulation of melanoblasts and melanoma. (**A**) Main regulated signaling pathways in *NF1*-low expressing metastatic melanoma. (**B**) Main regulated signaling pathways in *NF1*-low expressing tumor cell lines. (**C**) Venn diagram including *NF1*-low expressing metastatic melanoma, *NF1*-mutated melanoblasts, and *NF1*-low expressing tumor cell lines. (**D**) Common regulated signaling pathways in *NF1*-mutated melanoblasts and *NF1*-low expressing metastatic melanoma.

Similarly, we addressed the same question in the panel of tumor cell lines from the Cancer Cell Line Encyclopedia (CCLE). We filtered NF1-low and -high expressing cell lines in cBioportal and compared the two groups for gene regulation. The PKA and Paxillin pathways were redundant with the metastatic melanoma samples (Figure 2B). Integrins and Rho GTPases were also regulated, as we observed in hiPSCs samples, arguing for a more general role of NF1 in proliferating cells. In addition, three other pathways known to play crucial roles in transformation and tumor progression were found: Notch, Hippo, and PTEN. Evidence for an NF1 role in the transforming activity of the Notch pathway has been gathered in the context of Schwann cells transformation [57]. The modulation of the Hippo pathway has been reported to be mediated by NF1 loss in neurofibroma [58]. Despite being major tumor suppressors, PTEN and NF1 may not play redundant functions. Indeed, the concurrent loss of PTEN and NF1 in different tumor settings has been reported [59,60].

Last, we wanted to focus on the 263 genes which were regulated in both NF1-mutated melanoblasts and in NF1-low expressing metastatic melanoma (Figure 2C) because genes involved in melanocyte development are likely to be reactivated during melanoma progression [23,61]. The genes likely regulated by NF1 were involved in common signalings. Again, we found IL-6/8 and senescence/UPR signalings pathways (Figure 2D). Indeed, the Unfolded Protein Response (UPR) pathway plays a role in the cellular equilibrium between senescence and apoptosis [62]. Although not deeply investigated, NF1 could play a role in this pathway. In an Nf1-mutated mouse model of malignant peripheral nerve sheath tumors (MPNSTs), increased levels of UPR-associated genes (p-eIF2α, XPB1s, and GRP78) have been shown [63]. VEGF signaling, which we found regulated in NF1-mutated melanoblasts, is also associated with melanoma progression [64]. The endothelin pathway seems to play a role in melanoma. Recently, it was described how endothelin signaling promoted melanoma tumorigenesis driven by constitutively active GNAQ [65]. Additionally, the inhibition of EDNRB receptor signaling synergizes with MAPK pathway inhibitors in BRAF-mutated melanoma [66].

Finally, we mentioned above the redundant role of cAMP/PKA signaling during melanogenesis [13]. The implication of NF1 in this pathway has also been studied. Loss of NF1 leads to the activation of the cAMP/PKA pathway, which consequently phosphorylates the melanocyte-associated transcription factor MITF [46]. Such post-translational modifications of MITF leading to varying expression levels have been described in tumor cell subpopulations which respond differently to melanoma treatments [67,68].

4. Conclusions

In conclusion, we here describe transcriptomic signatures found not only in metastatic melanoma tumor cells but also in melanocyte progenitors, melanoblasts, in the case of an *NF1* partial loss of function. These signatures included the activation of VEGF, senescence/secretome, endothelin, and cAMP/PKA signaling pathways. More clinical research focusing on *NF1*-mutated melanoma, one of the four molecular subgroups classified by The Cancer Genome Atlas, is expected since no efficient targeted therapy has so far been available, unlike for the *BRAF*-mutated subgroup (BRAF/MEK inhibitors) or *NRAS*-mutated subgroup (MEK inhibitors clinical trials).

Author Contributions: Conceptualization; methodology; formal analysis; visualization; writing—original draft preparation: L.L.; writing—review and editing; funding acquisition: J.U. Both the authors have read and agreed to the published version of the manuscript.

Funding: This research was funded by the Deutsche Forschungsgemeinschaft (DFG, German Research Foundation)—Project number 259332240/RTG 2099.

Institutional Review Board Statement: The study was conducted according to the guidelines of the Declaration of Helsinki, and approved by the Ethics Committee of University Medical Center Mannheim, Mannheim, Germany approval no. 2009-350N-MA or of University Ulm, Ulm, Germany, approval A 185/09.

Informed Consent Statement: Informed consent was obtained from all subjects involved in the study.

Data Availability Statement: RNAseq data are available upon request.

Acknowledgments: We thank the DKFZ Genomics and Proteomics Core Facility for sequencing experiments and Agnes Hotz–Wagenblatt from the Core Facility Omics IT and Data management (ODCF) for data analysis support.

Conflicts of Interest: The authors declare no conflict of interest.

References

1. Larribère, L.; Kuphal, S.; Sachpekidis, C.; Sachindra; Hüser, L.; Bosserhoff, A.; Utikal, J. Targeted Therapy-Resistant Melanoma Cells Acquire Transcriptomic Similarities with Human Melanoblasts. *Cancers* **2018**, *10*, 451. [CrossRef] [PubMed]
2. Ferner, R.E. Neurofibromatosis 1. *Eur. J. Hum. Genet.* **2007**, *15*, 131–138. [CrossRef] [PubMed]
3. Deo, M.; Huang, J.L.-Y.; Fuchs, H.; de Angelis, M.H.; Van Raamsdonk, C.D. Differential effects of neurofibromin gene dosage on melanocyte development. *J. Investig. Dermatol.* **2013**, *133*, 49–58. [CrossRef] [PubMed]
4. Deo, M.; Huang, J.L.-Y.; Van Raamsdonk, C.D. Genetic interactions between neurofibromin and endothelin receptor B in mice. *PLoS ONE* **2013**, *8*, e59931. [CrossRef] [PubMed]
5. Diwakar, G.; Zhang, D.; Jiang, S.; Hornyak, T.J. Neurofibromin as a regulator of melanocyte development and differentiation. *J. Cell Sci.* **2008**, *121*, 167–177. [CrossRef] [PubMed]
6. Wehrle-Haller, B.; Meller, M.; Weston, J.A. Analysis of melanocyte precursors in Nf1 mutants reveals that MGF/KIT signaling promotes directed cell migration independent of its function in cell survival. *Dev. Biol.* **2001**, *232*, 471–483. [CrossRef]
7. Friedman, J.M.; Birch, P.H. Type 1 neurofibromatosis: A descriptive analysis of the disorder in 1728 patients. *Am. J. Med. Genet.* **1997**, *70*, 138–143. [CrossRef]
8. Gutmann, D.H.; Aylsworth, A.; Carey, J.C.; Korf, B.; Marks, J.; Pyeritz, R.E.; Rubenstein, A.; Viskochil, D. The diagnostic evaluation and multidisciplinary management of neurofibromatosis 1 and neurofibromatosis 2. *JAMA* **1997**, *278*, 51–57. [CrossRef]
9. De Schepper, S.; Maertens, O.; Callens, T.; Naeyaert, J.-M.; Lambert, J.; Messiaen, L. Somatic mutation analysis in NF1 café au lait spots reveals two NF1 hits in the melanocytes. *J. Investig. Dermatol.* **2008**, *128*, 1050–1053. [CrossRef]
10. Bos, J.L. Ras Oncogenes in Human Cancer: A Review ras Oncogenes in Human Cancer: A Review. *Cancer Rese* **1989**, *49*, 4682–4689.
11. Powell, M.B.; Hyman, P.; Bell, O.D.; Balmain, A.; Brown, K.; Alberts, D.; Bowden, G.T. Hyperpigmentation and melanocytic hyperplasia in transgenic mice expressing the human T24 Ha-ras gene regulated by a mouse tyrosinase promoter. *Mol. Carcinog.* **1995**, *12*, 82–90. [CrossRef]
12. Hemesath, T.J.; Price, E.R.; Takemoto, C.; Badalian, T.; Fisher, D.E. MAP kinase links the transcription factor Microphthalmia to c-Kit signalling in melanocytes. *Nature* **1998**, *391*, 298–301. [CrossRef] [PubMed]
13. Bertolotto, C.; Abbe, P.; Hemesath, T.J.; Bille, K.; Fisher, D.E.; Ortonne, J.P.; Ballotti, R. Microphthalmia gene product as a signal transducer in cAMP-induced differentiation of melanocytes. *J. Cell Biol.* **1998**, *142*, 827–835. [CrossRef]
14. Larribère, L.; Cakrapradipta Wibowo, Y.; Patil, N.; Abba, M.; Tundidor, I.; Aguiñón Olivares, R.G.; Allgayer, H.; Utikal, J. NF1-RAC1 axis regulates migration of the melanocytic lineage. *Transl. Oncol.* **2020**, *13*, 100858. [CrossRef]
15. Gregory, P.E.; Gutmann, D.H.; Mitchell, A.; Park, S.; Boguski, M.; Jacks, T.; Wood, D.L.; Jove, R.; Collins, F.S. Neurofibromatosis type 1 gene product (neurofibromin) associates with microtubules. *Somat. Cell Mol. Genet.* **1993**, *19*, 265–274. [CrossRef]
16. Lin, Y.-L.; Lei, Y.-T.; Hong, C.-J.; Hsueh, Y.-P. Syndecan-2 induces filopodia and dendritic spine formation via the neurofibromin-PKA-Ena/VASP pathway. *J. Cell Biol.* **2007**, *177*, 829–841. [CrossRef]
17. Kweha, F.; Zheng, M.; Kurenovaa, E.; Wallacec, M.; Golubovskayad, V.; Cance, W.G. Neurofibromin physically interacts with the N-terminal domain of focal adhesion kinase. *Mol. Carcinog.* **2009**, *48*, 1005–1017. [CrossRef]
18. Thomas, A.J.; Erickson, C.A. The making of a melanocyte: The specification of melanoblasts from the neural crest. *Pigment Cell Melanoma Res.* **2008**, *21*, 598–610. [CrossRef]
19. Lugassy, C.; Lazar, V.; Dessen, P.; van den Oord, J.J.; Winnepenninckx, V.; Spatz, A.; Bagot, M.; Bensussan, A.; Janin, A.; Eggermont, A.M.; et al. Gene expression profiling of human angiotropic primary melanoma: Selection of 15 differentially expressed genes potentially involved in extravascular migratory metastasis. *Eur. J. Cancer* **2011**, *47*, 1267–1275. [CrossRef]
20. Lugassy, C.; Zadran, S.; Bentolila, L.A.; Wadehra, M.; Prakash, R.; Carmichael, S.T.; Kleinman, H.K.; Péault, B.; Larue, L.; Barnhill, R.L. Angiotropism, Pericytic Mimicry and Extravascular Migratory Metastasis in Melanoma: An Alternative to Intravascular Cancer Dissemination. *Cancer Microenviron.* **2014**, *7*, 139–152. [CrossRef] [PubMed]
21. Larribere, L.; Utikal, J. De- and re-differentiation of the melanocytic lineage. *Eur. J. Cell Biol.* **2013**, *93*, 30–35. [CrossRef] [PubMed]
22. Larribère, L.; Utikal, J. Stem Cell-Derived Models of Neural Crest Are Essential to Understand Melanoma Progression and Therapy Resistance. *Front. Mol. Neurosci.* **2019**, *12*, 111. [CrossRef] [PubMed]
23. Linck-Paulus, L.; Lämmerhirt, L.; Völler, D.; Meyer, K.; Engelmann, J.C.; Spang, R.; Eichner, N.; Meister, G.; Kuphal, S.; Bosserhoff, A.K. Learning from Embryogenesis—A Comparative Expression Analysis in Melanoblast Differentiation and Tumorigenesis Reveals miRNAs Driving Melanoma Development. *J. Clin. Med.* **2021**, *10*, 2259. [CrossRef] [PubMed]
24. Akbani, R.; Akdemir, K.; Aksoy, A. Genomic Classification of Cutaneous Melanoma. *Cell* **2015**, *161*, 1681–1696. [CrossRef] [PubMed]
25. Krauthammer, M.; Kong, Y.; Bacchiocchi, A.; Evans, P.; Pornputtapong, N.; Wu, C.; Mccusker, J.P.; Ma, S.; Cheng, E.; Straub, R.; et al. Exome sequencing identifies recurrent mutations in NF1 and RASopathy genes in sun-exposed melanomas. *Nat. Genet.* **2015**, *47*, 996–1002. [CrossRef]
26. Cirenajwis, H.; Lauss, M.; Ekedahl, H.; Törngren, T.; Kvist, A.; Saal, L.H.; Olsson, H.; Staaf, J.; Carneiro, A.; Ingvar, C.; et al. NF1-mutated melanoma tumors harbor distinct clinical and biological characteristics. *Mol. Oncol.* **2017**, *11*, 438–451. [CrossRef]
27. Palmieri, G.; Colombino, M.; Casula, M.; Manca, A.; Mandalà, M.; Cossu, A. Molecular Pathways in Melanomagenesis: What We Learned from Next-Generation Sequencing Approaches. *Curr. Oncol. Rep.* **2018**, *20*, 86. [CrossRef]
28. Nissan, M.H.; Pratilas, C.; Jones, A.M.; Ramirez, R.; Won, H.; Liu, C.; Tiwari, S.; Kong, L.; Hanrahan, A.J.; Yao, Z.; et al. Loss of NF1 in cutaneous melanoma is associated with RAS activation and MEK dependence. *Cancer Res.* **2014**, *74*, 2340–2350. [CrossRef]

29. Whittaker, S.R.; Theurillat, J.-P.; Van Allen, E.; Wagle, N.; Hsiao, J.; Cowley, G.S.; Schadendorf, D.; Root, D.E.; Garraway, L. A genome-scale RNA interference screen implicates NF1 loss in resistance to RAF inhibition. *Cancer Discov.* **2013**, *3*, 350–362. [CrossRef]
30. Maertens, O.; Johnson, B.; Hollstein, P.; Frederick, D.T.; Cooper, Z.A.; Messiaen, L.; Bronson, R.T.; McMahon, M.; Granter, S.; Flaherty, K.; et al. Elucidating distinct roles for NF1 in melanomagenesis. *Cancer Discov.* **2013**, *3*, 338–349. [CrossRef]
31. Larribere, L.; Wu, H.; Novak, D.; Galach, M.; Bernhardt, M.; Orouji, E.; Weina, K.; Knappe, N.; Sachpekidis, C.; Umansky, L.; et al. NF1 loss induces senescence during human melanocyte differentiation in an iPSC-based model. *Pigment Cell Melanoma Res.* **2015**, *28*, 407–416. [CrossRef]
32. Brannan, C.I.; Perkins, A.S.; Vogel, K.S.; Ratner, N.; Nordlund, M.L.; Reid, S.W.; Buchberg, A.M.; Jenkins, N.A.; Parada, L.F.; Copeland, N.G. Targeted disruption of the neurofibromatosis type-1 gene leads to developmental abnormalities in heart and various neural crest-derived tissues. *Genes Dev.* **1994**, *8*, 1019–1029. [CrossRef] [PubMed]
33. Mossahebi-Mohammadi, M.; Quan, M.; Zhang, J.S.; Li, X. FGF Signaling Pathway: A Key Regulator of Stem Cell Pluripotency. *Front. Cell Dev. Biol.* **2020**, *8*, 79. [CrossRef]
34. Upadhyaya, M.; Spurlock, G.; Thomas, L.; Thomas, N.S.T.; Richards, M.; Mautner, V.-F.; Cooper, D.N.; Guha, A.; Yan, J. Microarray-based copy number analysis of neurofibromatosis type-1 (NF1)-associated malignant peripheral nerve sheath tumors reveals a role for Rho-GTPase pathway genes in NF1 tumorigenesis. *Hum. Mutat.* **2012**, *33*, 763–776. [CrossRef]
35. Shu, X.; Pei, D. The function and regulation of mesenchymal-to-epithelial transition in somatic cell reprogramming. *Curr. Opin. Genet. Dev.* **2014**, *28*, 32–37. [CrossRef] [PubMed]
36. Arima, Y.; Hayashi, H.; Kamata, K.; Goto, T.M.; Sasaki, M.; Kuramochi, A.; Saya, H. Decreased expression of neurofibromin contributes to epithelial-mesenchymal transition in neurofibromatosis type 1. *Exp. Dermatol.* **2010**, *19*, e136–e141. [CrossRef]
37. Kim, J.; Novak, D.; Sachpekidis, C.; Utikal, J.; Larribère, L. STAT3 Relays a Differential Response to Melanoma-Associated NRAS Mutations. *Cancers* **2020**, *12*, 119. [CrossRef]
38. Kuilman, T.; Peeper, D.S. Senescence-messaging secretome: SMS-ing cellular stress. *Nat. Rev. Cancer* **2009**, *9*, 81–94. [CrossRef]
39. Allouche, J.; Bellon, N.; Saidani, M.; Stanchina-Chatrousse, L.; Masson, Y.; Patwardhan, A.; Gilles-Marsens, F.; Delevoye, C.; Domingues, S.; Nissan, X.; et al. In vitro modeling of hyperpigmentation associated to neurofibromatosis type 1 using melanocytes derived from human embryonic stem cells. *Proc. Natl. Acad. Sci. USA* **2015**, *112*, 201501032. [CrossRef]
40. Zhang, H.; Hudson, F.Z.; Xu, Z.; Tritz, R.; Rojas, M.; Patel, C.; Haigh, S.B.; Bordán, Z.; Ingram, D.A.; Fulton, D.J.; et al. Neurofibromin deficiency induces endothelial cell proliferation and retinal neovascularization. *Investig. Ophthalmol. Vis. Sci.* **2018**, *59*, 2520–2528. [CrossRef]
41. Worzfeld, T.; Wettschureck, N.; Offermanns, S. G12/G13-mediated signalling in mammalian physiology and disease. *Trends Pharmacol. Sci.* **2008**, *29*, 582–589. [CrossRef]
42. Kedzierski, R.M.; Yanagisawa, M. Endothelin system: The double-edged sword in health and disease. *Annu. Rev. Pharmacol. Toxicol.* **2001**, *41*, 851–876. [CrossRef] [PubMed]
43. Bouallegue, A.; Bou Daou, G.; Srivastava, A. Endothelin-1-Induced Signaling Pathways in Vascular Smooth Muscle Cells. *Curr. Vasc. Pharmacol.* **2006**, *5*, 45–52. [CrossRef]
44. Sugden, P.; Clerk, A. Endothelin Signalling in the Cardiac Myocyte and its Pathophysiological Relevance. *Curr. Vasc. Pharmacol.* **2005**, *3*, 343–351. [CrossRef]
45. Larribere, L.; Utikal, J. Update on GNA Alterations in Cancer: Implications for Uveal Melanoma Treatment. *Cancers* **2020**, *12*, 1524. [CrossRef]
46. Larribere, L.; Utikal, J. Multiple roles of NF1 in the melanocyte lineage. *Pigment Cell Melanoma Res.* **2016**. [CrossRef]
47. Rossant, J. Mouse mutants and cardiac development: New molecular insights into cardiogenesis. *Circ. Res.* **1996**, *78*, 349–353. [CrossRef]
48. Cerami, E.; Gao, J.; Dogrusoz, U.; Gross, B.E.; Sumer, S.O.; Aksoy, B.A.; Jacobsen, A.; Byrne, C.J.; Heuer, M.L.; Larsson, E.; et al. The cBio Cancer Genomics Portal: An open platform for exploring multidimensional cancer genomics data. *Cancer Discov.* **2012**, *2*, 401–404. [CrossRef]
49. Gao, J.; Aksoy, B.B.A.; Dogrusoz, U.; Dresdner, G.; Gross, B.; Sumer, S.O.; Sun, Y.; Jacobsen, A.; Sinha, R.; Larsson, E.; et al. Integrative analysis of complex cancer genomics and clinical profiles using the cBioPortal. *Sci. Signal.* **2013**, *6*, pl1. [CrossRef] [PubMed]
50. Rodríguez, C.I.; Setaluri, V. Cyclic AMP (cAMP) signaling in melanocytes and melanoma. *Arch. Biochem. Biophys.* **2014**, *563*, 22–27. [CrossRef]
51. Holcomb, N.C.; Bautista, R.M.; Jarrett, S.G.; Carter, K.M.; Gober, M.K.; D'Orazio, J.A. cAMP-mediated regulation of melanocyte genomic instability: A melanoma-preventive strategy. In *Advances in Protein Chemistry and Structural Biology*; Academic Press Inc.: Cambridge, MA, USA, 2019; Volume 115, pp. 247–295.
52. Johannessen, C.M.; Johnson, L.A.; Piccioni, F.; Townes, A.; Frederick, D.T.; Donahue, M.K.; Narayan, R.; Flaherty, K.T.; Wargo, J.A.; Root, D.E.; et al. A melanocyte lineage program confers resistance to MAP kinase pathway inhibition. *Nature* **2013**, *504*, 138–142. [CrossRef] [PubMed]
53. Natale, C.A.; Li, J.; Zhang, J.; Dahal, A.; Dentchev, T.; Stanger, B.Z.; Ridky, T.W. Activation of G protein-coupled estrogen receptor signaling inhibits melanoma and improves response to immune checkpoint blockade. *eLife* **2018**, *7*, e31770. [CrossRef]

54. Ranzani, M.; Alifrangis, C.; Perna, D.; Dutton-Regester, K.; Pritchard, A.; Wong, K.; Rashid, M.; Robles-Espinoza, C.D.; Hayward, N.K.; McDermott, U.; et al. BRAF/NRAS wild-type melanoma, NF1 status and sensitivity to trametinib. *Pigment Cell Melanoma Res.* **2015**, *28*, 117–119. [CrossRef]
55. Hamamura, K.; Furukawa, K.; Hayashi, T.; Hattori, T.; Nakano, J.; Nakashima, H.; Okuda, T.; Mizutani, H.; Hattori, H.; Ueda, M.; et al. Ganglioside GD3 promotes cell growth and invasion through p130Cas and paxillin in malignant melanoma cells. *Proc. Natl. Acad. Sci. USA* **2005**, *102*, 11041–11046. [CrossRef] [PubMed]
56. López-Colomé, A.M.; Lee-Rivera, I.; Benavides-Hidalgo, R.; López, E. Paxillin: A crossroad in pathological cell migration. *J. Hematol. Oncol.* **2017**, *10*, 50. [CrossRef] [PubMed]
57. Li, Y.; Rao, P.K.; Wen, R.; Song, Y.; Muir, D.; Wallace, P.; Van Horne, S.J.; Tennekoon, G.I.; Kadesch, T. Notch and Schwann cell transformation. *Oncogene* **2004**, *23*, 1146–1152. [CrossRef]
58. Chen, Z.; Mo, J.; Brosseau, J.P.; Shipman, T.; Wang, Y.; Liao, C.P.; Cooper, J.M.; Allaway, R.J.; Gosline, S.J.C.; Guinney, J.; et al. Spatiotemporal loss of NF1 in schwann cell lineage leads to different types of cutaneous neurofibroma susceptible to modification by the hippo pathway. *Cancer Discov.* **2019**, *9*, 114–129. [CrossRef] [PubMed]
59. Keng, V.W.; Rahrmann, E.P.; Watson, A.L.; Tschida, B.R.; Moertel, C.L.; Jessen, W.J.; Rizvi, T.A.; Collins, M.H.; Ratner, N.; Largaespada, D.A. PTEN and NF1 inactivation in Schwann cells produces a severe phenotype in the peripheral nervous system that promotes the development and malignant progression of peripheral nerve sheath tumors. *Cancer Res.* **2012**, *72*, 3405–3413. [CrossRef]
60. Dankort, D.; Curley, D.P.; Cartlidge, R.A.; Nelson, B.; Karnezis, A.N.; Damsky, W.E.; You, M.J.; DePinho, R.A.; McMahon, M.; Bosenberg, M. Braf(V600E) cooperates with Pten loss to induce metastatic melanoma. *Nat. Genet.* **2009**, *41*, 544–552. [CrossRef]
61. Liu, J.; Fukunaga-Kalabis, M.; Li, L.; Herlyn, M. Developmental pathways activated in melanocytes and melanoma. *Arch. Biochem. Biophys.* **2014**, *563*, 13–21. [CrossRef]
62. Pluquet, O.; Pourtier, A.; Abbadie, C. The unfolded protein response and cellular senescence. A review in the theme: Cellular mechanisms of endoplasmic reticulum stress signaling in health and disease. *Am. J. Physiol. Cell Physiol.* **2015**, *308*, 415–425. [CrossRef]
63. De Raedt, T.; Walton, Z.; Yecies, J.L.; Li, D.; Chen, Y.; Malone, C.F.; Maertens, O.; Jeong, S.M.; Bronson, R.T.; Lebleu, V.; et al. Exploiting cancer cell vulnerabilities to develop a combination therapy for ras-driven tumors. *Cancer Cell* **2011**, *20*, 400–413. [CrossRef] [PubMed]
64. Ni, C.S.; Sun, B.C.; Dong, X.Y.; Sun, T.; Zhao, N.; Liu, Y.R.; Gu, Q. Promoting melanoma growth and metastasis by enhancing VEGF expression. *Wspolczesna Onkol.* **2012**, *16*, 526–531. [CrossRef] [PubMed]
65. Jain, F.; Longakit, A.; Huang, J.L.Y.; Van Raamsdonk, C.D. Endothelin signaling promotes melanoma tumorigenesis driven by constitutively active GNAQ. *Pigment Cell Melanoma Res.* **2020**, *33*, 834–849. [CrossRef]
66. Schäfer, A.; Haenig, B.; Erupathil, J.; Strickner, P.; Sabato, D.; Welford, R.W.D.; Klaeylé, L.; Simon, E.; Krepler, C.; Brafford, P.; et al. Inhibition of endothelin-B receptor signaling synergizes with MAPK pathway inhibitors in BRAF mutated melanoma. *Oncogene* **2021**, *40*, 1659–1673. [CrossRef] [PubMed]
67. Ennen, M.; Eline Keime, C.; Gambi, G.; Kieny, A.; Coassolo, S.; Thibault-Carpentier, C.; Margerin-Schaller, F.; Davidson, G.; Vagne, C.; Lipsker, D.; et al. MITF-High and MITF-Low Cells and a Novel Subpopulation Expressing Genes of Both Cell States Contribute to Intra-and Intertumoral Heterogeneity of Primary Melanoma. *Clin. Cancer Res.* **2017**, *23*, 7097–7107. [CrossRef]
68. Müller, J.; Krijgsman, O.; Tsoi, J.; Robert, L.; Hugo, W.; Song, C.; Kong, X.; Possik, P.A.; Cornelissen-Steijger, P.D.M.; Foppen, M.H.G.; et al. Low MITF/AXL ratio predicts early resistance to multiple targeted drugs in melanoma. *Nat. Commun.* **2014**, *5*, 5712. [CrossRef]

MDPI
St. Alban-Anlage 66
4052 Basel
Switzerland
Tel. +41 61 683 77 34
Fax +41 61 302 89 18
www.mdpi.com

Journal of Clinical Medicine Editorial Office
E-mail: jcm@mdpi.com
www.mdpi.com/journal/jcm

www.ingramcontent.com/pod-product-compliance
Lightning Source LLC
LaVergne TN
LVHW070610100526
838202LV00012B/607